Annotated Atlas of Electrocardiography

CONTEMPORARY CARDIOLOGY

CHRISTOPHER P. CANNON

SERIES EDITOR

1. MANAGEMENT OF ACUTE CORONARY SYNDROMES
   Edited by Christopher P. Cannon, 1999
2. MINIMALLY INVASIVE CARDIAC SURGERY
   Edited by Mehmet C. Oz and Daniel J. Goldstein, 1999
3. ANNOTATED ATLAS OF ELECTROCARDIOGRAPHY
   By Thomas M. Blake, 1999
4. PLATELET GLYCOPROTEIN IIB/IIIA INHIBITORS IN CARDIOVASCULAR DISEASE
   By A. Michael Lincoff and Eric J. Topol, 1999

Annotated Atlas of Electrocardiography

A Guide to Confident Interpretation

Thomas M. Blake, MD

Professor of Medicine Emeritus
University of Mississippi School of Medicine

HUMANA PRESS Totowa, New Jersey

999 Riverview Drive, Suite 208
Totowa, New Jersey 07512

This publication is printed on acid-free paper. ∞
ANSI Z39.48-1984 (American National Standards Institute)
Permanence of Paper for Printed Library Materials.

For additional copies, pricing for bulk purchases, and/or information about other Humana titles, contact Humana at the above address or at any of the following numbers: Tel.: 973-256-1699; Fax: 973-256-8341; E-mail: humana@humanapr.com or visit our Website: http://humanapress.com

Cover design by Patricia F. Cleary.

ISBN 0-89603-762-2

Printed in the United States of America. 10 9 8 7 6 5 4 3 2 1

Library of Congress Cataloging-in-Publication Data

Blake, Thomas M. (Thomas Mathews), 1920–
Annotated atlas of electrocardiography : a guide to confident interpretation / Thomas M. Blake.
p. cm.
Includes bibliographical references and index.
ISBN 0-89603-762-2 (hardcover : alk. paper). --ISBN 0-89603-768-1 (softcover : ak. paper)
1.Electrocardiography--Atlases. I. Title.
[DNLM: 1. Electrocardiography atlases. 2. Heart Diseases-diagnosis atlases. WG 17B636a 1999]
RC683.E5B547 1999
616.1'207547'0222--dc21
DNLM/DLC for Library of Congress 98-36685
CIP

Preface

The purpose of *Annotated Atlas of Electrocardiography* is to promote awareness of electrocardiography as the practice of medicine, based on the same knowledge of anatomy, physiology, and pathology that underlies all clinical activity; examination of an electrocardiogram is very much like physical examination. For those considering the subject for the first time, it will provide a foundation for experience, and, it is hoped, a stimulus to want to learn more. Those already familiar with a pattern approach, and a vocabulary that does not translate easily to signs and symptoms, and who are not satisfied, will be reassured that there is more to it than that.

A medical student watching a doctor listen to a patient's heart with a stethoscope knows exactly what data are being acquired and how they are being processed. That same student watching that same doctor interpret an electrocardiogram may not understand either what data are being acquired or how they are being processed, but should. It is important to know how we know what we know.[5]

The practice of electrocardiography is easy, just as the practice of any other branch of medicine is easy; all that is needed is to know how, and to be experienced. After Vesalius had introduced scientific methods to the study of anatomy, someone observed that Galen had held medicine back a thousand years. Someone else replied that it wasn't Galen who had held things back, but doctors who had accepted tradition (the state of the art?) without questioning anything. Dr. Semmelweiss lost his job for proposing that doctors wash their hands in an antiseptic solution before delivering babies. Tradition is important in eletrocardiography, but questioning is in order, too. Most books on the subject consist largely of pictures of tracings, with the clinical setting described—an "external" approach. If one knows the patient, it is difficult to see the tracing objectively. Physical examination is not entirely objective, either, when the history is known, but the doctor is still responsible for evaluating the findings, and their relation to history and lab, as objectively as possible. Medical students all learn the vocabulary of electrocardiography in their first year, and are shown tracings later as part of patient presentations, but not often are they taught the methods needed to analyze them. The approach in this book is to examine the tracing first, and convert the findings to the vocabulary of clinical medicine. Only then can they be coordinated with information from history, physical, and other laboratory studies.

It is a pleasure to acknowledge the professional counsel of faculty colleagues Drs. Kenneth R. Bennett, Angel Markov, Charles K. Moore, Khidir Osman, Douglas A. Wolfe, and, especially, Drs. Patrick H.Lehan, Gaston Rodriguez, and Thomas N. Skelton, the input of medical students, house officers, Fellows, and technicians, and the technical support of Mr. William Buhner in Computer Graphics, Mrs. Faye Johnson of the Computer Laboratory, and Mr. Rickey Shields, Mr. Russell Burnett, and the staff of Middle South Computer Exchange. The support of Mr. Thomas Lanigan of Humana Press and his patient and capable staff has been invaluable.

Thomas M. Blake, MD
JACKSON, MISSISSIPPI

Contents

1 Introduction

Contents

Introduction

I have a faculty friend who says that details of curriculum and teaching methods are unimportant; when medical students decide what they want to learn, they'll learn it. The more experience I have the more I recognize the wisdom in this view. It is as applicable to electrocardiography as to any other discipline, of course, but with a difference; neither criteria for competence in electrocardiography, nor guidelines for its practice, are standard. There are calls from time to time for adequate training ("teaching" would be a better word) by qualified and experienced physicians, but criteria for what is adequate are not given. Familiarity with the current cardiology literature sometimes seems to be the only test of qualification, and numbers of tracings the only measure of experience. Standards for completeness and usefulness of the interpretation are not mentioned, and explanation is not often required.

Nobody would expect medical students to put what they know about anatomy, physiology, and pathology into clinical practice without having been shown how to apply it, how to take a history and do a physical examination, but comparable methods for application of the basic sciences to orderly analysis of electrocardiograms are not taught. No certifying agency would approve a chart system that notes only diagnoses without a record of the findings on which they are based, but no documentation of findings, or of reasoning, is required of those who interpret electrocardiograms, and there are no rules for determining acceptability of their conclusions. Everybody knows the vocabulary, and the prevailing view seems to be that interpretation is just a matter of pattern recognition, a situation that does not stimulate many to want to learn.

This paradox led to *The Practice of Electrocardiography,* a textbook with definitions, methods, and criteria for each step of the process, from recording to interpretation.[1] That book includes a few illustrative tracings, but its subject is methods, how to analyze a tracing, decide what it means, and express the result in language that makes it useful to another doctor. To try to do this by showing tracings would be like teaching physical examination by showing patients, reading by showing printed pages, or how to play a piano by playing one.

Once a logical approach has been mastered, though, a set of tracings, selected to demonstrate the variations that can be expected in each component, and the complexity of their interrelations, each accompanied by a brief discussion, can be useful as an introduction to clinical experience; hence this book, an atlas, an annotated workbook. Think of it as serving the same purpose as the set of tissue sections issued to students in the course in Pathology. Their textbooks have pictures, but to look at a picture in a book is not the same as examining a slide, studying different fields under different magnifications, and going back and looking again after having read the next page. The same is true in electrocardiography. Pictures in textbooks show classic examples of single abnormalities, but this is not always what is seen in practice. Right bundle branch block, for instance, may be an isolated abnormality, but also may be found in the same tracing with atrial fibrillation, and/or a myocardial infarct, and not all examples of right bundle block, even when uncomplicated, look like all others.

Target Audience

A premise that must be identified early is that all doctors should be capable of analyzing and interpreting EKGs, to the same extent that they can analyze and interpret chest X-rays. Only in this way can the completeness and adequacy of the official report be subjected to the same critical evaluation as the X-ray report, or any other consultant's note. Given that, what this collection has to offer depends upon the role, experience, and motivation of the user. For a medical or nursing student, it is intended to stimulate interest, and encourage building confidence and a firm foundation for experience. Those who are more advanced can benefit by comparing their findings and interpretations to those recorded and discussed here, considering the reason for any discrepancy, and deciding for themselves what is "right." Experienced practitioners, especially those who have depended largely on pattern recognition, can get insight, and find examples of some unusual forms. All, especially technicians and those responsible for teaching and supervising them, should gain an increased appreciation of the importance to the patient of technical skills. The browser may enjoy it at any level.

Electrocardiography and Physical Examination

Examination of an electocardiogram is much like physical examination (Fig. 1–1); in each, four methods are used to identify features that will be correlated with information from the history and other sources to produce a diagnosis. In one, Temperature, Pulse, Respiration, and Blood Pressure are noted, and Inspection, Palpation, Percussion, and Auscultation are applied the head, chest, abdomen and,extremities. In the other, Rates and Intervals are estimated, and the Orientation, Duration, Amplitude, and Contour of P, QRS, ST, and T are determined. The difference between them is the ease with which the relevance of the findings is recognized.

The connection between the findings on physical examination, and the structural and functional characteristics they represent, is clear, and their relation to each other, and to the history, is obvious. Findings in the electrocardiogram are more abstract, representing the course through time and space of a single theoretical point as it departs from and returns to, or fails to return to, another, fixed, point in a medium with certain characteristics. They are just as real as murmurs and blood pressure, but must be converted to the language of the history and physical to be meaningful, much as a computer program written for one disc operating system is converted to run on another. A hundred years of laboratory study and clinical correlation have made it possible to do this, but the bottom line always reflects judgment.

Sometimes the findings in a tracing, by themselves, can establish a diagnosis objectively. Atrial fibrillation or second degree AV block are examples. More often the meaning of the findings depends, to some extent, on clinical judgment, and this is influenced by their stability or instability, and by the interpreter's experience and knowledge of the clinical setting. Interpretation of electrocardiograms is the practice of medicine, and the first rule for that, as everyone knows, is to do no harm. The doctor is supposed to do the right thing, even when the data on which decisions must be based are incomplete,[4] and this requires that the reasoning behind decisions be known and understood to the extent possible.

The Clinical Nature of Electrocardiography

Though based on sound principles of anatomy and physiology, and a hundred years' experience, in practice electrocardiography is, of all clinical disciplines, the most subject to judgment. Its usefulness depends on interpretation, and this is communicated from one doctor to another in the report; *the EKG report is to the electrocardiographer what a scalpel is to a surgeon, the ultimate interface with the patient.* The most basic assumption in verbal communication is that everyone involved attributes the same meaning to the symbols it employs, words; i.e., speaks the same language. This has not always been

EKG Compared to Physical Examination

History	*Physical*	*Lab (EKG)*
Chief Complaint	TPR and BP	Rates and Intervals
Present illness	IPPA	ODAC
Systems review	Head	P
Past history	Chest	QRS
Personal history	Abdomen	ST
Et cetera	Extremities	T
↓	↓	↓
Impression	Impression	Interpretation
Topography	Topography	Mechanism
Etiology	Etiology	Structure
Manifestations	Manifestations	Function

The language of the history and physical examination is the same as that of anatomy, physiology, and pathology; understood by all doctors. The relation of findings to the patient, to signs and symptoms, is obvious.

The language of electrocardiography is unique, and must be translated to that of clinical medicine to be useful.

⇓

Diagnosis

Information from all three sources, history, physical, and lab, is processed, and as each new piece of information is considered, thinking adjusts automatically to assimilate it. The process works much like a word-processing program, and leads to a summary statement that tells what the problem is, where it is, and what brought it about; manifestations, topography, and etiology.

Fig. 1-1

recognized in electrocardiography, so the definitions in Appendix I are offered to satisfy this requirement.

How to Use This Book

Some understanding of anatomy, physiology, and electrocardiography is assumed. The book can be used most effectively as a supplement to the text described above, but it can be helpful in conjunction with any EKG book in which the terminology is defined clearly and used consistently; all aim at the same result, and achieve it with different degrees of success. Shown a classic example of an acute myocardial infarct, for instance, or a PVC, not many doctors would disagree about the interpretation. However, when asked to explain exactly how they know it, their responses would vary widely, and, when the findings are less than classic, their reports may be made meaningless by such modifiers as "possible," "consistent with," or "cannot rule out." To rely on experience as the sole basis for authority is to say "Trust me; that's what an infarct, or a PVC, looks like," an approach that may satisfy a patient, but is not very helpful to one who wants to learn. Confidence comes with understanding how we know what we know, precisely which features of the line on the graph tell us that it represents an infarct, what it is about that beat that tells that it originated in the ventricular myocardium.

Having read this introduction and determined into which of the user categories you fall, the next step is to review the "Summary of Rules, Assumptions, Methods, and Criteria for an Interpretation of EKGs" in Chapter 2. Neither these nor the definitions in Appendix I are very controversial, but must be understood as the rules of the game. If you choose not to accept one or more of them, write down your alternative, apply it consistently, and be prepared to justify your choice, at least to yourself. *Don't memorize anything*, but be aware that definitions and principles, though fundamental, are not agreed upon by all practitioners. If you are looking for a specific subject, use the index; if browsing, or testing yourself, describe tracings according to the methods outlined in Chapter 2 and compare your findings and conclusions to those in the box beneath each tracing. You are the one who decides what is in the patient's best interest. A good way to test the validity of your work, to determine whether you are "right", is to be sure that all abnormalities noted in your description are accounted for in the interpretation, and that the interpretation is justified in the description. It helps to mark questionable findings as you go. Numbers in parentheses refer to pages in *The Practice of Electrocardiography*[1] where the subject is discussed in more detail, The bibliography there will lead to the literature. The index can be used to find other examples of a feature.

About the Tracings

With only a few exceptions, neither the reasons these tracings were ordered, the clinical setting, nor what effect the interpretations may have had, is known. This is a problem faced by most who interpret electrocardiograms for others, and is a limiting factor in how helpful they can be. It underscores the importance of being sure what information there is in the tracing itself, of stating it clearly, and of documenting the features that explain it. Whether the interpretation is "right" is a matter of judgment, and the primary doctor is the final arbiter of that. It is always possible to imply the same thing in different words, and to interpret the same findings as having different meanings. Risk to the patient is minimized if there is good communication between the doctor who orders the tracing and the one who interprets it. Comparison to previous tracings, the more the better, is part of every interpretation. Serial changes cannot be shown very well in a book of this size, but there is often information in the difference between two tracings that is not inherent in either alone.

The tracings are in the usual twelve-lead format, recorded at twenty-five millimeters (mm) per second with one millivolt (mV) producing a deflection of ten millimeters. The grid has been eliminated to maximize visibility of detail, but the time lines in the margin are standard, representing 0.04, 0.20, and 3.0 seconds. A pair of calipers in one's hand helps. Most photocopiers will permit restoration to original size if that is desired.

Chapter 3 includes a tutorial and a summary.

2 Methods

CONTENTS

Methods

Management of a patient's problems is based on their assessment by three methods: history, physical examination, and laboratory study. In most instances, the results of laboratory study are supplied by technicians as facts, often numbers, to be put into context by the same doctor who took the history, did the physical examination, and ordered the test, but at other times lab results represent the opinion of a second doctor. Reports of X-ray studies, tissue sections, and electrocardiograms are in this second category; in effect, consultation notes.

This is recognized by radiologists and pathologists, who document the findings leading to their interpretations, but only rarely by those who interpret electrocardiograms; explanation is not part of the usual EKG report. All three groups study structures and functions well known to the doctors to whom they report. A chest X-ray is an easily recognizable picture of these, and a tissue section is a slice of the unknown itself, but an electrocardiogram is only a representation of their effect on the position in space of a hypothetical point in a series of instants. Radiologists and pathologists work in language common to all doctors, and the relevance to the patient of their reports is easy to evaluate, but electrocardiographers work in a jargon whose meaning is not obvious to all concerned, and their reports must translate electrical events into the vocabulary of clinical medicine.

Another factor is the very important role played by those who prepare material for study. In the case of X-rays and tissue sections, they are usually technologists who have been trained for their work, are employed by the doctors who interpret it, and understand their contributions to patient care; only seldom are all three of these qualifications found in EKG technicians.

All medical students are taught how to take a history and do a physical examination, and doctors are required to record their findings in both categories (albeit sometimes only briefly). Comparable documentary support for the interpretation of electrocardiograms depends upon comparable methods for their analysis, and instruction in these is not part of most medical school curricula; introduction to them is the subject of this chapter. Their use depends upon you. See Fig. 1-1, "EKG Compared to Physical Examination." The worksheet in *Fig. 2-1* identifies the findings to be evaluated in detail and is comparable to the form for physical examination learned by secondyear medical students in the course on physical diagnosis. The versions in *Figs. 2-2, 2-3,* and *2-4* can be compared to the changes in patient writeups with increasing experience.

The short form for the physical examination of the tracing is *not* something to be memorized; repetition will make it second nature. It serves not only as a guide for acquisition of data but also as an outline for their display in a fixed order, documenting the findings and explaining the interpretation.

EKG WORKSHEET

Patient Information

(1) Name a ______ ID Number b ______ Date and time tracing made c ______

Mechanism

(2) Rates/minute and intervals in hundredths of a second.

Atria: **a** ______ Vents: **b** ______ PR: **c** ______ QRS: **d** ______ QT: **e** ______

(3) Pacemaker for atria: **a** ______ AV conduction: **b** ______ Pacemaker for ventricles: **c** ______

Structure

(4) Atria (P): ______

(5) Vents (QRS): frontal **a** ___° RV1:SV1 **b** ___ : ___ Transition **c** ______ RV6:SV6 **d** ___ : ___ Contour **e** ______

Function

(6) ST: Displacement (the position of a point, J) **a** ______

Contour (the shape of a line) **b** ______

(7) T: Frontal **a** ____°, Precordial **b** ____V1, ____V2, ____V3, ____V4, ____V5, ____V6

(8) U: not remarkable ( ), other______

Other

(9) QRS-T angle: Frontal **a** ______°, Horizontal **b** ______°

(10) Change since tracing of date/time: ______ , ______

Interpretation

(11) Mechanism: ______

(12) Structure: ______

(13) Function: ______

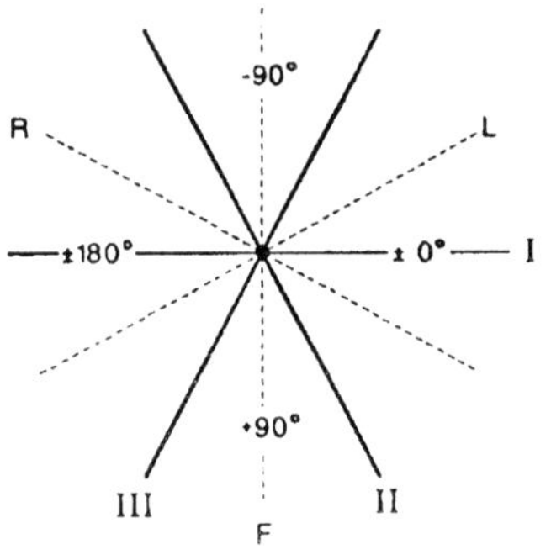

All leads are labeled at their positive poles

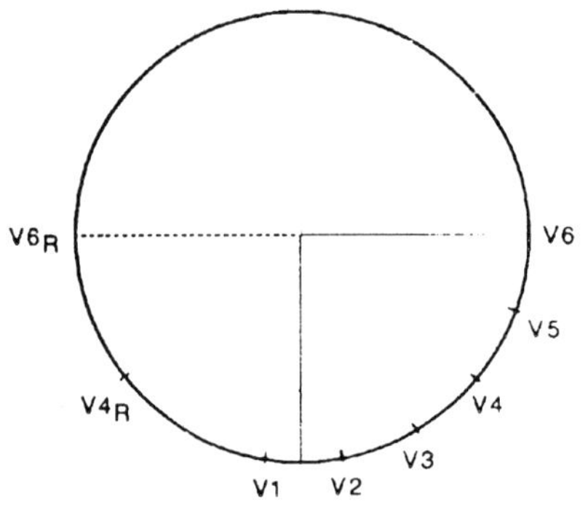

Interpreted by: ______, Date: ______

Fig. 2-1 Order for analysis of an electrocardiogram.

Description

A rate V rate PR duration QRS duration QT duration Mechanism

QRS: Frontal axis R:S V1 transition R:S V6 Contour

ST: displacement

ST: contour

T: Frontal axis positive/negative/amplitude/contour V1-6

Ad hoc: P, U, change since previous tracing, etc.

Interpretation

(1) Mechanism: atria, ventricles, and relation between them
(2) Structure: P and QRS
(3) Function: ST-T-U

Signed:____________________, Date:_________, Time:_________

Fig. 2-2 Short form for describing an EKG, intermediate version.

A V PR QRS QT Mechanism

MFQRS R:SV1, Tz, R:SV6, Contour

ST displacement

ST contour

MFT V1, V2, V3, V4, V5, V6

Interpretation:____________________

Signed:_____________, Date/time:___

Fig. 2-3 Short form, minimal version.

80 80 20 08 40 sinus

+30 1:10 V4 10:0 normal

none

normal

+60 negative V1 positive V2-6

(1) Sinus mechanism, rate 80
(2) Within normal limits

Signed:_____________, Date/time:___

Fig. 2-4 Example of short form completed.

Summary of Rules, Assumptions, Methods, and Criteria for EKG Interpretation

1. Interpretation of an electrocardiogram, conversion of the information in it to language relevant to signs and symptoms, is the practice of medicine; judgment is always a factor, but it must be based on objective, documented data.
2. This process requires that (a) the vocabulary of the method be defined clearly, (b) definitions are used consistently, and (c) each step is treated as specifically as possible. The difference between what is seen, and what it is interpreted to mean, must be plain.
3. Einthoven's hypotheses are basic to all electrocardiography. They have been validated by nearly a hundred years of experience, and are assumed to be operative unless there is proof to the contrary. They can be summarized usefully. (a) The heart acts electrically as a single dipole, or generator, (b) in the center of a volume conductor (the thorax and abdomen) of equal conductivity throughout. (c) The shoulders and symphysis pubis form an equilateral triangle about this, and (d) the arms and legs act as linear conductors attached to the body at these apices.
4. Two other facts are almost as basic: (a) the ventricles are activated *simultaneously* in a radial direction, i.e., from endo cardium to epicardium; and (b) the nature of the recorder, a galvanometer, is such that there is only *one point in play*, a point that moves in time and space, reflecting the *net* result of *all* electrical activity in the body. Its position at any instant can be represented as the tip of an arrow originating at the center of this system, an instantaneous vector, or "axis." When this points toward the positive pole of a lead, an upstroke is written in that lead; away from it, a downstroke.
5. There are two criteria for acceptability of an interpretation, completeness and adequacy. It is complete if it covers mechanism, structure, and function, and adequate if it does this as precisely as possible in words that relate the findings to signs and symptoms. Caveats (e.g., "possible," "cannot rule out," and "consistent with") are inappropriate. Three levels of confidence are recognized: suggestive, probable, and actionable. Helpful discussion may be added as a comment, and there are no clear rules for language here.

   Definitions are listed in Appendix I.

3 A Guide to Use of the Collection

Contents

Each tracing in the Collection has been analyzed (rates and intervals, and orientation, duration, amplitude, and contour of P, QRS, and ST-T-U) and the findings documented and reassembled as an interpretation with three elements, mechanism, structure, and function, stated in the language of the history and physical examination, not in EKG jargon. Their usefulness depends on direct relevance to the three components of a diagnosis: topography, etiology, and manifestations. With so many parts, and so many ways to indicate most of them, no mutually exclusive classification is completely satisfactory. *Fig. 3-1* and the list below, however, offer a framework for evaluation of the information in each. The QRS is the stable part of the ventricular complex, ST is intermediate, and T/U most sensitive; a "shift to the right" implies diminishing specificity, much as a "shift to the left" does in a white cell differential (43).* Use the index for cross references.

Consider

1. Rates and intervals
2. P/*f*: origin of atrial excitation, atrial enlargement
3. PR: long (AV block), short (pre-excitation ?), A/V relation
4. QRS: Initial: pre-excitation, myocardial infarction
   Mid/diffuse: left ventricular hypertrophy, left bundle branch block, right ventricular enlargement
   Terminal: RBBB, fascicular block, hypothermia

*Numbers in parentheses refer to pages in *The Practice of Electrocardiography*[1].

7. ST: displacement, contour (injury ?)
8. T/U: orientation, duration (QT), amplitude, contour, (coronary insufficiency? left ventricular overload? drug or electrolyte effect/imbalance?, nonspecific?)

A Tutorial: *The Mechanism*

The mechanism of the heartbeat is always defined first in an EKG report. This definition indicates the focus from which atrial excitation proceeds, its rate and its rhythm, the same for the ventricles, and the causal relation, if any, between them. It is usually called "the rhythm." On physical examination, atrial activity is judged by its effect on the ventricles (not many of us use the jugular venous pulse), but in the EKG it is observed directly, and may occur at the same time as ventricular activity. When it can be identified, it is as a P or an *f* wave (see below). If it cannot be identified, this must be noted. You will rarely be called upon to interpret a tracing that shows no ventricular activity, but atrial activity may not be visible even though present.

The reason for defining mechanism in such detail is that in the traditional jargon of electrocardiography "rhythm" and "heart" relate to the ventricles alone, but that is not being as precise as possible; atria and ventricles may function independently or in various combinations. It may make a difference, for instance, that, even when the ventricles are being driven satisfactorily by an artificial pacemaker, there is atrial fibrillation. Ectopy may not be even suspected when the ventricular rhythm is regular at a rate of 80, but there may be atrial activity at a rate

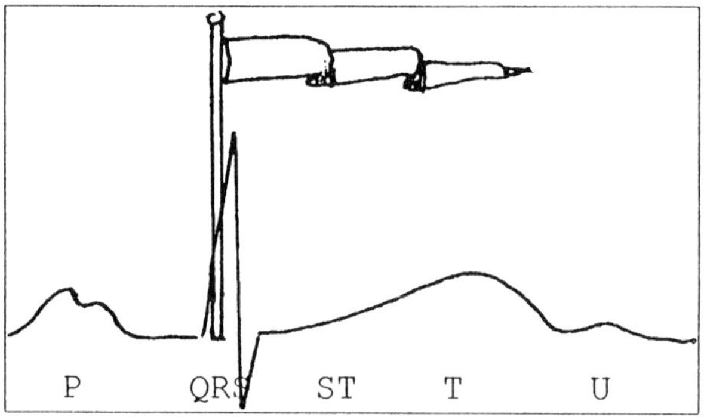

Fig. 3-1 The sensitivity-specificity of QRS-T is like a pennant on a pole. (Modified from Fig. 2-9 in *The Practice of Electrocardiography*[1].)

of 320. Regular ventricular activity at rate 40 may be of sinus origin with normal AV conduction, the sinus rate may be 80 with 2:1 AV block, or there may be complete AV block with junctional or ventricular escape, or some other explanation. Accurate knowledge of these, or other alternatives, depends on findings in the EKG documenting the rate and origin of atrial and ventricular beats. The rhythm of each is accepted as regular (within the limits of sinus arrhythmia) unless specified otherwise. In practice, QRS rate is observed first, and atrial rate is assumed to be the same; if it is not, this will become apparent as soon as the PR interval is evaluated, the next step, and notation of the atrial rate can be changed accordingly. To say that there is a PR is to say that P gave rise to the QRS that follows.

The name for the mechanism usually combines all three components, and those in common use do not always make perfect sense, often failing to distinguish among what is present, how it got to be that way, and what sustains it, and between atria and ventricles. Analysis of the relation between atria and ventricles in series of beats was the first clinical application of electrocardiography and is in the forefront of its application now. It should be pursued with all the precision possible.

A Tutorial: *Examination of One Heartbeat*

Atrial Activity (Fig. 3-2)

If atrial activity is identifiable (19), usually in Lead II or V1, it is as either *f* waves (irregular, unpredictable, fibrillary)(10) or P waves (regular, predictable, discrete) (70). The most important feature of a P is its presence; second, its orientation as an indication of its origin (28) (usually leftward, caudad, and initially ventrad and terminally dorsad when of sinus origin); and last its morphology, pointing to abnormality of one or both atria (29).

PR Interval (Fig. 3-3)

To enter a value for PR is to say that the impulse that produced the P traversed the AV junction and gave rise to the QRS (10,20, ±149). The time required for this, the PR interval, measured from the beginning of P to the beginning of QRS (8), is usually about 0.20 sec (Å0.04 sec) (21). It can be too long, first degree AV block (27, 150), but no minimum duration can be specified.

QRS Orientation

The orientation of QRS as a whole, its "axis" in the frontal leads, and its "transition" in V1-6, is part of the description of every tracing. It treats ventricular depolarization as an instantaneous event, though, rather than the time-consuming, complicated process that it is (34, 37), and, by itself, has little clinical application. The comparable finding on physical examination is the position of the patient (e.g., supine or seated). Like the axis, this is noted in every case, but, unlike the axis, not always even reported, much less accorded much significance by itself.

QRS Duration

The width of QRS (22) is a measure of the time required for ventricular depolarization. It cannot be too narrow, normal is the fastest possible, but if it is 0.12 sec or more, it is abnormal and must be explained. When this is the case, the key is usually in the contour (see below). If there is no abnormality of contour; i.e., if the complex consists of straight lines and sharp angles, widening may be evidence of poisoning, as with potassium (231), antiarrhythmics (231), or antidepressants (230).

QRS Amplitude (Voltage) (Fig. 3-4)

There are many, many ways in which QRS voltage may be modified (228), and a variety of definitions for low and high (41, 193, 228). It is assessed in every tracing, but the only time it is likely to present a problem is when the simplistic assumption

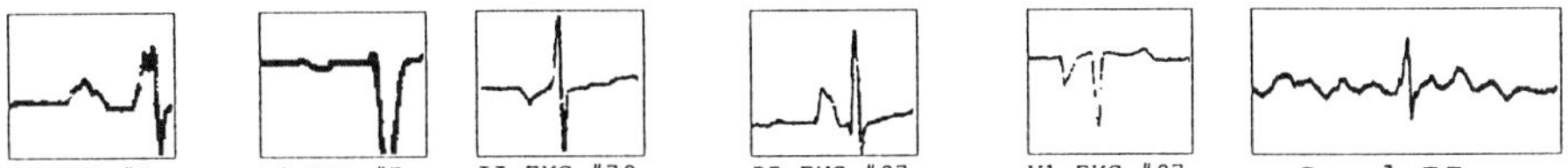

Fig. 3-2 Atrial Activity

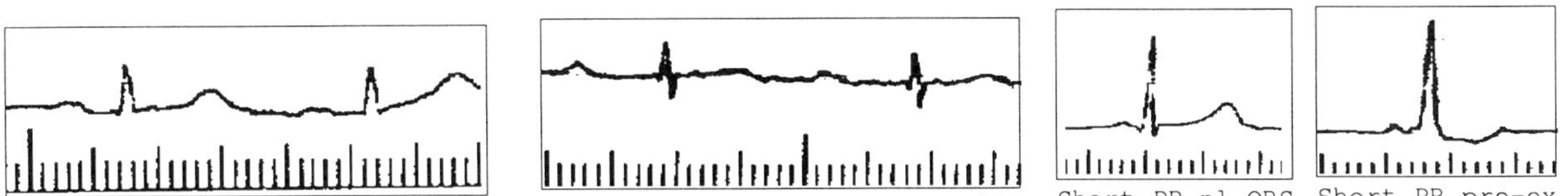

Fig. 3-3 PR Interval

is made that high voltage represents left ventricular hypertrophy (however high and hypertrophy are defined). There are almost as many definitions for the anatomic reality needed for validation of the EKG numbers as for the numbers used to define "high" (192,198). A similar, but less frequent, problem is equating low voltage with pericardial effusion (228). QRS voltage is notoriously inconstant (see inset), and, when it is the only presumably abnormal finding, has little if any clinical importance.

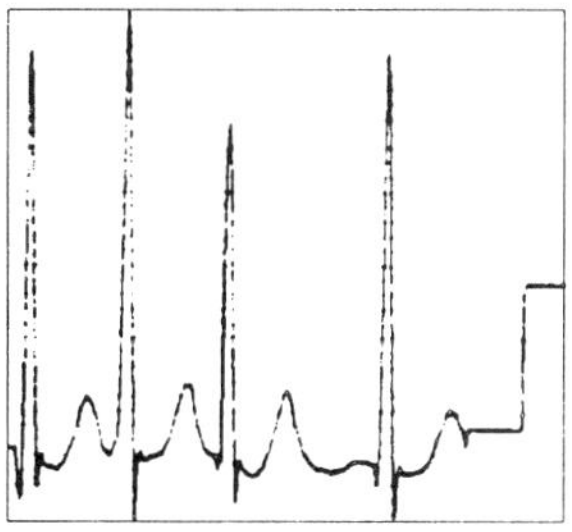

Fig. 3-4 QRS Amplitude

QRS Contour (Fig. 3-5)

Orientation, duration, and amplitude are mutually exclusive, independent variables. Orientation and amplitude can be expressed objectively in numbers that define the position at any instant of the moving point that the tracing represents, and so can the duration of each of its components (Q, R, S) as an indication of the rate at which this motion occurs. The shape of the graph that results is a function of all three, and varies with the point on the body (the position of the positive pole of the lead) from which it is recorded. Shapes are described by adjectives, not numbers.

The normal QRS contour is characterized by straight lines and sharp angles. Abnormality is often associated with widening of at least part of the complex, and may involve the initial forces selectively, as with myocardial infarction (173) and pre-excitation (155); only the terminal ones, as with right bundle branch block (159), left fascicular block (162), and hypothermia (237); or the whole complex, as with left bundle branch block (160). Fascicular block changes orientation of the late forces, but need not change either duration or contour. Other explanations are possible for all of these. There is some notching (42) in most tracings.

ST-T (Figs. 3-6, 3-7)

ST-T (44) may be normal in orientation, duration (QT), amplitude, and contour (below) or abnormal in any or all of these in any combination. ST may be elevated and arched, for instance, 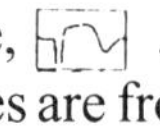 , or depressed and sagging, 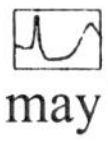 (both examples are from EKG 73). T amplitude may be normal, low, or tall; its contour defies precise description (48). See Fig. 3-6.

The level of the J *point* above or below the baseline defines ST displacement (elevation/depression) (9) (see "The tracing and its components" in Appendix

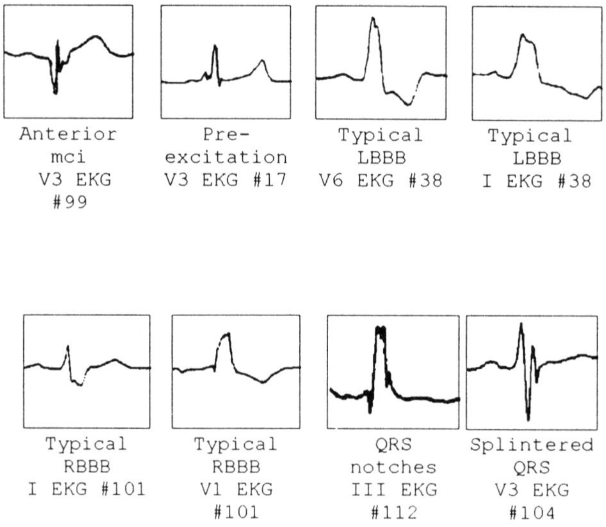

Fig. 3-5 QRS Contour

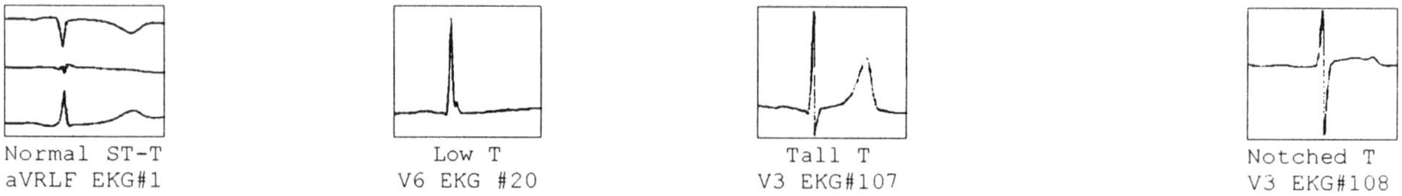

Fig. 3-6 T Contour

I) and the course of the *line* between this point and the apex of T is described as the ST contour. In the normal, the trace departs from the baseline at an increasingly rapid rate till it reaches the peak of T, as in Fig. 3-7 A, B, and E. If J and the peak of T are the same distance from the baseline, as in Fig. 3-7 D and F, ST is flat (or arched or sagging) (45, 202). Description of ST requires judgment and adjectives, and there are no absolutes. It cannot be accomplished entirely by computer programs, but, nevertheless, must be evaluated before interpretation is attempted. Displacement and contour are separate findings, a concept that can be illustrated by projecting a line from the apex of T back through QRS as in the diagrams in Fig. 3-7. If it reaches the B point, the contour is normal; if not, probably abnormal.

The Collection

Try to recognize an electrocardiogram for exactly what it is, a graphic representation of electrical activity in the heart, a *symbol*. It contains information that can be extracted by orderly analysis. Its elements must be considered, individually and collectively, and the findings reassembled to produce an interpretation, a report, whose usefulness depends on its relevance to information obtained from history, physical examination, and other laboratory studies. This requires precise definitions of not only the findings in the tracing, but also of the methods used to determine them, the limitations inherent in these methods, and the clinical reality thought to explain them. Dr. Wilson pointed out that electrocardiographic abnormalities are findings, not diseases[8], and Dr. Hayakawa emphasized that the symbol is not the thing symbolized [5].

The tracing contains information in three mutually exclusive categories, mechanism, structure, and function, and one or more of these may be normal while the others are abnormal; the mechanism, for instance, may be sinus in a tracing that shows an acute infarct and bundle branch block. Awareness of

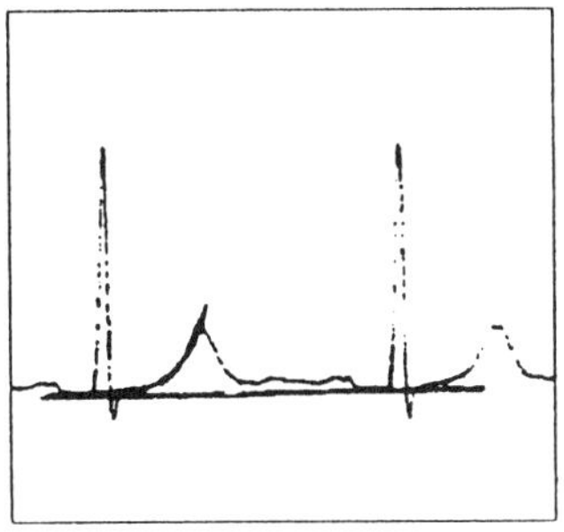

A Normal ST-T V5 EKG #2

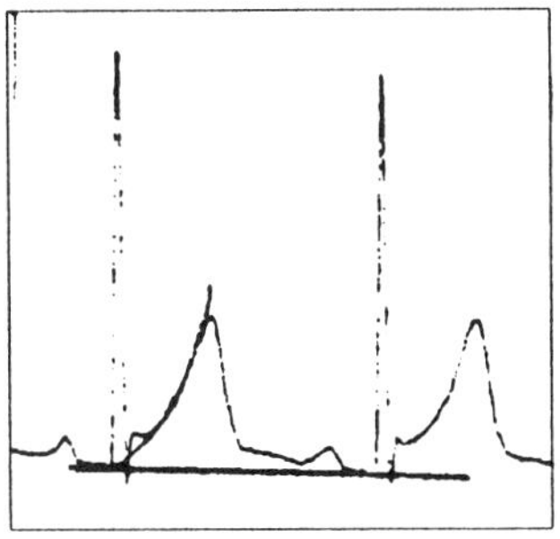

B Elevated J, normal ST-T, "Early repolarization" V5 EKG #21

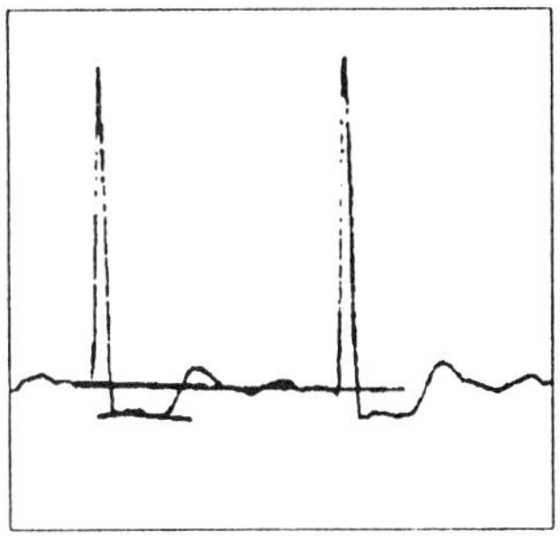

C Subendocardial injury as with coronary insuf. V5 EKG #55

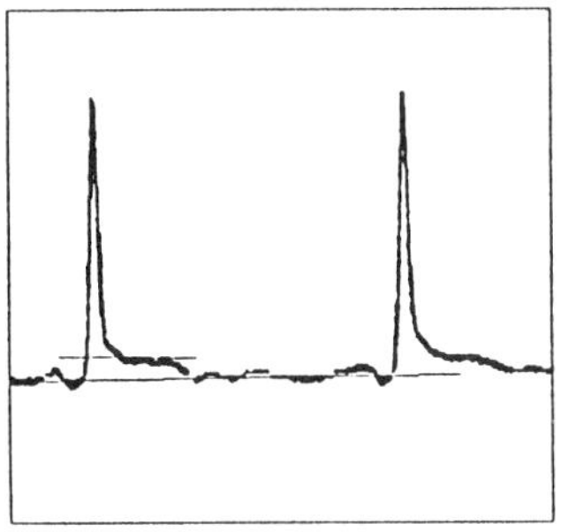

D Subepicardial injury as with pericarditis V% EKG #86

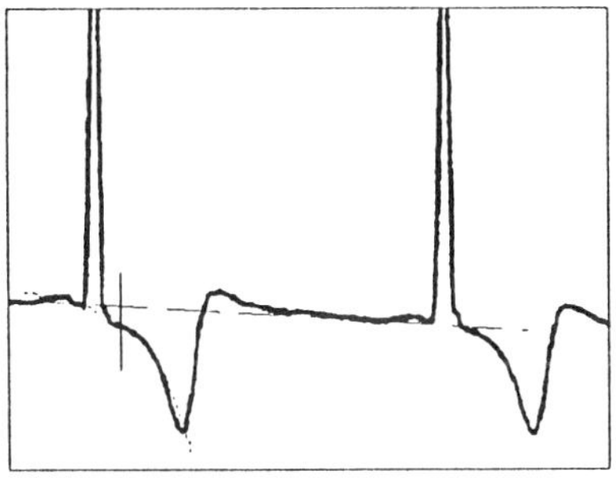

E Normal ST-T opposite QRS, as with left ventricular overload V5 EKG #67

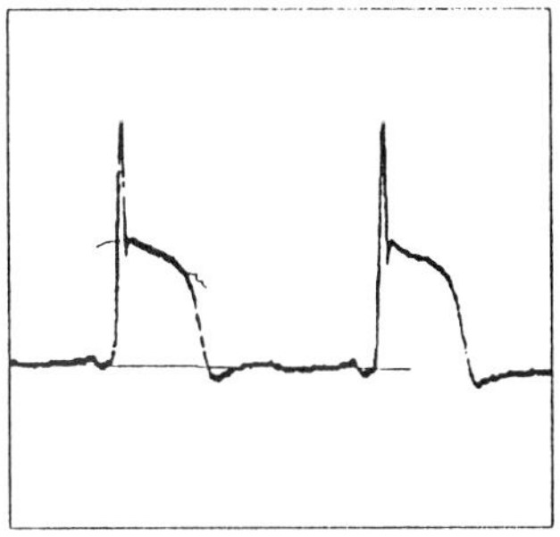

F ST elevation as with acute myocardial infarct V5 EKG #42

Fig. 3-7

the limitations of the method is necessary, including especially the range of normal for each component, and can come only with experience; complete analysis of every tracing, not just the feature that seems most important at the moment, is essential.

As a starting point, the first six tracings in this collection are normal in all respects; after that most include more than one abnormality. As a critical reader, you should ask how I know they are normal: "Who says so?" One response would be to cite authority derived from experience with hundreds of students and over a million tracings. Experience does count, and is a factor, but that approach is counter to the whole idea of electrocardiography as the practice of medicine; practitioners should understand the derivation of the decisions for which they are responsible. To that end, a better answer to your question is to describe the findings and my reasoning, leaving it up to you to decide whether I am right...just as I would explain a diagnosis of any clinical entity by describing the findings on which it is based. These are documented beneath each tracing. They were determined by the methods detailed in Chapter 2 of the textbook[1], and summarized in Chapter 2 of this one. Each is subject to modification within the limits of those methods. You may or may not agree; if you disagree, you should be able to say why. The final decision is yours.

Numbers in parentheses in the text below each tracing refer to pages in the *The Practice of Electrocardiography*[1] where more discussion will be found, and leads to the larger literature.

The Collection of Electrocardiograms

Contents

Note: Numbers in parentheses in the text of the Collection refer to pages in *The Practice of Electrocardiography*[1]. Abbreviations are defined in Appendix 2.

EKG 170	Right Atrial Enlargement, Pulmonary Emphysema
EKG 171	Old Lateral Myocardial Infarct (or crossed arm leads)
EKG 172	Old Inferior Myocardial Infarct: Evidence obliterated by transposition of left arm and leg leads
EKG 173	Precordial Leads on the Right: Within normal limits, but incomplete
EKG 174	Atrial Fibrillation; Digitalis Effect, Coronary Insufficiency; Left Ventricular Hypertrophy
EKG 175	Artifact Called Infarct, Precordial Leads in Reverse Order
EKG 176	Inferior Myocardial Infarct can be Masked by Crossed Left Arm and Leg Leads
EKG 177	Sinus Pauses, Bigeminy
EKG 178	Atypical IV Conduction Defect, Old Anterior Myocardial Infarct, Peri-Infarction Block? Etc.?
EKG 179	Crossed Left Arm and Leg Leads Simulate Inferior Myocardial Infarct
EKG 180	Crossed Arm Leads, Precordial Leads in Reverse Order
EKG 181	Acute Anterior Myocardial Infarct, Evolutionary Change
EKG 182	Artificial Atrial and Ventricular Pacemakers, Capturing Regularly (DDD)
EKG 183	QRS-Triggered Artificial Ventricular Pacemaker, Functioning Properly (VVT)
EKG 184	Time and Three Dimensions
EKG 185	Sinus Mechanism, Rate 230
EKG 186	Atrial Flutter, Effect of Adenosine
EKG 187	Duchenne Muscular Dystrophy
EKG 188	Simulator
EKG 189	Agonal
EKG 190	Cardiac Transplant, Two Sets of P Waves
EKG 191	Positive Exercise Test
EKG 192	AV Block in an Infant
EKG 193	P "Mitrale"
EKG 194	P "Congenitale"
EKG 195	Left Atrial Enlargement, Left Ventricular Overload
EKG 196	Left Bundle Branch Block, Anterior Myocardial Infarct
EKG 197	Mid-Precordial ST-T-U Pattern as with Coronary Insufficiency
EKG 198	Computer Called Infarct in an Infant
EKG 199	Artifact Mimics Ventricular Tachycardia
EKG 200	Muscle Tremor Simulates VT/VF

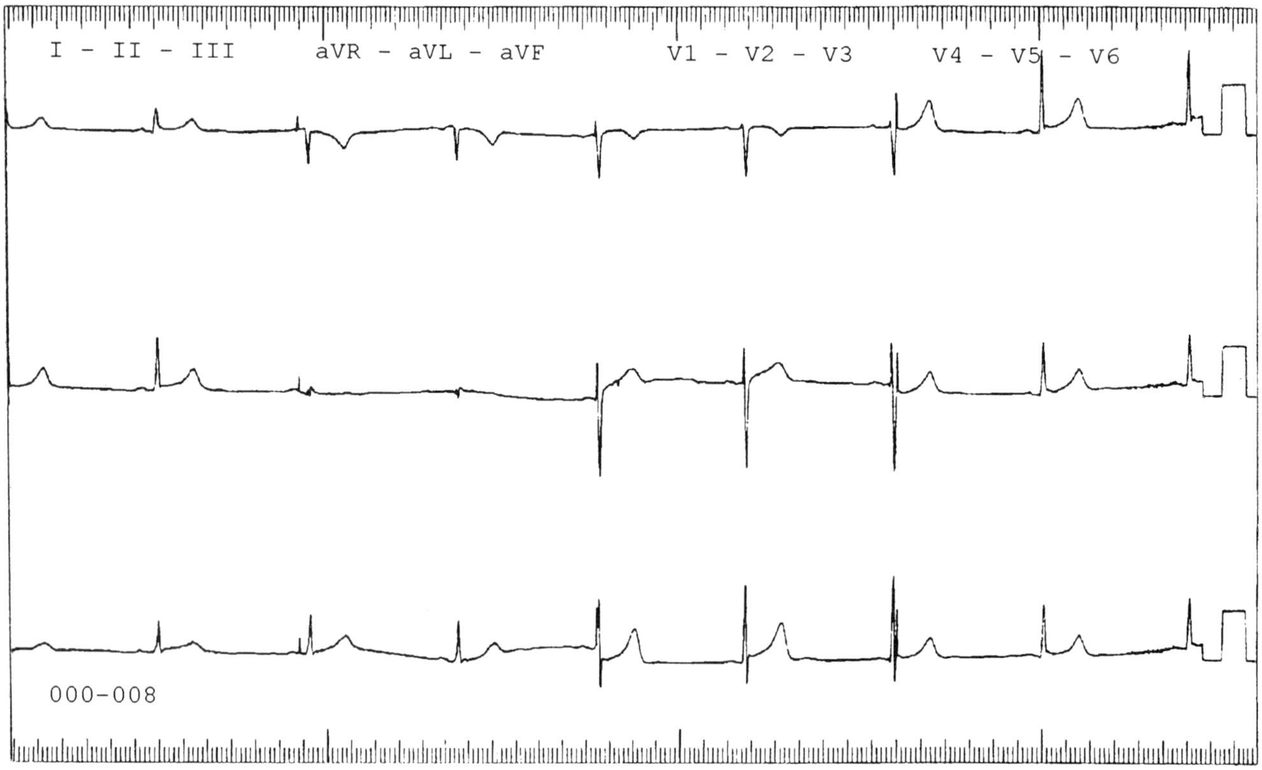

Within Normal Limits

Neutral, B point, baseline

```
55    55    16    08    40      sinus
+60   1:10    V2½   10:0    normal
              none
              normal
+60  negative V1,  positive V2-6

(1) Sinus mechanism, rate 55
(2) Within normal limits
```

Begin at the beginning. Between beats, when there is no electrical activity, the components of Einthoven's dipole (85) coincide to define a single point, Wilson's "central terminal of zero potential" (88), in the center of the chest at the level of the fourth intercostal space anteriorly. The EKG machine, a galvanometer, measures the difference in potential between two points, and when there is only one point there is no difference in potential, no voltage. The machine identifies this as its default level and places it at the center of the chart. As the paper moves, a flat line is written, the theoretical baseline. In a perfect tracing, this is the level in the interval between the U wave of one beat and the P of the next, and, for practical purposes, of the PQ segment, J point, and TU segment. Pragmatically, though, the trace is not perfectly steady, and the most nearly reproducible representation of neutral is the point that defines the beginning of QRS, the B point (8). Recognizing that it takes two points to determine a line, the baseline connects the B points of two contiguous beats in as nearly flat a section of the lead as possible (9, 221). All measurements are to or from the B point, or above or below the baseline. Position of the trace above this level means that the net force at that instant is directed toward the positive pole of the lead; negative, away from it.

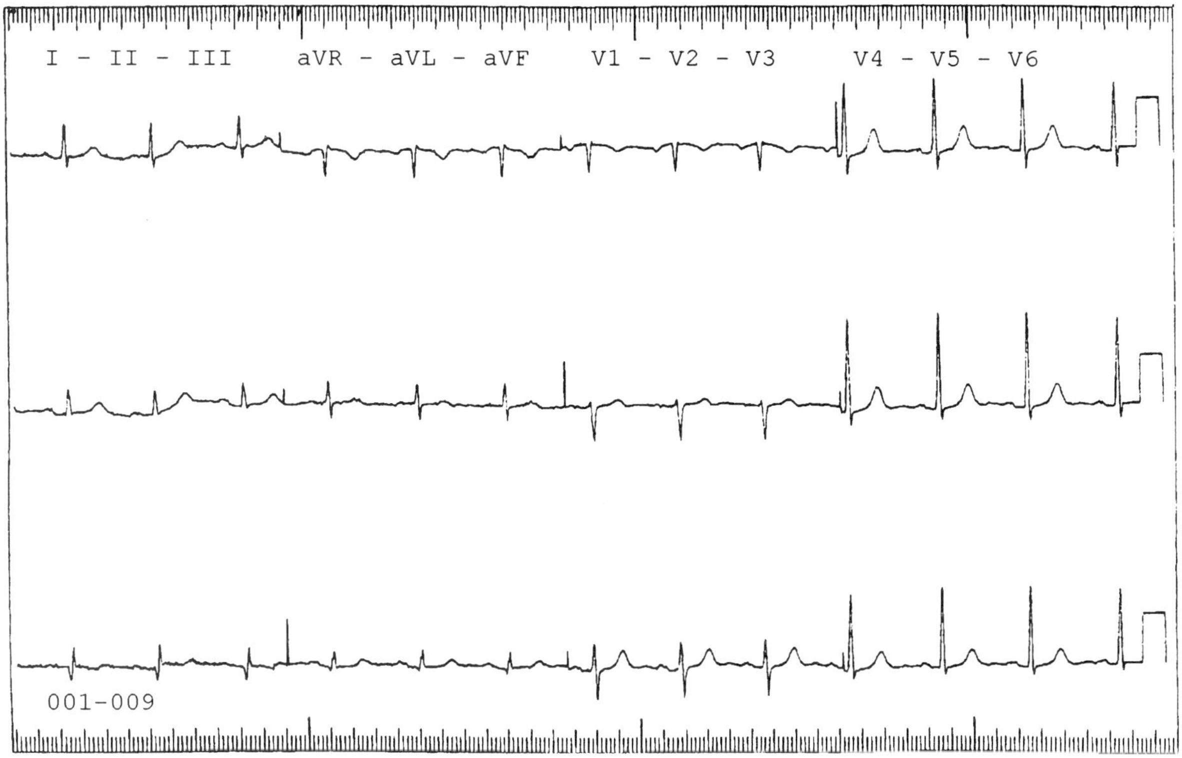

Within Normal Limits

Rates and Intervals

```
75    75    20    08    40      Sinus
+45    0:5    V3    15:1      normal
               none
              normal
+45   negative V1   positive V2-6

(1) Sinus mechanism, rate 75
(2) Within normal limits
```

Paper speed is 25 mm/sec(s). Rates are in beats per minute; intervals, in hundredths of a second. Time is indicated on an original by the background millimeter grid (12, 103), and in these tracings, by marks in the upper and lower margins, at 0.04, 0.20, and 3.0 s. It is helpful to have calipers in hand, but most rates and intervals can be estimated satisfactorily by inspection, recognizing reasonable limits of the method. The rhythm, both atrial and ventricular, is always relevant but rarely mentioned, in contrast with the axis, which is rarely important but nearly always noted. It is assumed to be (approximately) regular (123) unless stated otherwise. Intervals are measured to or from the B point (8), and all vary inversely with rate. Each is measured in the lead in which it is longest *and* can be identified with confidence. The limiting factor is deciding where P begins and where QRS and T end. The upper limits of normal are about 0.20 s (±0.04) for PR, 0.08 (±0.02) for QRS, and 0.40 (±0.04) for QT. No useful values can be given for lower limits. The QTc, included in most computer headers, represents an attempt to "correct" the measured QT for rate, but is of little value (24).

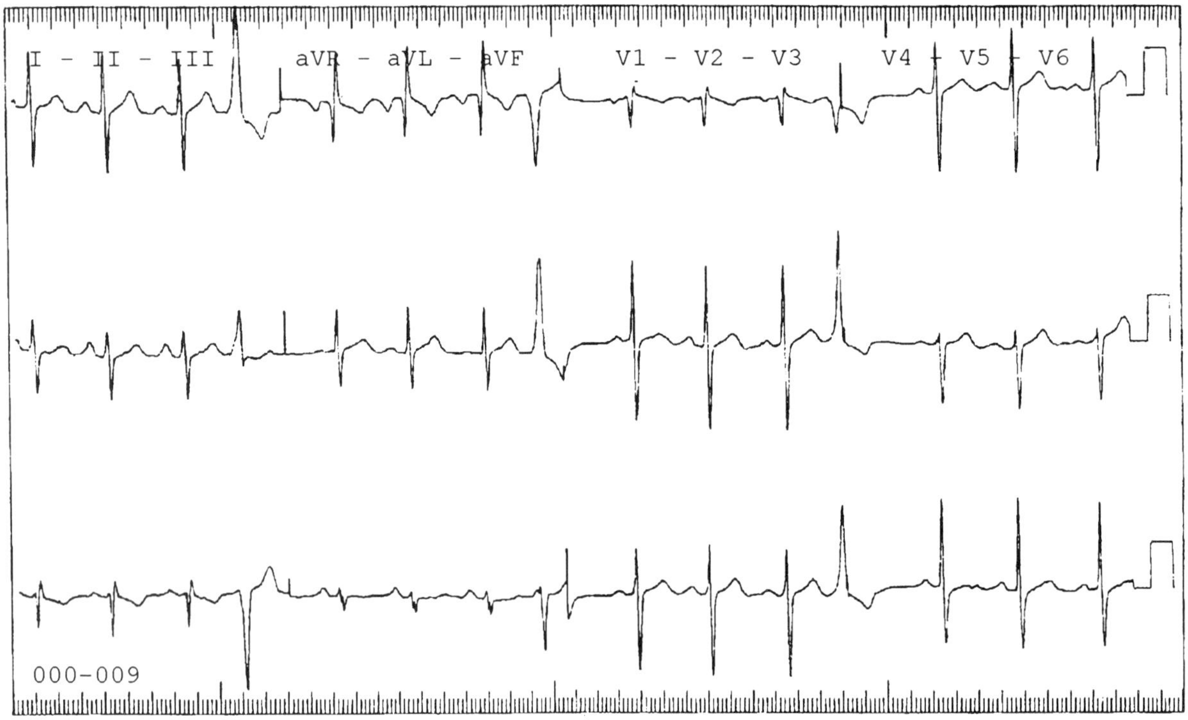

Within Normal Limits

Orientation, Axis

```
90   90   20   06   36    sinus/PVCs
--   1:6:2  V2-6  20:10    normal
              none
             normal
±0     neg V1 low         pos V2-6

(1) Sinus mechanism, rate 90,
    with PVC's
(2) Within normal limits
```

Orientation of QRS in the frontal plane is known as the electrical axis of the heart, the mean frontal QRS, or just "the axis" (34, 115, 226). In the horizontal plane, orientation is sometimes noted as early or late transition (38). Its counterpart on physical examination is the position of the patient (e.g., supine). Like the position of the patient, it is considered in every tracing, but, unlike the position of the patient, it is usually identified, and even offered as an interpretation ("left axis deviation"), even though neither "axis," the method by which it was determined, nor the range of normal is clear It has been known for many years that the axis "per se" has little clinical value.[2,3] It is a finding, much as the white cell count or the blood pressure is a finding, and its meaning can be evaluated only when the features above are known, and in the context of all other findings (226).

Orientation of the QRS as a whole, of each of its components individually, and of any other wave, is a function of its area, not just its amplitude (34). The computer called the axis in this tracing -90°, but a better assessment is that it is indeterminate "S1,2,3" (35, 88, 227), which recognizes the limits of the method.

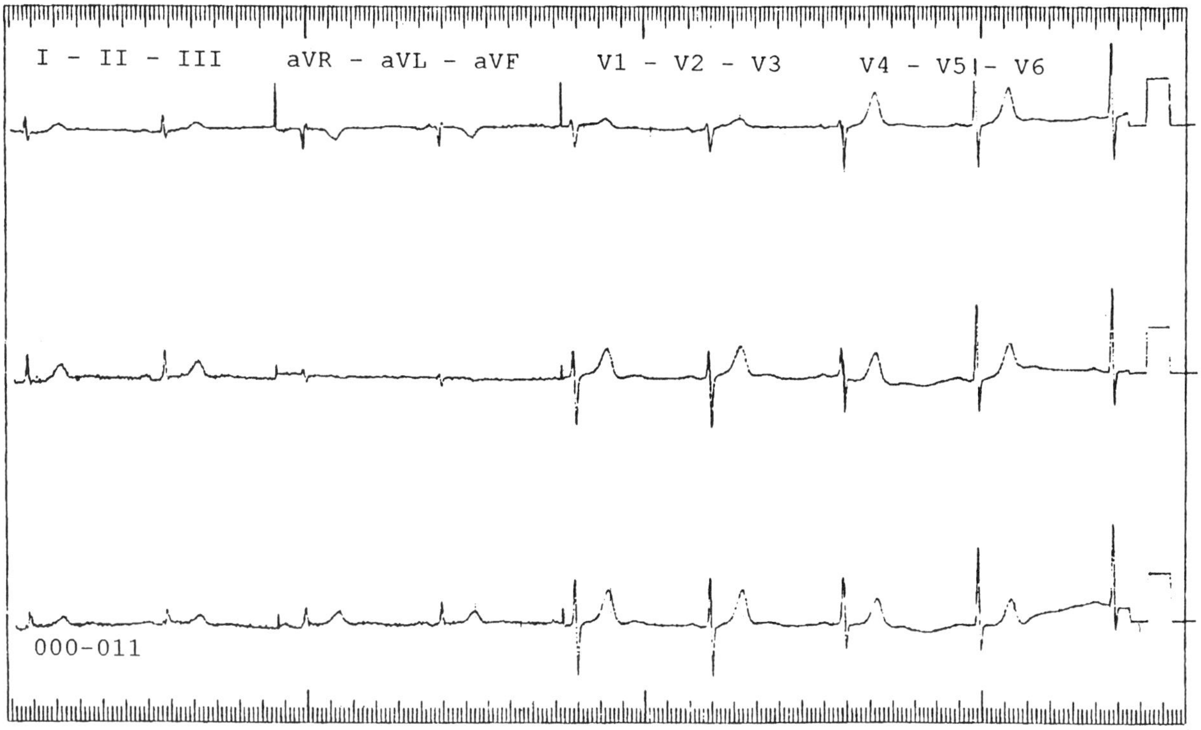

Within Normal Limits

Duration

```
50   50   20   08   40     sinus
+60  1:5   V3   15:5       normal
              none
             normal
+60         positive V1-6

(1) Sinus mechanism, rate 50
(2) Within normal limits
```

Duration of intervals and complexes was discussed with EKG 2, and in this tracing, as in that one, all are normal. The duration of P cannot be estimated usefully, but that of QRS is an important feature (75), representing the time needed for excitation of the ventricles. The atria are depolarized sequentially, and abnormality of both can be seen in a single tracing, but the ventricles are depolarized simultaneously, endocardium to epicardium (76), and to call abnormality in both is beyond the limits of the method for a single tracing. As with all intervals, the B point is a given; estimation of duration depends on choice of a point for the other end (29). For QRS, that means J, and the fact that J is really a shoulder rather than a point (119) limits the accuracy of this step. QRS duration ranges from about 0.04 s in infants to 0.10 s in adults, ±0.02 s. It cannot be too short, normal being the fastest possible, but can be lengthened in several ways besides bundle branch block (168), including pre-excitation and poisoning, as with antidepressants, antiarrhythmics, and potassium. If QRS is wide, its contour, and the duration of PR, are especially important; bundle branch block and pre-excitation both affect contour, but bundle branch block does not change PR. Poisoning is not likely to change either.

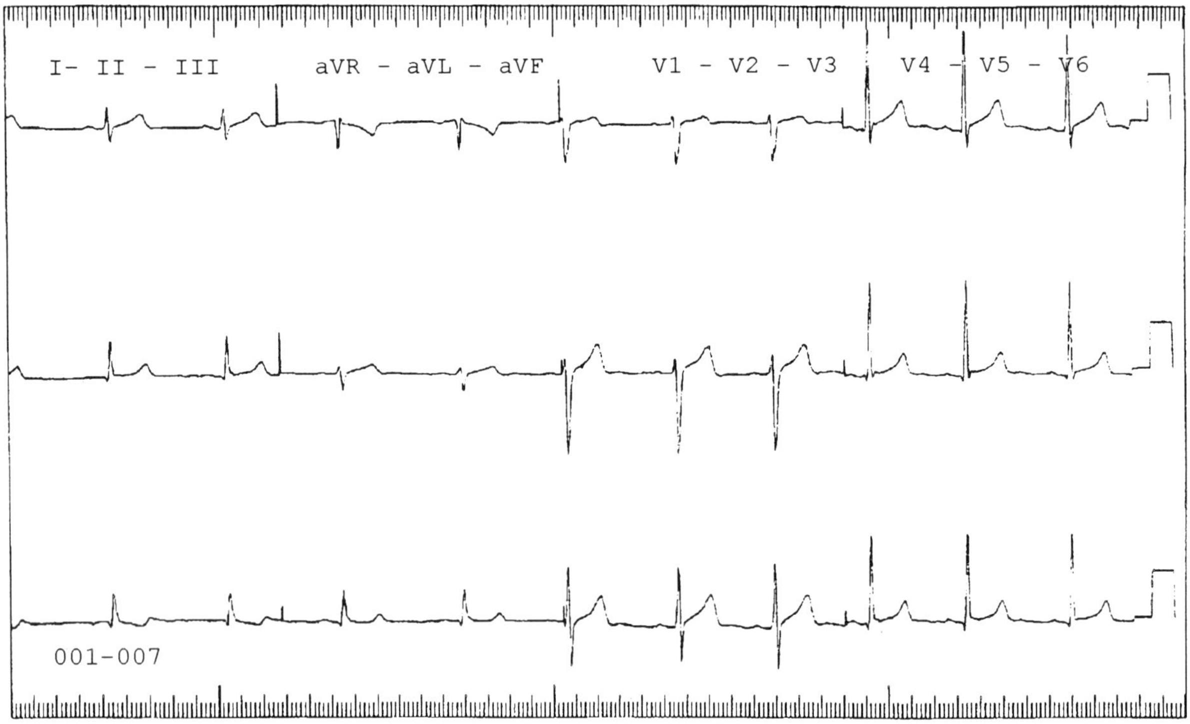

Within Normal Limits

Amplitude (voltage)

65	65	20	08	40	sinus
+75	2:8	V2½	20:0		normal
		none			
		normal			
+15		Positive V1-6			low V1

(1) Sinus mechanism, rate 65
(2) Within normal limits

With the exception of QRS, amplitude (voltage) is not often useful as an isolated finding in any component of the tracing, but it may be for QRS (39), and is estimated, at least in the horizontal plane, as part of routine analysis. T voltage is evaluated as high or low in proportion to QRS (50). P and U are too small and/or ill-defined for quantitative measurement; and as with T, description of them often combines amplitude and contour, e.g., small, prominent, peaked, notched.

QRS voltage becomes a problem for the patient in two settings. When perceived as high, it may be equated with left ventricular hypertrophy (195), low, with pericardial effusion (228), but neither of these is justified; voltage is influenced by many, many factors (229), and one can choose from a wide range of definitions of low and high. Its usefulness depends on correlation with reality, and there are as many criteria for the anatomic reality of left ventricular hypertrophy as there are for high QRS voltage.

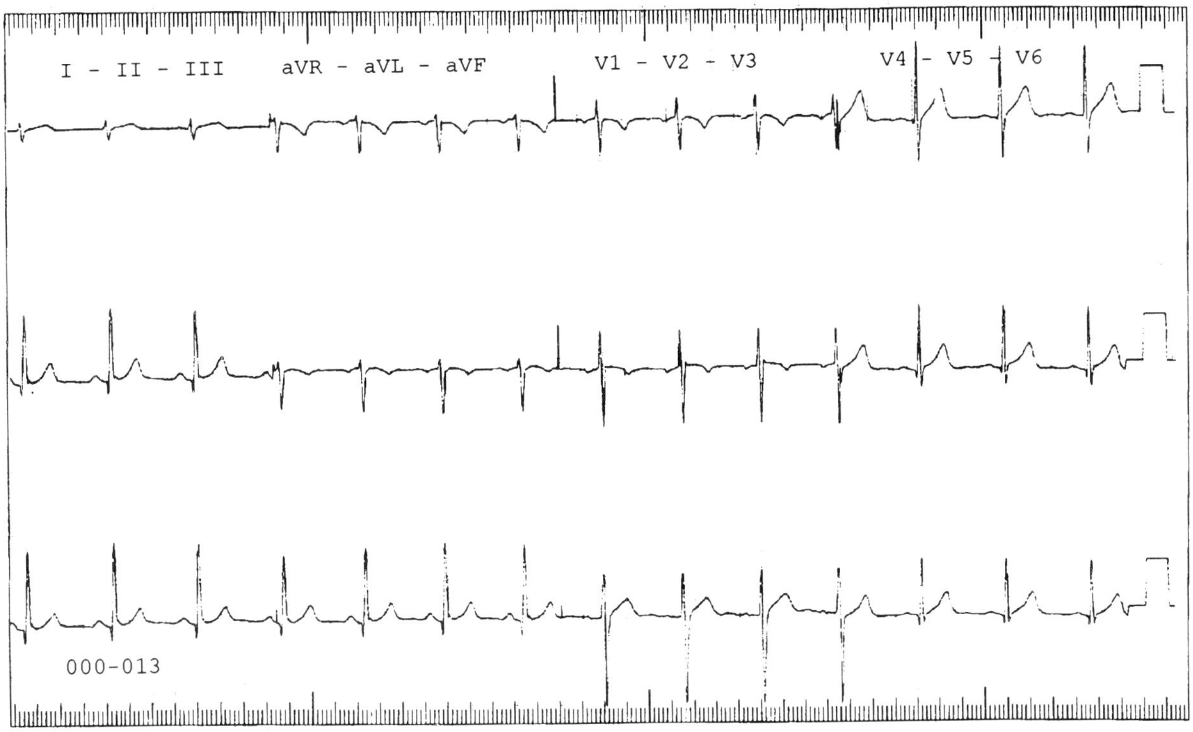

Within Normal Limits

Contour

85 85 16 08 36 sinus
+90 3:6 V3½ 12:1 normal
none
normal
+75 neg V1-2 pos V3-6

(1) Sinus mechanism, rate 85
(2) Within normal limits

A P wave is a little bump in the tracing whose predictable rhythm and recurrence correlate it with atrial depolarization. When normal, it is a small, more or less rounded wave, typically positive in Lead II, often with a small notch just past its mid-point, and initially positive and terminally negative in V1 (10, 27).

QRS is composed of sharp angles and straight lines (27, 41). In leads in which it is tall, as in II, III, aVF, and V5-6 here, it is often introduced by a clean, sharp, narrow Q.

ST-T represents ventricular repolarization. Seen in a lead to which it is nearly parallel, it departs from the baseline at an increasingly rapid rate, reaches maximum amplitude near its end, and returns quickly to the baseline. aVR and V6 are good examples in this case. The difference between ST and T is much like that between night and day; in some ways it is easy, but there is not a precise point at which one ends and the other begins (43).

U is a small, long, smooth wave that follows T and, as in this tracing, is not always identifiable. See the index for examples.

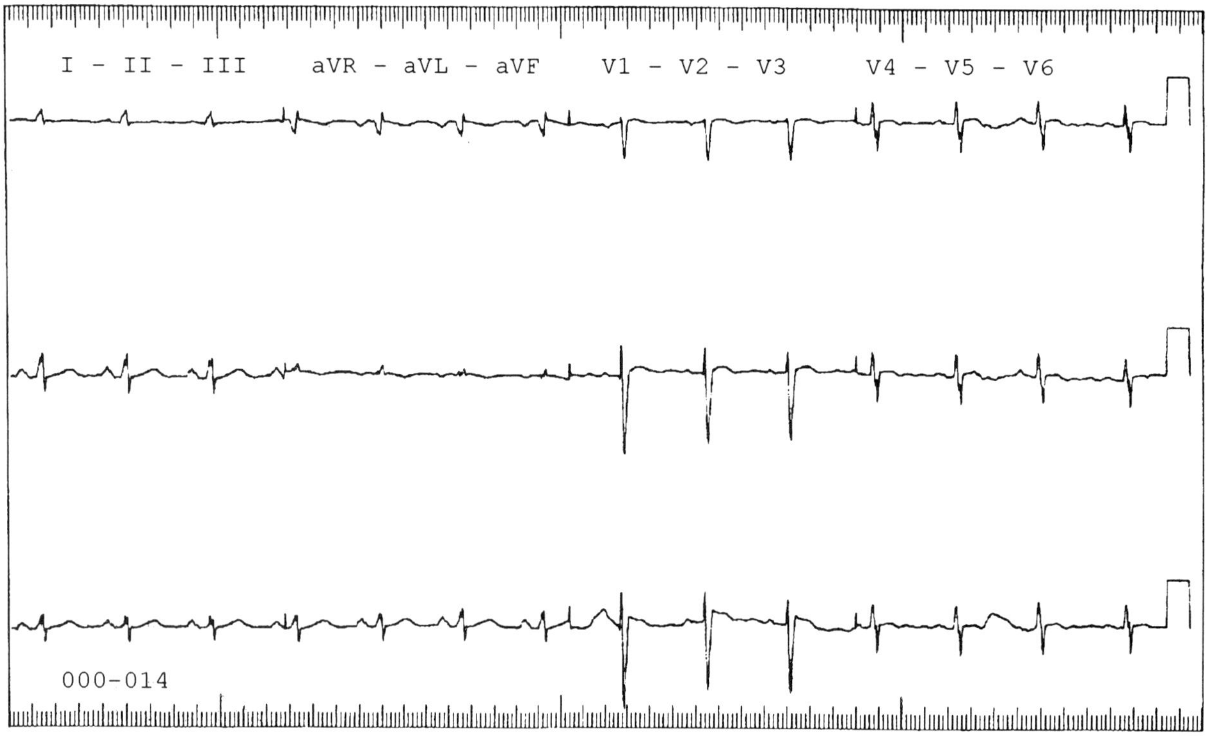

Probably within Normal Limits

(At worst, only small ST-T abnormalities)

80 80 16 08 40 sinus
?+45 1:6 V4-6 6:5 normal
none
related to T
?+75 isoelectric V1-6

(1) Sinus mechanism, rate 80
(2) Probably WNL, at worst only small ST-T abnormalities

This tracing might be called abnormal because precordial T voltage is low, but T must be evaluated in relation to QRS (52), and QRS is nearly equally biphasic in all leads so that its net amplitude is low. Expressed differently, the precordial QRS transition is wide and to the left, "late" (38), and in the frontal projection QRS orientation is arbitrary. These findings are within the limits of normal.

This tracing is included chiefly for comparison with EKGs 9, 10, and 11 from the same person at different times. In this one there are P waves (27,70), i.e., evidence of organized atrial depolarization, and their orientation to the left and caudad (positive in Lead II), and terminally dorsad (negative in V1), and contour (note the notch in Lead II just past the summit) are typical of a sinus origin. See insets.

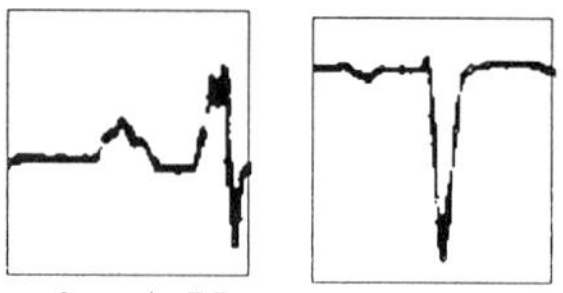

Lead II Lead V1

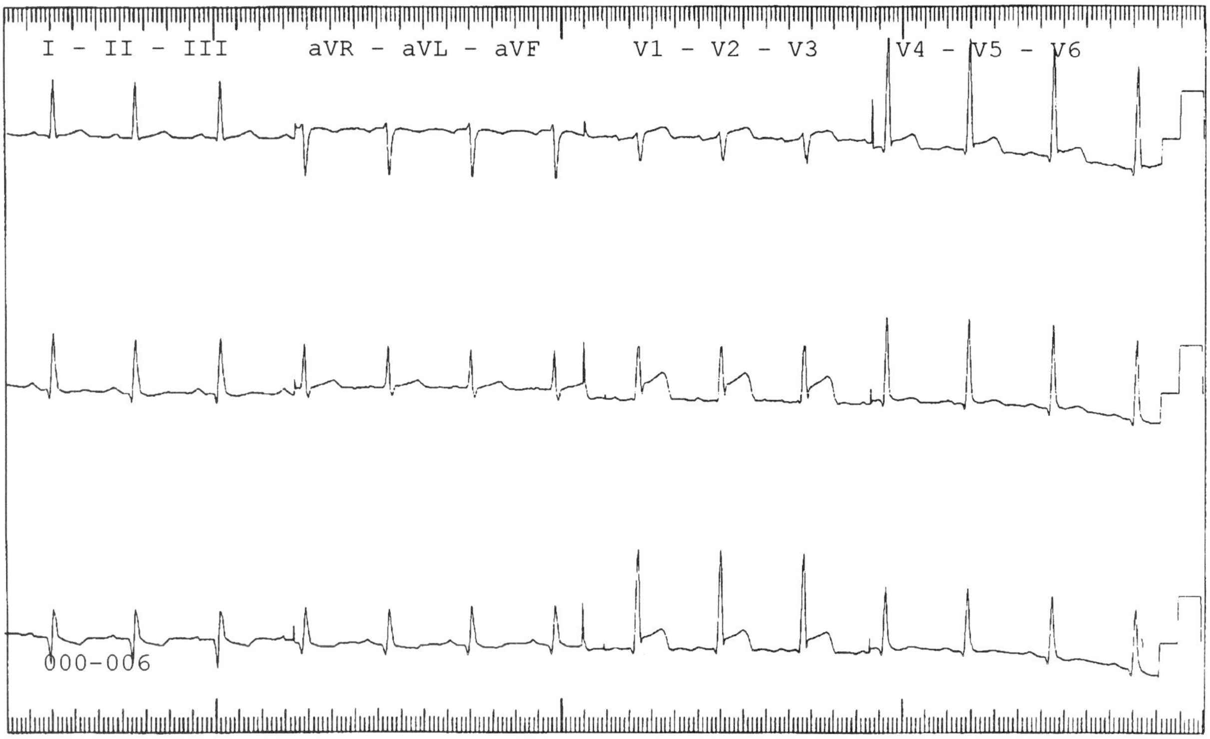

ST Displacement

Myocardial injury

There is marked ST displacement (the elevation in V2, for instance, is relatively large when considered as a fraction of QRS amplitude in the same lead), and its contour can be described as straightened. Directed anteriorly, perpendicular to the frontal plane, it does not show in frontal leads. T voltage, seen overall, is low. This pattern is abnormal, implying anterior, predominantly superficial, injury (202, 208). Mostly because ST displacement is very marked, it is more like that with a new infarct than pericarditis; see EKGs 54, 86, and 115. The prominence of Q2,3,F is at least a strong suggestion of an inferior infarct (173), but the ST evidence of injury (180) is not where it would be expected with an inferior infarct, and there is no QRS evidence of an anterior one.

85 85 20 08 36 sinus
+30 1:5 V1½ 10:0 Q2,3,F
elevated V2-4
straightened
±0,low +V1-5, low V5, ±V6

(1) Sinus mechanism, rate 85
(2) ST-T abnormalities, probably ant myocardial injury
(3) Old inferior myocardial infarct, probably

There is no doubt that there is myocardial injury, but no specific explanation for it is clear. How this is to be applied in management of the patient depends on the clinical setting and stability of the findings, information available to the doctor who ordered the study, but often not to the one who reports it.

EKG 9

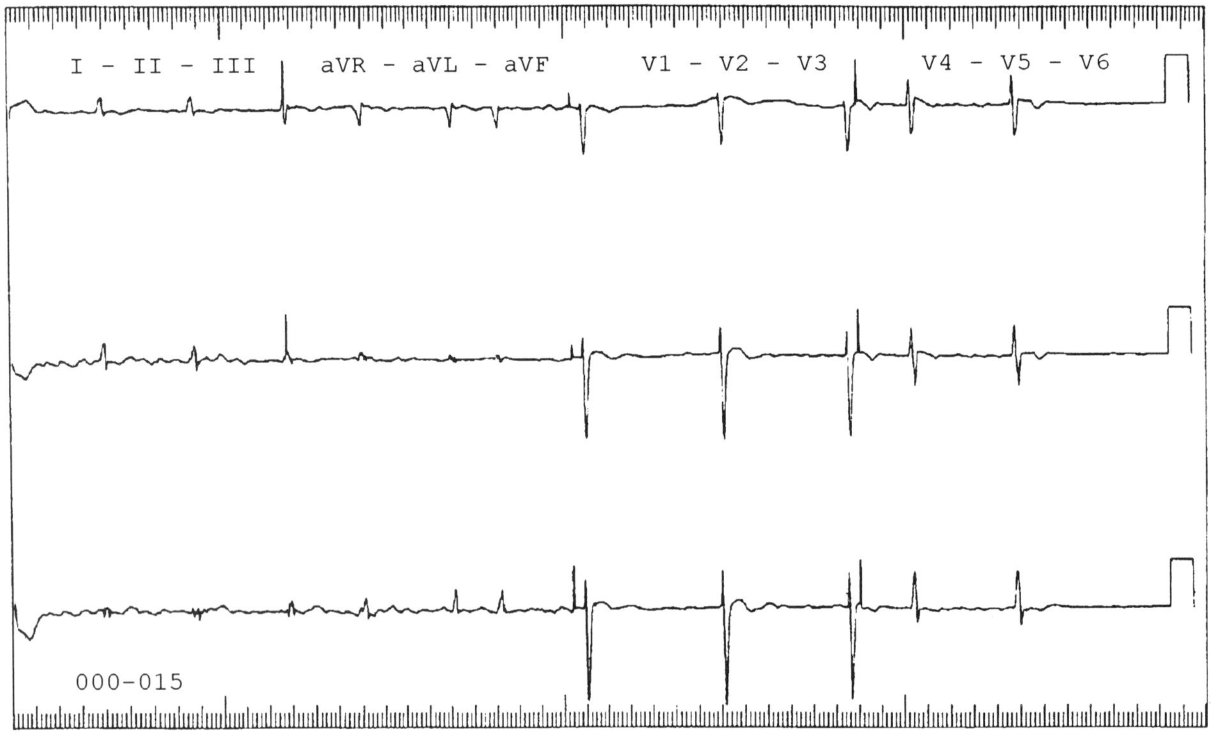

Atrial Fibrillation

```
--  75  --  08  --      see below
low +30  1:10  V4-5  8:2  normal
        slightly up V2-4
              arched
low     isoelectric  V1-6

(1) Atrial fibrillation, rate
    about 75, with PVC
(2) ST-T abns, nonspecific
```

This tracing shows nicely the typical pattern of atrial fibrillation, a word that almost describes itself when pronounced with a long "I". It is a picture of individual fibers at work and was once called "chaos cordis" (131). The trace is not the same between any two pairs of ventricular beats in a given lead, and this distinguishes it from the organized activity represented by P waves. The difference is emphasized by comparing this tracing to EKGs 7 and 10, showing a sinus mechanism and atrial flutter; all from the same patient. On physical examination, atrial activity is judged chiefly by its effect on the ventricles (not many of us are very good at evaluating its reflection in the jugular pulse), but in the EKG it is observed directly. The atria cannot function in an organized fashion at rates above about 300/min; beyond that, individual fibers, or groups of fibers, act independently, "fibrillate," producing f waves, and, with the exception of some instances of pre-excitation (EKG #150), second degree AV block is implicit. Like P waves, f waves represent atrial depolarization, but, unlike P waves, are totally unpredictable. Ventricular rhythm is typically irregular, but may not be (132). When atrial activity occurs during ventricular activity, the position of the trace at any instant represents both (121).

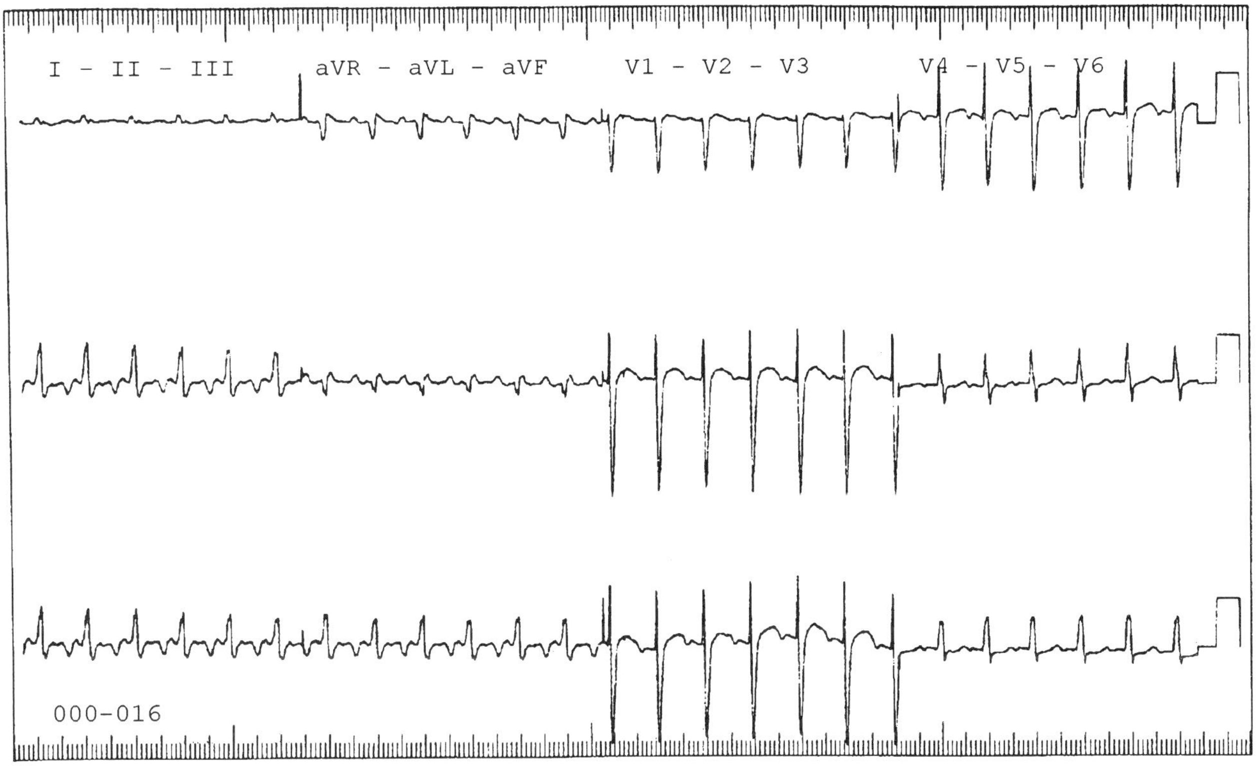

Atrial Flutter

```
300   150 --    08   ?28   see below
+75    1:10    V3-4    8:2    normal
        slightly up V2-4
            arched
??        ±V1        +V2-6 low

(1) Atrial flutter, 300/150
(2) ST-T abns, nonspecific
```

This tracing demonstrates the importance of identifying the rate and rhythm of the atria separately from those of the ventricles, the pacemaker for each, and the relation between these potentially independent systems. EKG 7 is from the same patient with a sinus mechanism, and makes it easy to see that there are two Ps for each QRS in this one; the first, continuous with the distal end of QRS. That it is really a P, negative in inferior leads, not an S, is an interpretation based on definition of the baseline (see Appendix I) and awareness that the position of the trace at any instant represents all electrical forces, not just ventricular or atrial. Atrial and ventricular activity may be in progress at the same time. EKG 9, from the same patient, but with atrial fibrillation, shows how arbitrary the difference between flutter and fibrillation, can be, as well as the difference between f waves and P waves. In flutter, there are P waves, but their rate is greater than the AV conduction system can process in the time between them, and the result is that they don't all get through to the ventricles; second degree AV block is implicit in the diagnosis of both flutter and fibrillation (129).

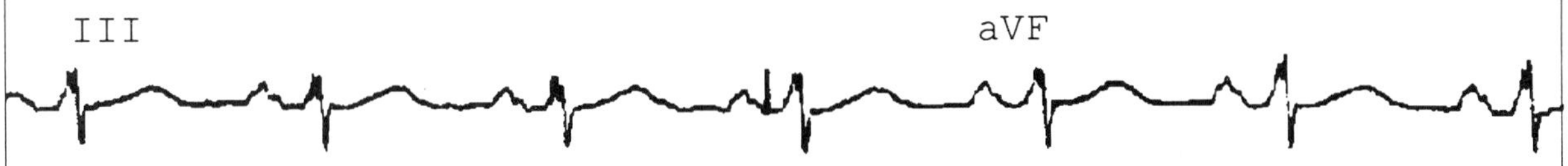

A Sinus mechanism, rate 80 (EKG #7)

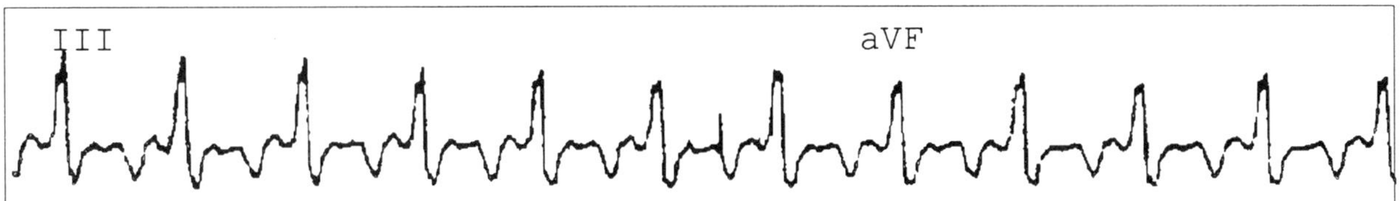

B Atrial flutter, 300/150 (EKG #10)

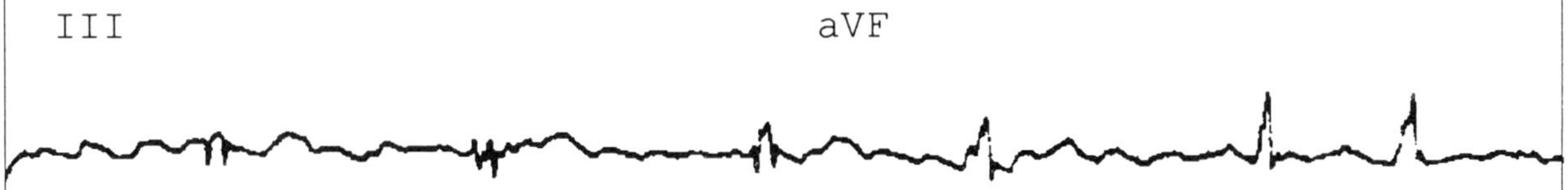

C Atrial fibrillation, rate about 75 (EKG #9)

Atrial Activity

Sinus, Flutter, and Fibrillation

These three tracings are from the same patient. **(A)** illustrates the feature of a P wave that makes it a P wave and not just a bump, its predictable repetition (though isolated P waves with PACs lack this); Its orientation, the direction in which the atria are activated, indicates its origin as high (sinus) or low.

In atrial flutter **(B)** as in a sinus mechanism, there are P waves, but their orientation is different, and they occur at a rate greater than even a normal AV conduction system can transmit one-to-one; there are two abnormalities in the tracing, "tachyatria" and (physiologic) second degree AV block, but only one in the patient, usurping atrial ectopy.

f waves **(C)** represent atrial depolarization, just as P waves do, but have neither of the features that make a P a P. Atrial fibrillation is characterized by continuous, chaotic (i.e., fibrillary) motion of the trace, and there is at least second degree AV block; without it there would be ventricular fibrillation, and it need not be named as a separate finding.

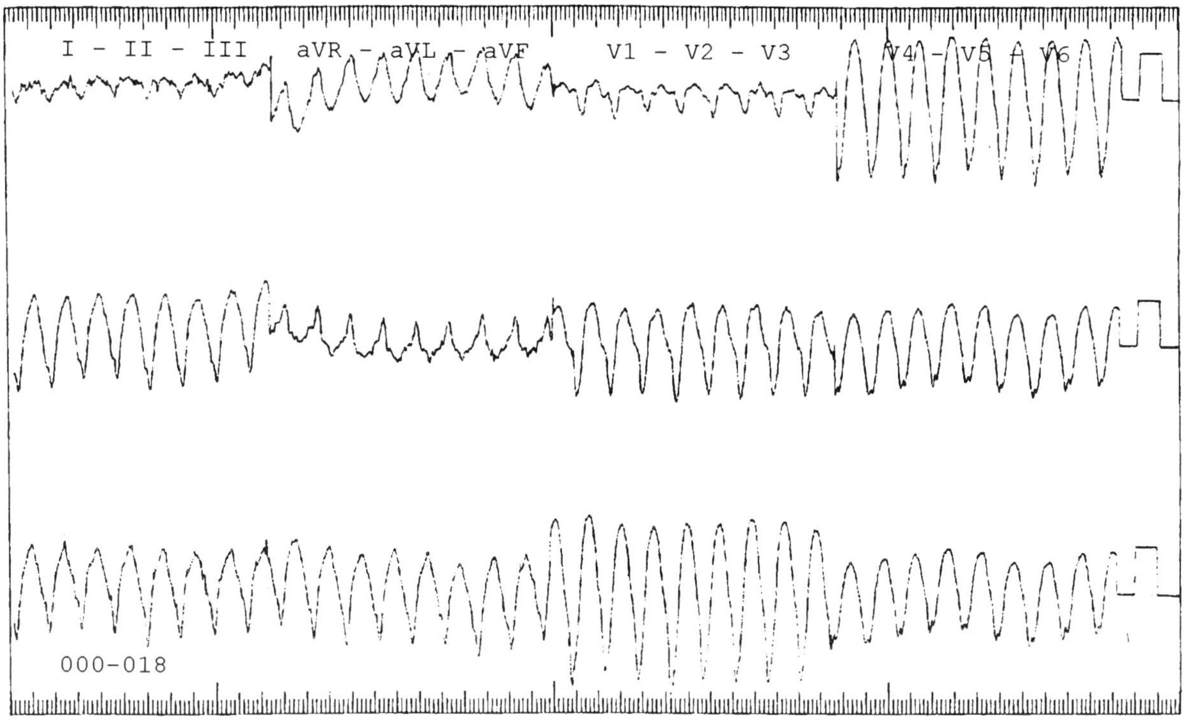

Ventricular Tachycardia (?)

```
--   200   --   16  ?32   see below
--   0:5   --   ?0:10    diff slur
        ?up 2,3,F and V2-6
         arched, insep T
?+90     ±V1     positive V2-6

(1) Ventricular tachycardia,
    probably, vs. SVT with IVCD
```

The computer is always helpful, but its readout depends upon not only those who write the programs but also the definitions used by those who choose the words, both groups composed of humans. The limits of the method are considerable (224). The readout for this tracing said the mechanism was atrial flutter. P waves are a part of atrial flutter, and, at least theoretically, there must be P's, at a rate slower than the ventricular rate, for the diagnosis of ventricular tachycardia, but no atrial activity is identifiable here.

What the tracing shows is two things: an ectopic mechanism (ventricular rate 200) with regular rhythm, and prolongation of intraventricular conduction time. An intraventricular pacemaker would explain both. A supraventricular one could explain the rate and rhythm just as easily, and there are several possible explanations for widening of QRS (168). The combination of usurping supraventricular ectopy and one of these, especially bundle branch block, is common. The things in this tracing that favor a ventricular origin are the QRS of the same sign all the way from V1 to V6, and its marked prolongation (144). Description of ST displacement is arbitrary. It depends upon the level of the baseline, which requires defining the beginning of QRS (9), and that is not clear.

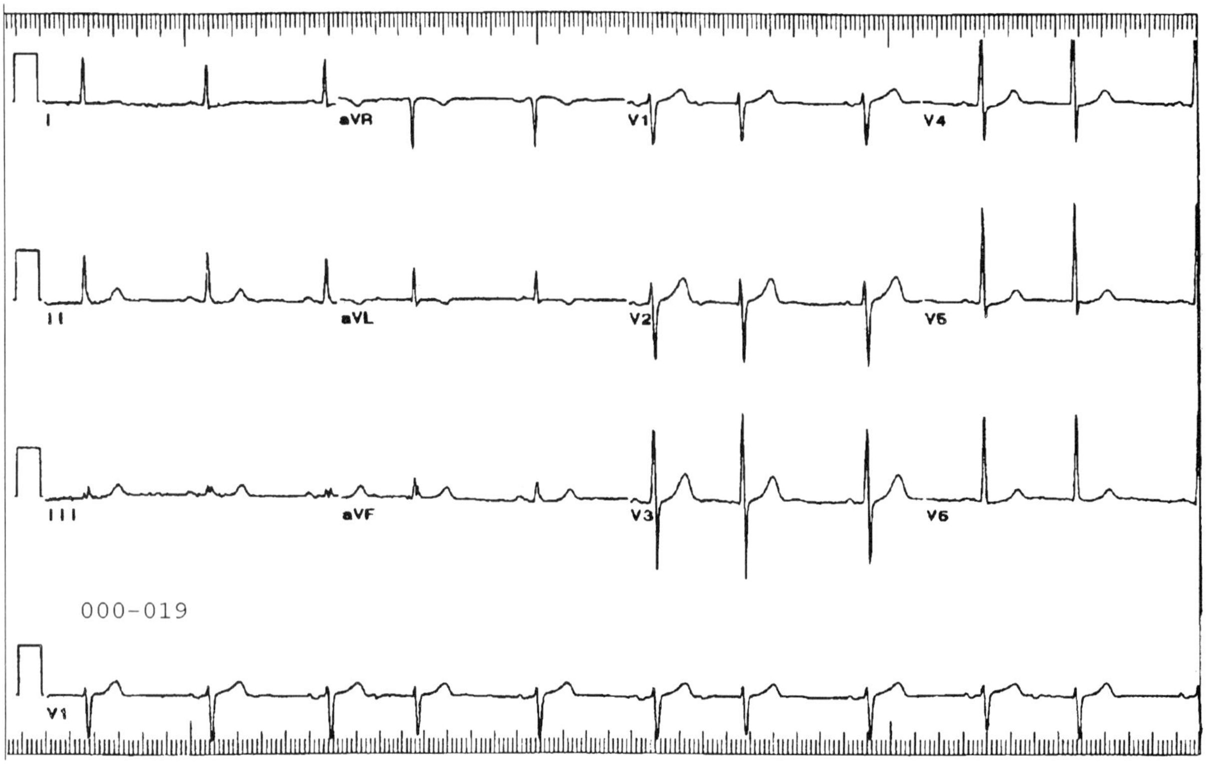

PACs with First Degree AV Block

```
65   65   16   08   36      see below
+30    2:8    V3    15:0     normal
                none
               normal
+90           positive V1-6

(1) Sinus mechanism, rate 65
(2) PAC's with 1° AV block
(3) Otherwise within nl limits
```

If a PAC occurs early enough following a conducted beat, the normal refractory state of the junctional apparatus can be enough to slow its passage. If it had occurred just a bit earlier, it would have been blocked (129). (Some would say "nonconducted," apparently expressing the judgment that block implies impairment of AV conduction, while nonconducted is evidence of the normal refractory period.) What the tracing shows objectively is failure of an atrial impulse to negotiate the AV junction. If one accepts that PACs are not abnormal, this tracing is not abnormal. The computer called the mechanism atrial fibrillation, but that is one of those things that can be "ruled out"; P waves and *f* waves are mutually exclusive. The tracing should be reported as within normal limits; especially in a 78-year-old with no clinical information.

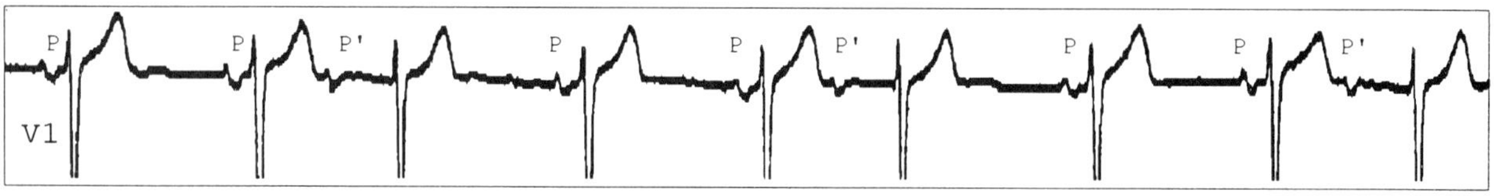

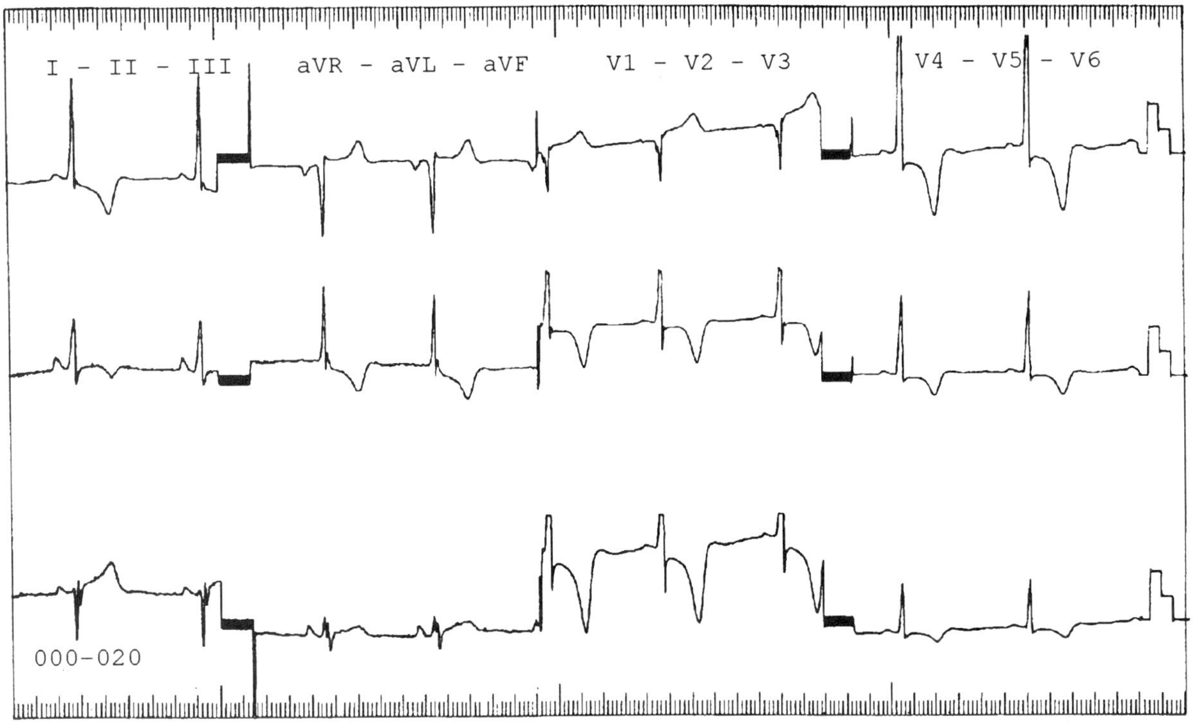

Idiopathic Hypertrophic Subaortic Stenosis

(IHSS, Asymmetric Septal Hypertrophy)

```
55    55    16     10     44        sinus
±0   0:20   V1½   (V5)40:0          early
                                    notch
     sl dn I,L,V2-6, up aVR,V1
           related to T
+165  +V1  neg V2-6,   deep, sym-
                    metrical V2-4

(1) Sinus mechanism, rate 65
(2) Left ventricular hypertrophy
(3) ST-T abns typical of cor in-
    suf and suggestive of LVO
```

This is a good example of the importance of recognizing both components of a problem; "insufficiency" and "ischemia" both identify discrepancy between supply and demand (137, 219). Etymologically, "ischemia" says impairment of supply; "insufficiency" does not take sides. This patient was an 18-yearold high school athlete with IHSS, and the deep, symmetrical mid-precordial T pattern typical of coronary insufficiency is probably explained by local increase in demand for blood (oxygen) rather than diminution of supply. Also, the pattern in the frontal plane suggests left ventricular overload, as would be expected in response to increase in resistance to outflow, effectively aortic stenosis. QRS evidence for left ventricular hypertrophy completes the picture. Note that the precordial leads were recorded at half gain.

The abnormality of initial QRS contour suggests scarring deep in the ventricular myocardium, a finding explained more commonly by infarction, or, in association with short PR, ventricular pre-excitation.

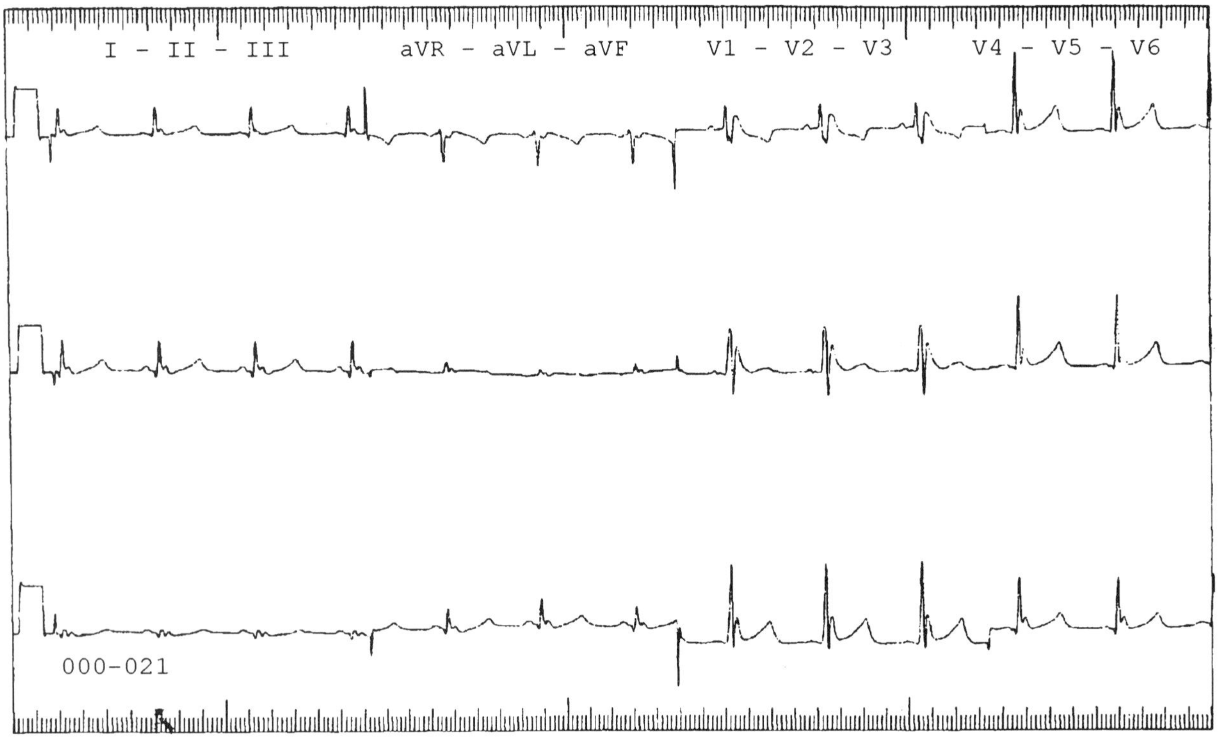

Hypothermia

```
75    75    12    12    44     sinus
+30   5:3   ?V1   10:0  late notch
           slightly up V3
           not remarkable
+45    neg V1,    flat    pos V3-6

(1) Sinus mechanism, rate 75
(2) Abnormal QRS duration and
    contour  (?hypothermia)
(3) Otherwise Within normal
    limits
```

Body temperature may be lowered to pathologic levels by several mechanisms other than exposure to cold; in this case, brain damage. The patient, a young man, was in good health prior to sustaining brain damage in an automobile accident shortly before admission to the ER. Details are lacking, but his temperature was off the bottom of the scale on the thermometer, i.e., below 94°F.

The critical finding is the prominent notch late in the wide QRS, seen best here in V3-5. This feature was emphasized by Osborn (237) and has come to be called an "Osborn wave." It is similar to "after potentials," described more recently, and may presage ventricular ectopy (217).

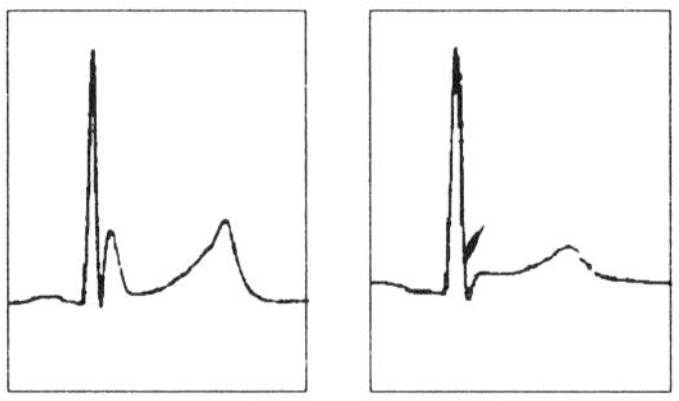

V4 donor   V5,recipient

The patient was brain dead, and his heart was transplanted. A tracing from the recipient, made a few hours later (inset), shows a normal QRS. See EKGs 119 and 123, in both of which the ST-T pattern of injury, also typical of hypothermia, shows better than in this one.

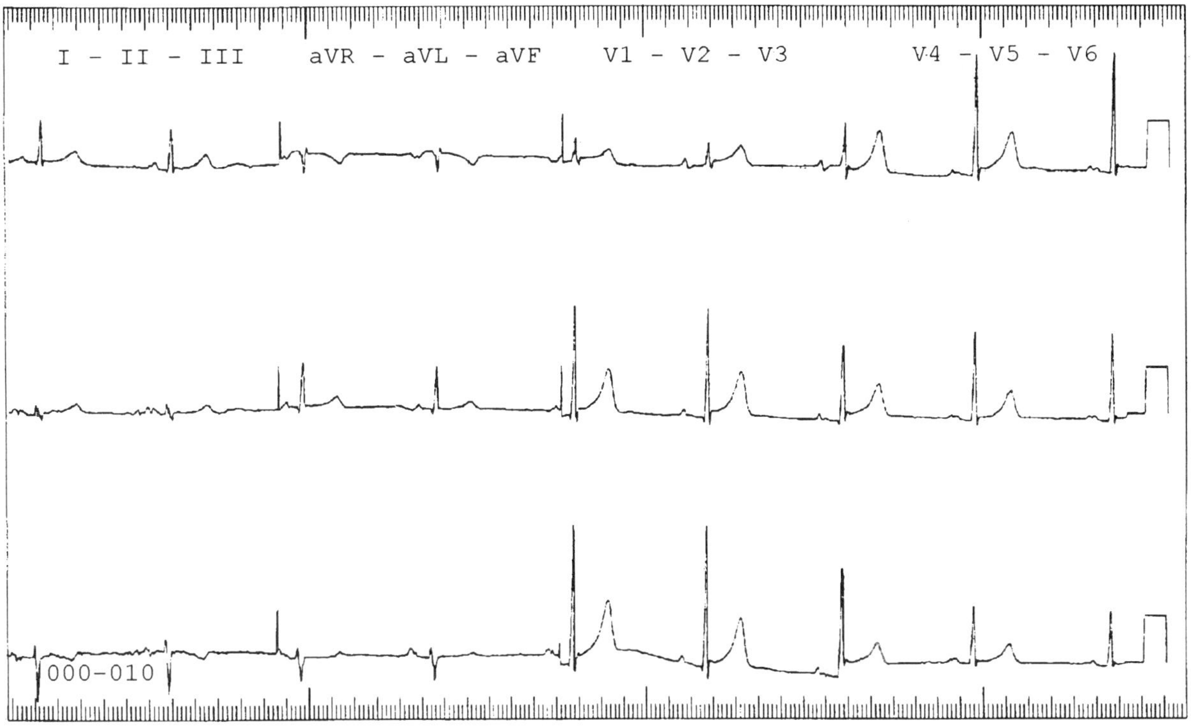

Early Repolarization

Within Normal Limits

```
50    50    20    08    44     sinus
-30    5:1    V1    10:0     normal
         slightly up V5-6
              normal
+15      positive V1-6

(1) Sinus mechanism, rate 50
(2) Within normal limits
```

ST displacement (orientation) is defined by the position of the J point above or below the baseline; its amplitude, as slight, moderate, or marked (as compared to the amplitude of the QRS in the same lead). ST contour can be described as normal, sagging/ arched, flat, or straightened (44). ST-T is a continuum, there is not a point at which ST ends and T begins, and assessment of ST contour involves the T wave. When ST is elevated in leads with a positive QRS, as in those from the left side of the chest, and T is tall, its contour remains normal, and, for some reason not entirely clear the pattern is widely known as "early repolarization" (45, 205). The term has no clinical implication but is often proposed as an interpretation. A similar ST-T pattern seen in right precordial leads, where QRS is negative and T is positive, is simply accepted as normal, and not mentioned. Compare to the pattern of pericarditis (EKGs 54, 86, and 115). Description of every component of every tracing will generate awareness of the range of forms each can take. Note the prominent notch in the normal P wave in Lead II, and the "early" precordial QRS transition (farther to the right than usual) with a prominent R in V1. It was probably this RV1 that the computer saw as evidence of a dorsal infarct (178).

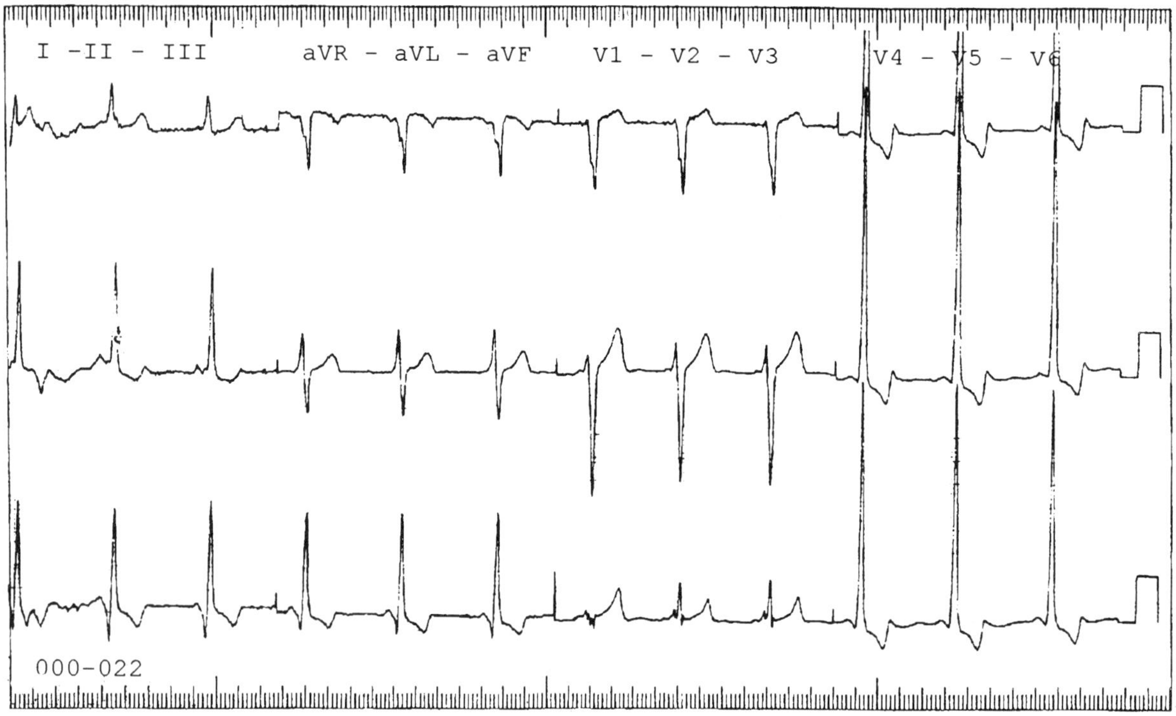

Ventricular Pre-excitation, Delta Wave, Left Ventricular Hypertrophy, and Strain (?)

Ventricular pre-excitation alone will usually explain all the findings in a tracing in which it is present, but it may also complicate, or even cancel, the effects of others. In this tracing, for instance, QRS amplitude suggests left ventricular hypertrophy, and the ST-T pattern typical of left ventricular overload supports that interpretation. The Q3 suggests an infarct. The problem is that these interpretations assume simultaneous radial depolarization of the ventricles (*see* page 8), and pre-excitation negates that. When there is pre-excitation, caution is needed in any further interpretation.

The idea of an anomalous wave, shaped like the Greek letter delta and sandwiched between P and QRS, is illustrated well in V3 (inset) (169).

See EKGs 64, 136, 137, and 142.

70 70 ?08 12+ 40 sinus
+60 1:15 2½ 50:0 early slur
none
related to T
-45 positive V1-3, negative V4-6

(1) Sinus mechanism, rate 70
(2) Ventricular pre-excitation
(3) Otherwise probably WNL

--evidence for left ventricular hypertrophy, and/or strain, is equivocal.

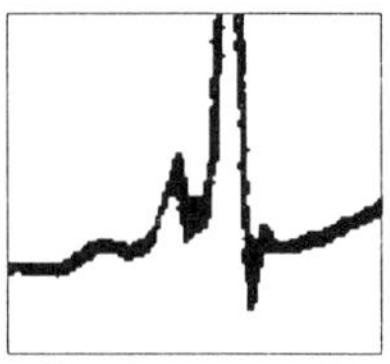

"Delta wave"
V3 above

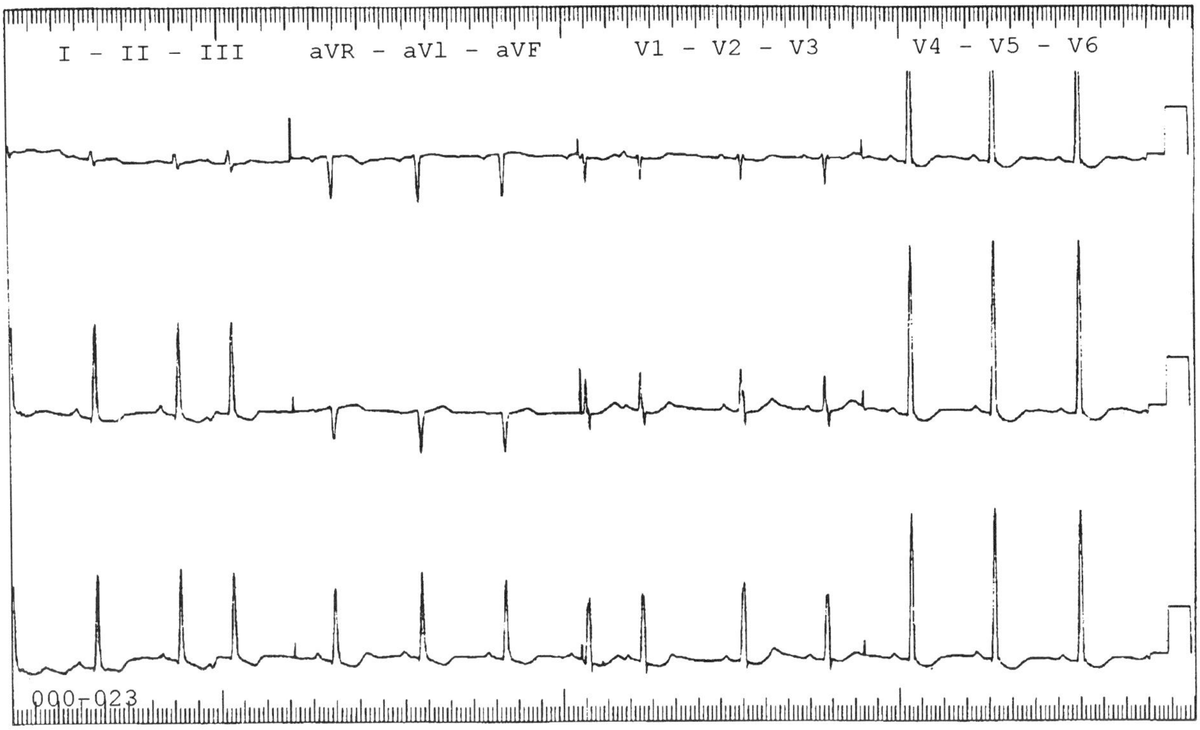

Digitalis Effect

85 85 16 08 36 sinus
+90 rSr 1:5:1 V1½ 30:0 normal
none
sagging
low ±V1, pos V2-3 low, ±V4-6

(1) Sinus mechanism, rate 85, with PAC's
(2) ST-T abnormalities, suggestive of digitalis effect

Digitalis is given for its effect; to say that the ST-T pattern suggests digitalis effect does not mean that the level is excessive. In toxic doses it can produce multifocal ectopy, AV block, and acceleration of a junctional pacemaker, but there are always alternative explanations for each of these. Digitalis, like ischemia, is exceedingly common as a factor in the production of EKG abnormalities, but the tracing shows only the abnormality, not its etiology. All ST-T abnormalities are nonspecific, but some do suggest explanations, and digitalis effect is one of these (229). It is shown well in V4-6, where T voltage is low and ST sags but is not depressed. The precise duration of QT is always arbitrary, but, especially in leads with low T voltage and sagging of ST, it appears short. Coronary insufficiency, often in the differential, has little effect on QT duration, and typically produces flattening and depression of ST in these leads. Patterns are not always typical, and digitalis effect and coronary insufficiency often coexist. Bear in mind that there is only one point on the paper, and its position at any instant reflects the net of everything that is happening. There is little correlation between therapeutic levels of digitalis and findings in the EKG.

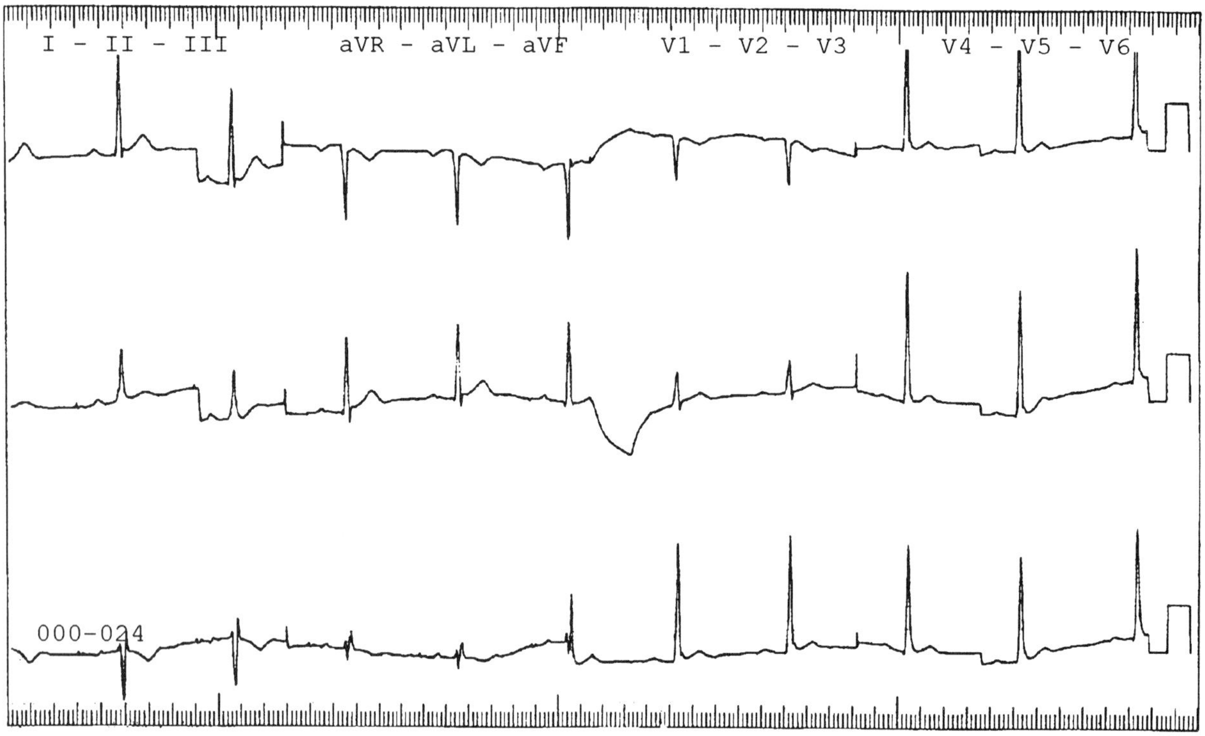

Short QT

60	60	20	10	40	sinus
±0	0:10	V1½	25:0		normal
		none			
		related to T			
-15	neg V1,		pos V2-6 low		

(1) Sinus mechanism, rate 60
(2) Probably WNL, at worst only small ST-T abnormalities

The duration of any interval is measured in the lead in which it is longest *and* in which its beginning *and* end can be estimated with confidence. Given the B point as the beginning (23, 202), the duration of QT is a function of where T ends, and this is not a point at all; the curve approaches the baseline asymptotically. It is all right for a computer program to define QT to a thousandth of a second, but this is about as useful as expressing temperature, blood pressure, or pulse rate to the third decimal place. Also, the lead in which it is measured makes a difference, and criteria used by computer programs are not often obvious. There are not many things that will shorten QT (202). Often it *looks* short in some, or most, leads, V1-6 in this case, but can easily be measured as within normal limits in others, Lead III here.

The QTc, or QT corrected, is a device intended to combine the measured value and the rate in one figure. It is derived by mathematic manipulation of the observed QT and the ventricular rate. Several formulae are available for this purpose, and it has little clinical value; computerized mathematics can't compensate for the fact that basic observation is approximate at best (24).

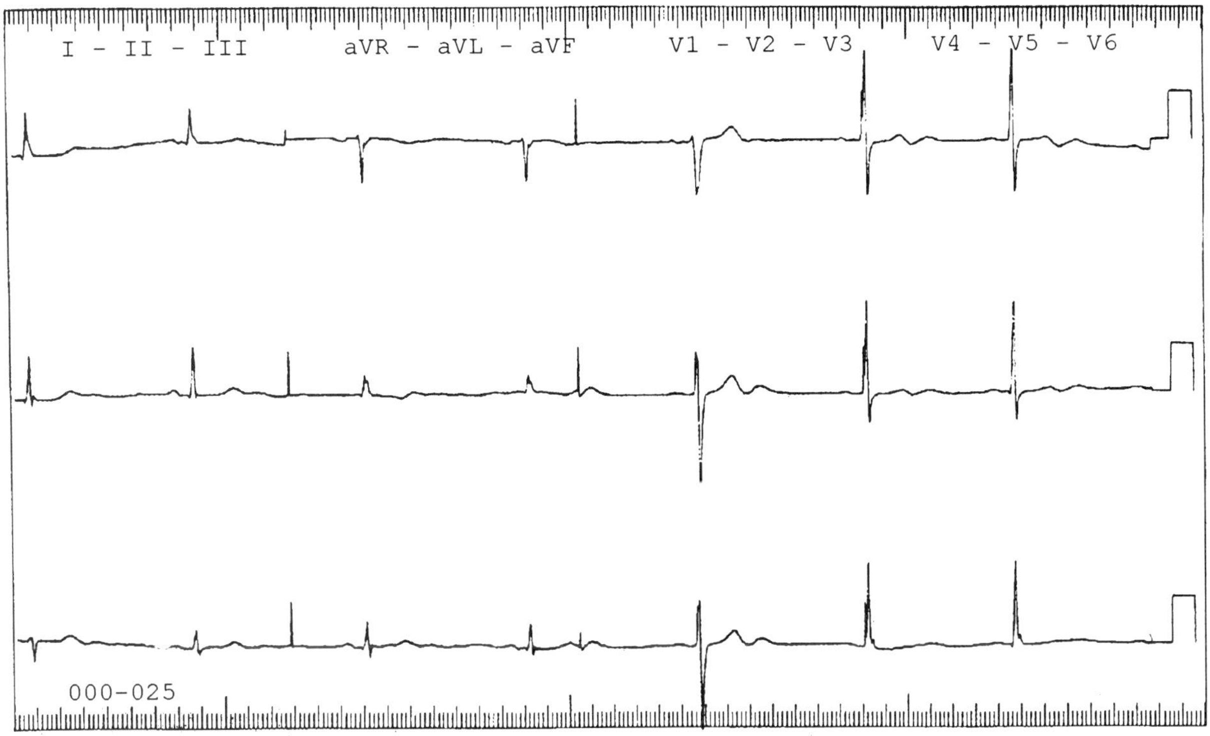

Prominent U Wave

45 45 20 10 44 sinus
+30 1:10 V3½ 15:0 normal
none
related to T
low pos V1-5, low V4-5, ±V6
U: prominent

(1) Sinus mechanism, rate 45
(2) ST-T-U abnormalities, non-specific

A U wave is part of the normal ventricular complex, but usually very small and less well understood than the other waves (51, 217). It is prominent in most leads in this tracing, but not abnormal. If it is considered in analysis of every tracing, the range of normal will become apparent and minor departures from that will not be over-interpreted.

U may be merged with T so that the value given for QT is inappropriate. In this case, for instance, the computer program called the QT interval 0.50 sec, with a "QTc" of 43 (24). When the observed QT is much longer than about 0.44 sec, no matter what the rate, there is a good chance that it is really a QU.

The only abnormality here is low T voltage, an abnormality, to be sure, but limited to the most sensitive and least specific part of the tracing (201). Its importance, if any, can be evaluated only in the whole picture, and this can be emphasized by adding to the report a comment to the effect that the abnormality is minimal, or that the tracing is not far from normal. Similarly, a ventricular rate this slow may raise a question of AV block, especially if the patient is old, and a note that AV conduction is normal is helpful.

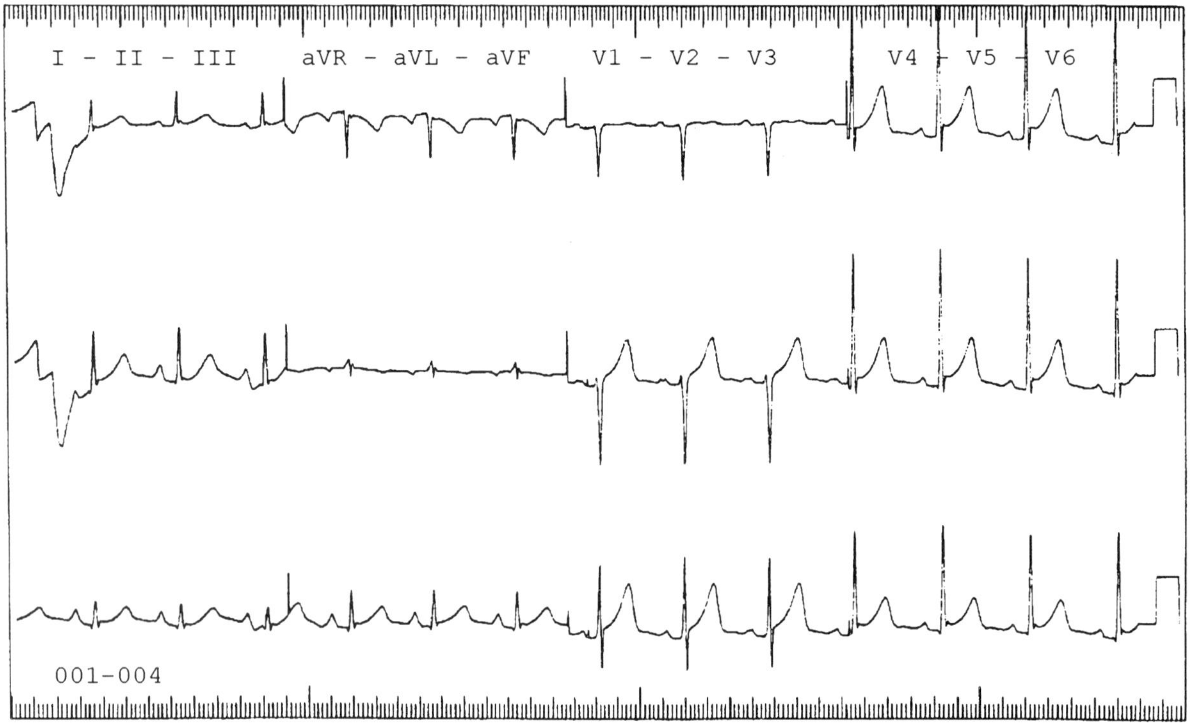

Early Repolarization

80 80 20 08 40 sinus
+60 0:10 V2½-3 20:0 normal
up II,aVF,V3-6, sl down aVR
normal
+60 ±V1 +V2-6

(1) Sinus mechanism, rate 80
(2) Within normal limits

This ST-T pattern is normal (45, 205). It differs from the more common picture in that T voltage is relatively great and the J point is not at the baseline but displaced in the same direction as T and QRS; in this case, elevated in leads II, aVF, and V2-6, and slightly depressed in aVR. ST contour is normal (if the curve from the peak of T is projected backward through QRS, it reaches the baseline at approximately the B point; see "A tutorial: Examination of one heartbeat..." in Chapter 3). As in V4-5 here, the QRS may end with a sharp rebound after having almost reached the baseline, or having passed it to make a tiny S. The term "early repolarization" apparently reflects the interpretation that, by the time the QRS is finished, repolarization has produced enough potential to position J apart from the baseline. The alternative is absolutely no ST displacement, and the limits of the method must be kept in mind. A variant of this picture, ST elevation in right precordial leads, where QRS is negative and T positive, is so common that it is not even mentioned, much less named. The difference between this pattern and that of subepicardial injury as with pericarditis is that with injury T voltage is lower so that ST contour is flattened (see EKGs 54, 86, and 115). The baseline artifact in Leads I and II is evidence of a loose connection to the right arm, and, probably, motion of that arm.

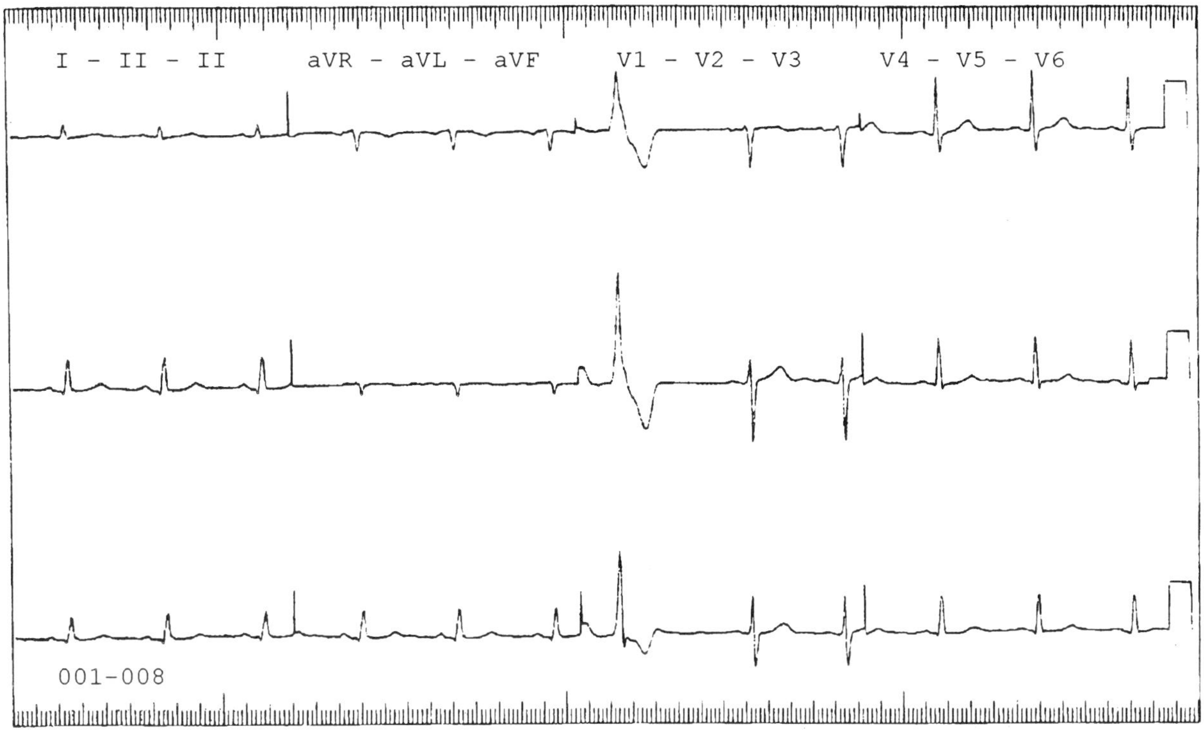

Premature Ventricular Contraction (PVC)

70	70	16	08	40	sinus
+75	1:8	V3	8:0		normal
		none			
		normal			
+60	±V1	positive V2-6			low V6

(1) Sinus mechanism, rate 70 with one PVC
(2) Within normal limits

Premature beats of ventricular origin can be called PVBs, or VPBs, beats instead of contractions, but this has little merit, and they are usually known as PVCs. One prominent cardiologist has written that the way to recognize them is that they look like PVCs. While this is almost always true, it does not say much to one who does not know what a PVC looks like; the name itself does that (142). A PVC occurs earlier than expected in the context of previous beats (premature) and produces a wide QRS of bizarre configuration with proportionately modified ST-T, indicating activation of the ventricular myocardium more slowly than normal and over pathways other than normal; normal is the fastest possible. A PVC may, or may not, be followed by a retrograde P in ST-T.

PVC's are sometimes called "extrasystoles," a term that is accurate only when they are interpolated (143) (EKG 130). They are so common in normals that, except when very frequent, multifocal, or occur in groups, they need not even be mentioned in the report. A premature beat of supraventricular origin, with aberrant ventricular conduction (169)(EKGs 58, 76), may be indistinguishable from a PVC, especially when there is atrial fibrillation and there is no premature P.

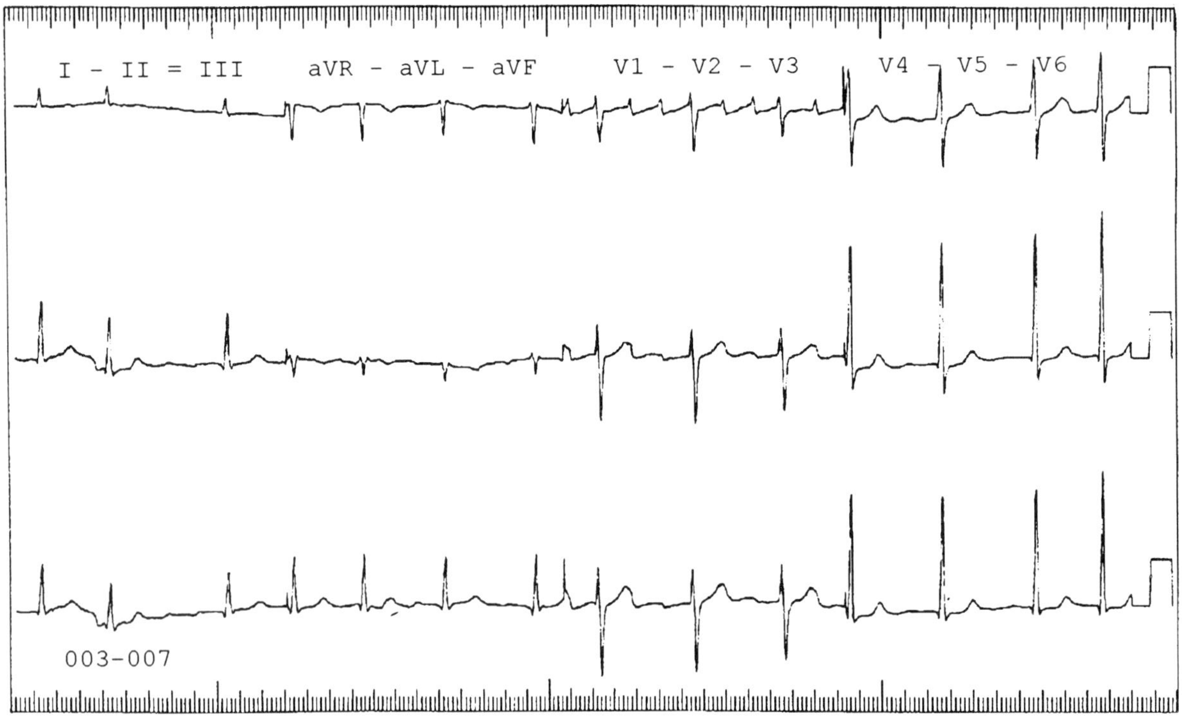

Atrial Ectopy

Flutter? Atrial Tachycardia with Block?

```
215   85   --   08   40     see below
+75   2:6    V4    25:1       normal
                 none
         some flattening
+90    ±V1         positive V2-6

(1) Atrial flutter, 215/85
(2) Otherwise within normal
    limits
```

There are P waves (27, 70), as distinct from *f* waves (10), but their origin (as indicated by their orientation, chiefly in the frontal plane), is not clear. There is second degree AV block by definition (152); all QRSs are of supraventricular origin (not wide) but not all atrial beats get through to the ventricles. This can be explained in this case by input into the AV conduction system at a rate greater than it can handle; it is not necessary to postulate impairment of AV conduction.

When second degree AV block occurs with atrial rate not much above what might be expected to be transmitted one-to-one, about 180-200, it raises the question of impairment of AV conduction in addition to excessive input. This picture is sometimes called "PAT with block" and attributed to digitalis excess, especially if P waves are directed caudad, suggesting repetitive depolarization, "automatic" atrial activity, rather than reentry (129). In typical flutter, P is negative in leads II, III, and aVF, and continuous atrial activity is assumed, "reentry."

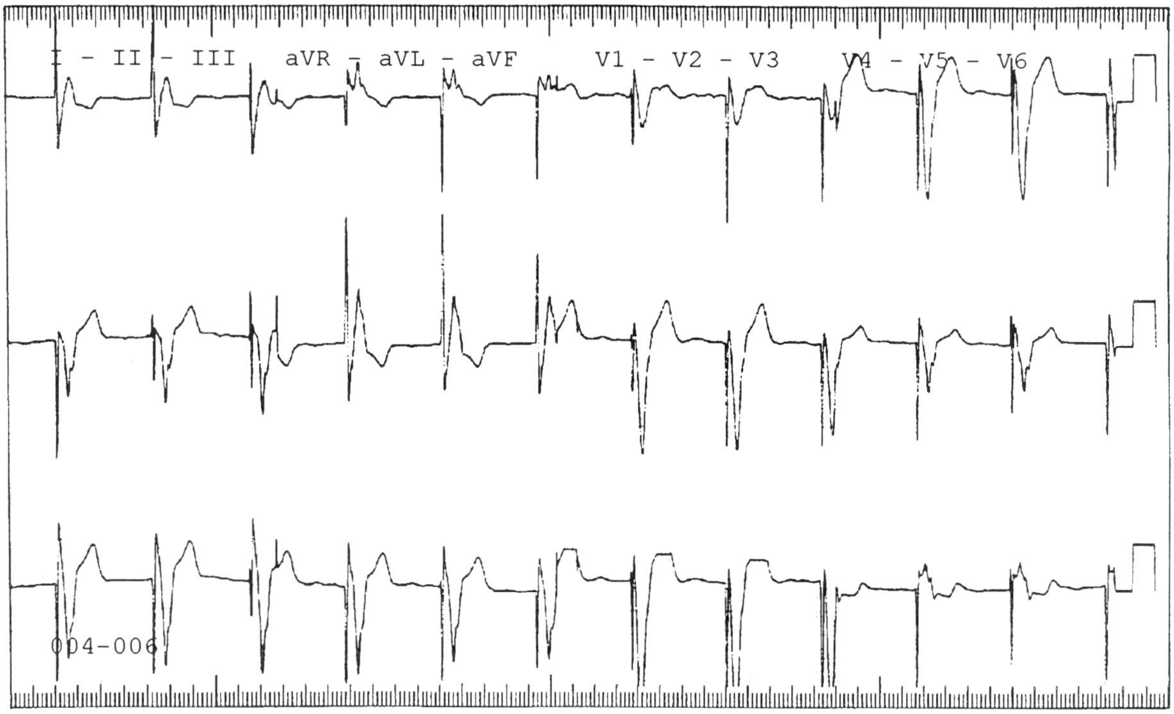

Atrial Fibrillation, Third Degree AV Block, Artificial Ventricular Pacemaker (VVI)

```
--   70   --   20  44     see below
-75   5:8  V5½  5:1    diff slur
        up V2-4, down V6
         not remarkable
+105  ±V1      pos V2-5      ±V6

(1) Atrial fibrillation
(2) 3° AV Block
(3) Artificial ventricular
    pacemaker capturing regu-
    larly, rate 70
```

It is important of identify all three components of the mechanism; atrial, ventricular, and the relation between them. Atrial fibrillation shows best in II, III, aVF, and V1. The absence of AV conduction, third degree, or complete, AV block, is indicated by the perfectly regular QRS rhythm. With complete AV block, the ventricles may be driven by a junctional focus, and if there is also an IV conduction defect distinction from an idioventricular one may be difficult, depending largely on rate (153). In this case, the spike initiating each QRS identifies an artificial pacemaker (V), its amplitude implies a unipolar system, and the QRS pattern of LBBB indicates origin in the right ventricle (140). Sensing also is ventricular (V) so that intrinsic ventricular activity will inhibit (I) the device.

When the ventricles are activated from a focus in the ventricular wall, there is no longer simultaneous radial depolarization (76), and neither QRS nor ST-T can be interpreted by the usual rules. Why is it important to know that there is atrial fibrillation when an artificial ventricular pacemaker is functioning properly?

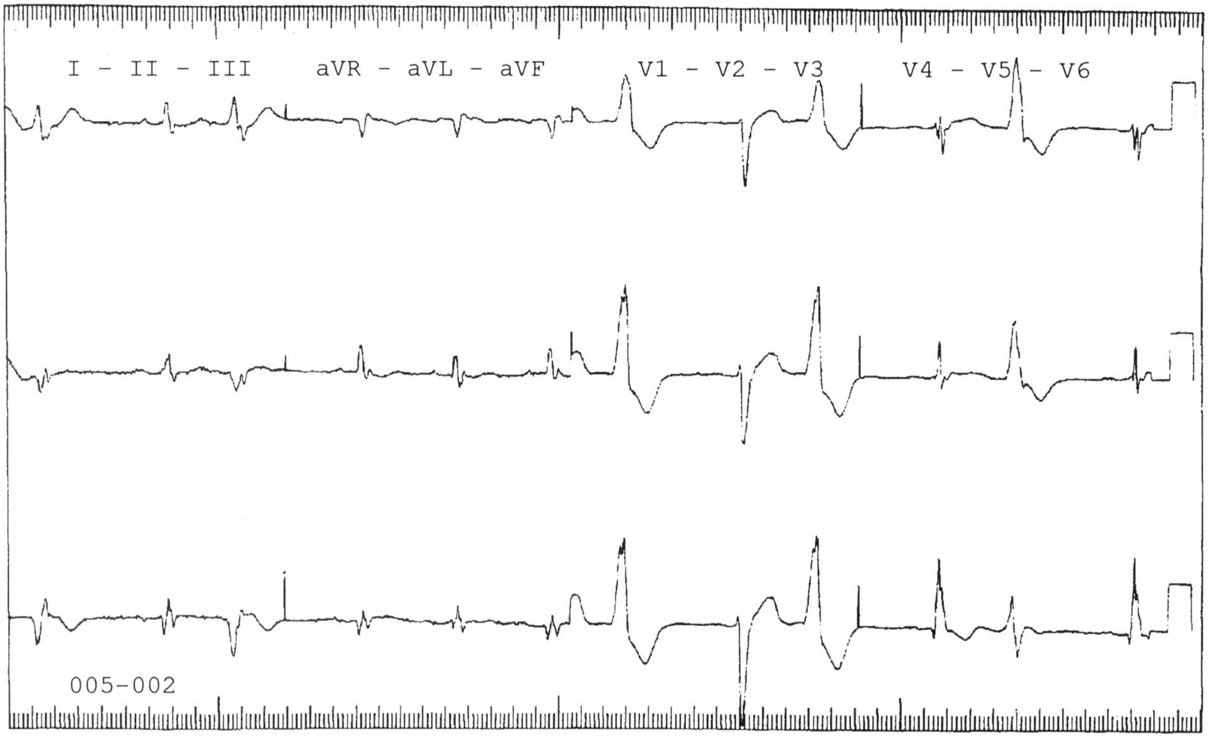

Premature Ventricular Contractions

Suggests Old Inferior Myocardial Infarct

70   70   20   10   40   sinus w PVC
?±0   1:15   V3½   15:0   Q3,F
none
related to T
low +30   pos V1-4   ±V5   neg V6

(1) Sinus mechanism, rate 70
(2) Frequent PVC's
(3) ST-T abns suggestive of left ventricular overload
(4) Suggests old inferior MCI

--Nothing looks new.

The basic mechanism is sinus; note that despite their small size, which limits description of contour, there is no doubt that there are P waves (10, 27). Precise duration of PR is arbitrary, but easily evaluated as not long.

There are frequent PVCs, their specific characteristics varying according to the view (lead), but all falling at the same interval after the preceding conducted beat, as nearly as that can be estimated, and presumably all coming from the same focus.

There is no ST displacement. T voltage is a little low, but its contour is not remarkable, and its only clear abnormality is its orientation nearly opposite QRS, suggesting left ventricular overload (187).

The Q wave in Leads III and aVF has to be noted as suggestive of an infarct, but is far from diagnostic, and nothing at all looks new. The first beat is a PVC. Its configuration is of little help in recognizing an infarct (180).

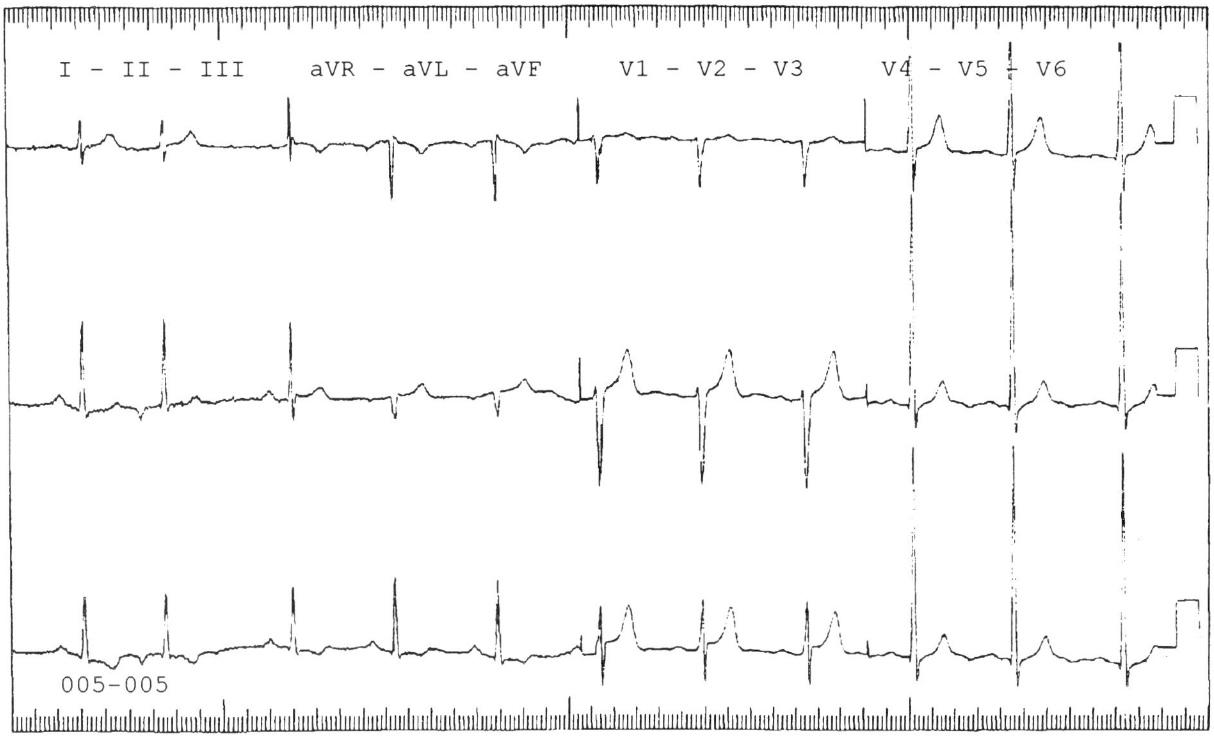

Premature Atrial Contraction

Suggests Left Ventricular Hypertrophy

```
65    65    20    08    40    sinus
+75   0:10   V3   45:0    normal
              none
          related to T
±0   ±V1,       positive V2-6

(1) Sinus mechanism, rate 65,
    with one PAC
(2) Suggests left ventricular
    hypertrophy
(3) Otherwise probably WNL, at
    worst only small ST-T abns
```

Neither their time of onset nor their configuration can be described precisely, but there is no question that there are P waves, one for each QRS. They are directed leftward and caudad with some initial ventrad component, though a terminal dorsad one is not identifiable. The mechanism is sinus, and PR is not long.

The second beat occurs early, is preceded by a P that is different from others in the same lead, and is followed by a QRS-T that is (substantially) the same as the others. These are the features that define a PAC (127), a beat originating early from an atrial focus. The PR interval with a PAC may be shorter than usual, or longer (EKG 13), depending on refractory periods and time after a conducted beat, and its QRS may vary a little with the same factors (ventricular aberration) (169). If the P is not obvious, a PAC with ventricular aberration may be mistaken for a PVC, and distinction is not always possible. When P is not identifiable, "premature beat of supraventricular origin" would be a better term, but it is acceptable to call them PACs.

EKG 27

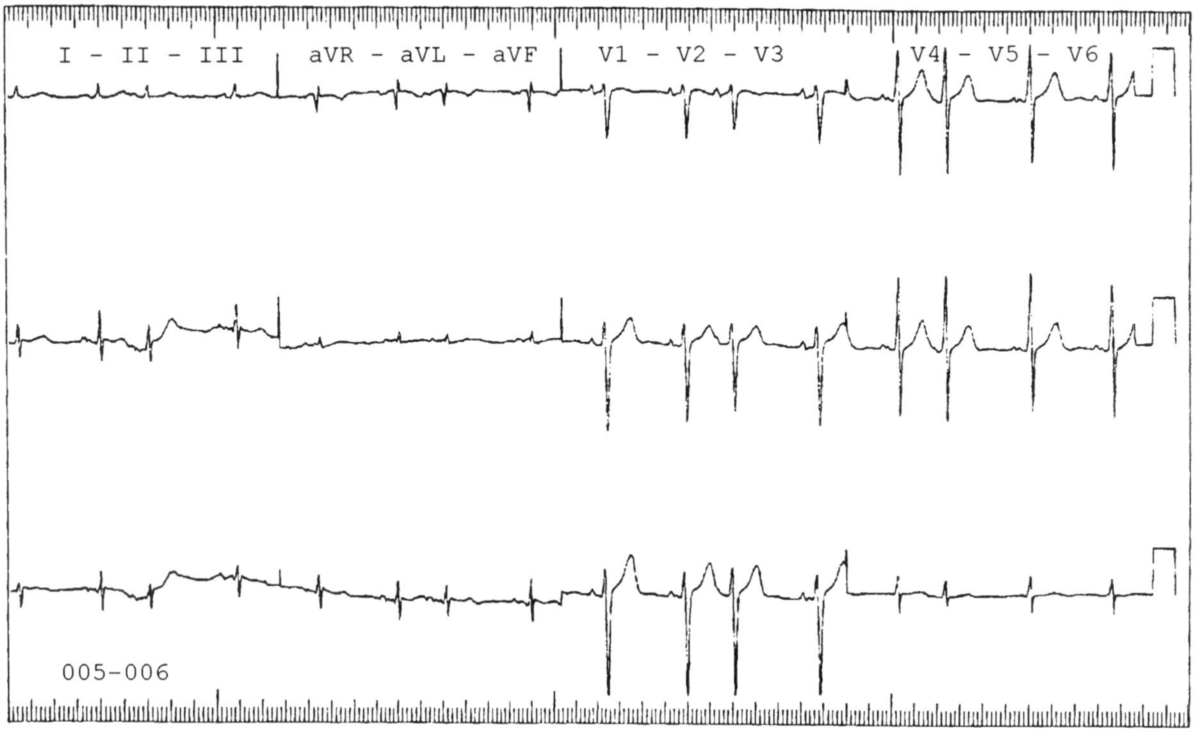

Premature Atrial Contractions (PACs), Low T Voltage

95 95 12 08 36 sinus
?±0 2:10 V4-5 4:3 normal
none
related to T
low ?+45 ±V1 pos V2-5 ±V6

(1) Sinus mechanism, rate 95, with PAC's
(2) Probably WNL, at worst only small ST-T abnormalities

Premature contractions of supraventricular origin are usually called PACs whether P is identifiable or not. The mechanism in this tracing is clearly sinus; P is directed to the left and down as indicated by its positivity in Lead II, and PV1 is initially positive with a hint of terminal negativity. The duration of PR is arbitrary, but not long. The premature QRSs are not wide, their ST-T is the same as in sinus beats, and, at least in some instances they are preceded by a P that is easily identifiable as such, even though its intrinsic characteristics are vague. Note the third beat in V1-2-3. Its P is not much different from the sinus one in V1; in V2, it is superimposed on the downstroke of T, and it is not even identifiable in V3...but the three leads are just different views of the same event. Failure to see something in one lead need not prove that it is not present.

In order to develop awareness of the limits of the method, every component must be described in every tracing, whether it seems important or not. The mean frontal QRS in this tracing, for instance, varies from beat to beat, and the right leg electrode is insecurely attached.

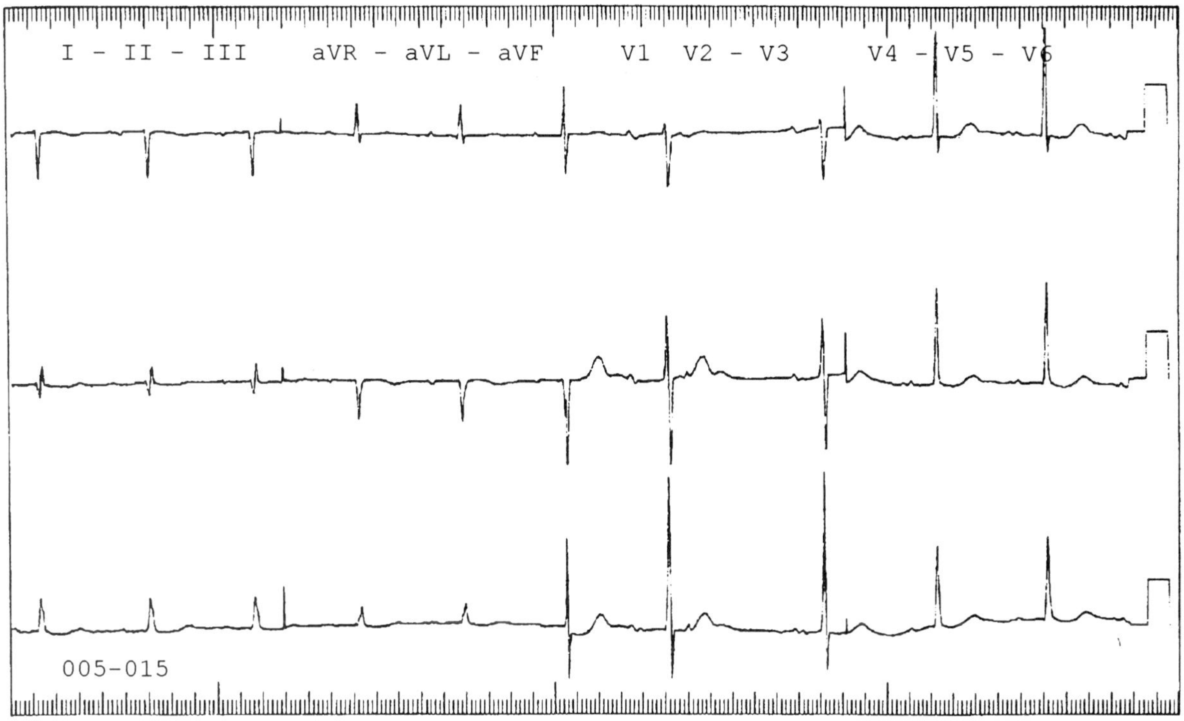

First Degree AV Block, Blocked PACs, Crossed Arm Leads

```
60    60    32    08   40      sinus
+45   1:10  V2    08   20:0   normal
                 none
             related to T
low +90       ±V1          +V2-6 low

(1) Sinus mechanism, rate 60
    with one blocked PAC
(2) First degree AV block
(3) Otherwise within normal
    limits

--T voltage is a little low,
  but not enough to call ab-
  normal by itself.
--Interpretation corrects for
  crossed arm leads.
```

As always, estimation of the length of PR is subject to interpretation, but it does not take much experience to recognize that it is long in this tracing (27, 150). Note the small P superimposed on ST in the first full beat in V1-2-3, a PAC that is "blocked"; i.e., not followed by a QRS. The AV conduction system was still refractory when the premature impulse reached it (129, 241). Blocked PACs are common even when AV conduction is normal, and any impairment of AV conduction makes them even more likely.

Transposition of arm leads is perhaps the most common technical error (104). Correction for it is easy (107), but, unrecognized, it may lead to an interpretation of an infarct (EKGs 152, 153). The keys are a negative P in Lead I (if there is not dextrocardia), and QRS directed apparently both rightward (negative in I) and leftward (positive in V6). What effect would it have on V leads (107)? Can crossing of right arm and leg leads be corrected as easily? Left (106)? Crossing of leg leads makes no difference; they are both attached to the same apex of Einthoven's triangle.

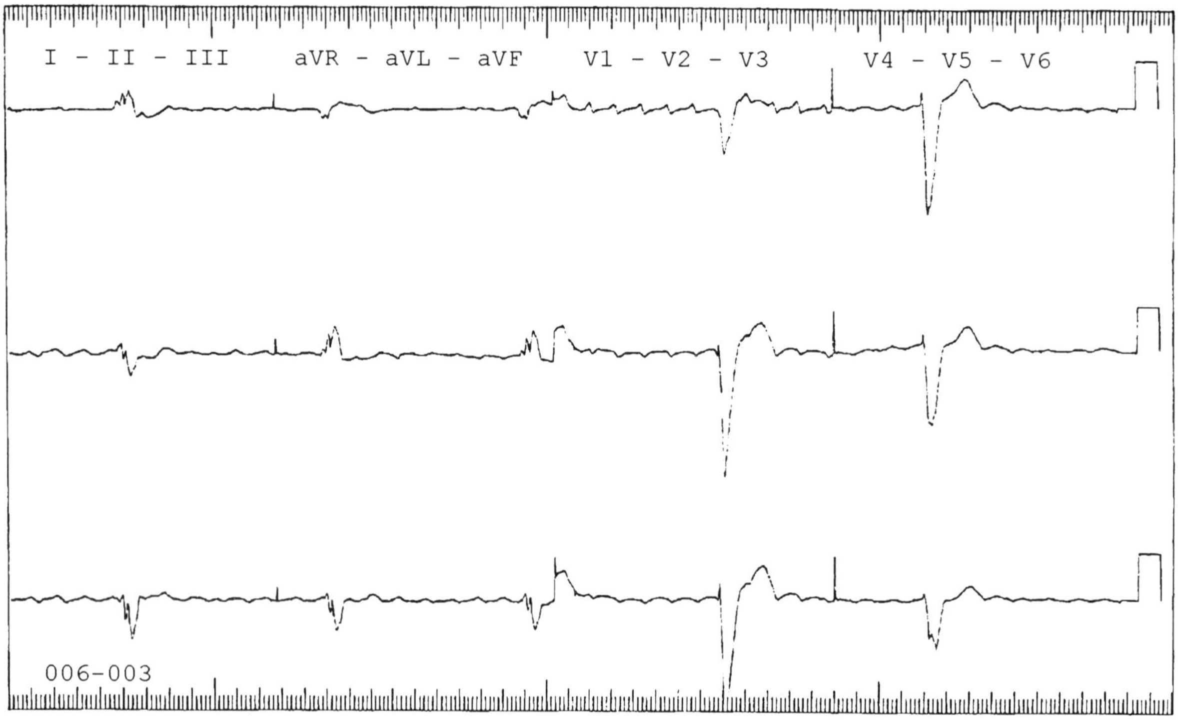

Atrial Tachycardia, Third Degree AV Block, Idioventricular Pacemaker (?)

```
250   --   35  20  54    see below
-45  0:10  --   1:10     diff slur
               none
         not remarkable
low        ±V1        positive V2-6

(1) Atrial tachycardia, 250
(2) 3° AV block
(3) Idioventricular pacemaker
    (or artificial?),rate 35
```

There is no single name for this mechanism as a whole, but if all three components are identified in the report, the doctor who knows the patient can use them effectively in determining a course of action. First, the atria. There are P waves, but their orientation is not clear. They may represent atrial reentry, classic flutter, but are separable from each other in V1, suggesting repetitive firing of a single focus. In either case, the atria are beating rapidly from an atrial focus, and the term in common use that comes closest to indicating this is atrial tachycardia...even though "cardia" does not separate atria from ventricles. AV block is complete; the ventricles must be dealt with separately (120). QRS rhythm is regular, and QRS duration means prolonged IV conduction time. An intrinsic ventricular origin would explain both, but the rate is a little fast for that, and slow for an artificial one, or for a junctional one with an IV conduction defect. The initial spike suggests an artificial pacemaker. Knowledge of the clinical setting would make these choices easy, but the EKG alone won't resolve them.

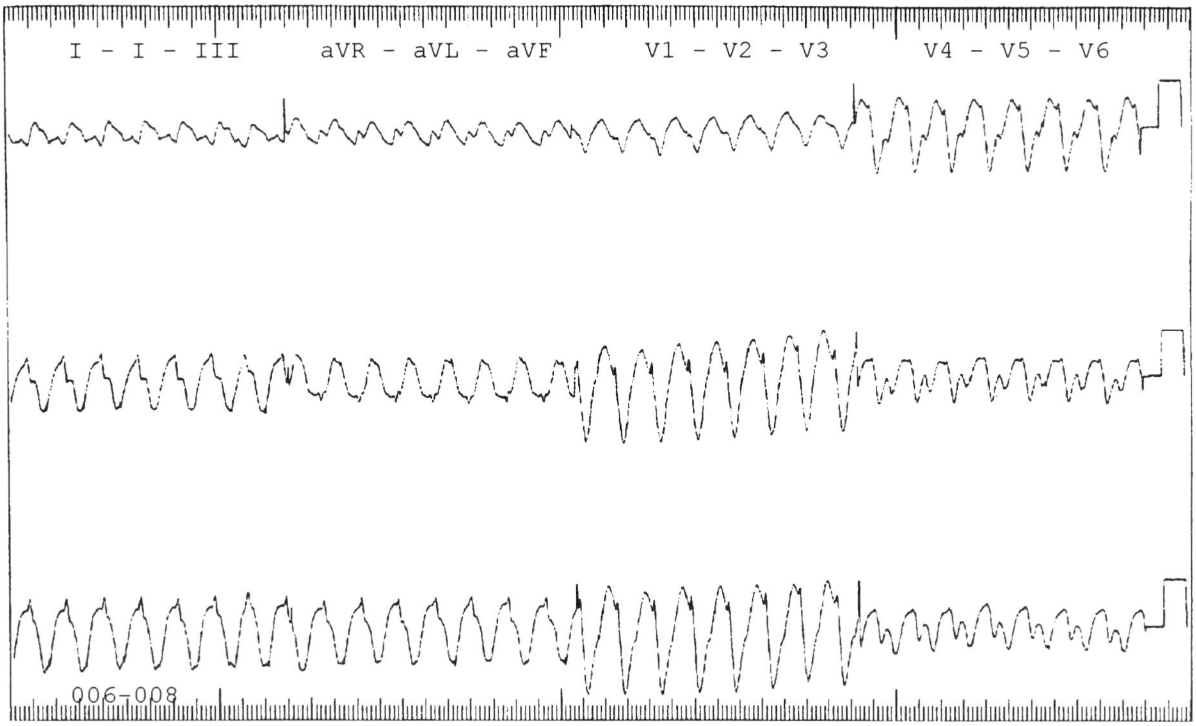

Ventricular Tachycardia (?)

It is clear that the ventricles are beating (or at least being activated) rapidly, but to give a specific rate is more informative than just to say fast, and to name the mechanism "ventricular tachycardia" says nothing about the atria, though "cardia" includes them. The presence of P waves at a rate slower than QRSs is an important criterion for the diagnosis of ventricular tachycardia, but atrial activity is not identifiable in this tracing. QRS rate and configuration could be explained as easily by an ectopic (not sinus) supraventricular (atrial or junctional) mechanism, with an IV conduction defect, as by a ventricular origin. Distinction between these possibilities on the basis of the electrocardiogram alone is not possible. The very wide QRS and its negativity in all precordial leads are in favor of a right ventricular origin, but a much more important factor in this case is the availability of a control tracing (inset) made when the mechanism was clearly supraventricular; specifically, sinus. Knowledge of other laboratory findings, and of the clinical setting, would make the choice much easier, at least at an actionable level.

```
--  185  --  20  ?32  see below
?-75  0:5  --  23  diffuse slur
      ?up 2,3,F, down V2-5?
      not coparable from T
?+90 low          positive V1-6

(1) Ectopic mechanism, rate 185,
    with regular rhythm, prob
    of ventricular origin,
    (vs atrial with left bundle
    branch block)

--no further interpretation is
  justified
```

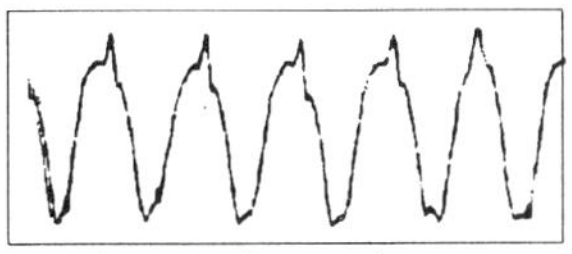

Lead III from above

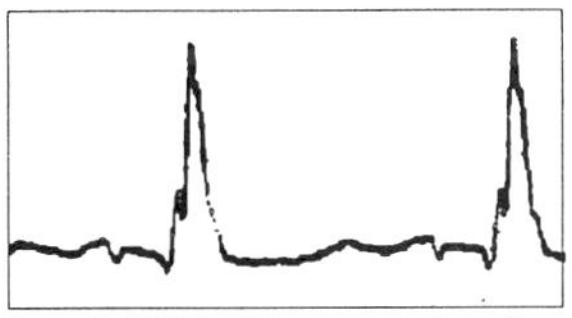

Lead III from control

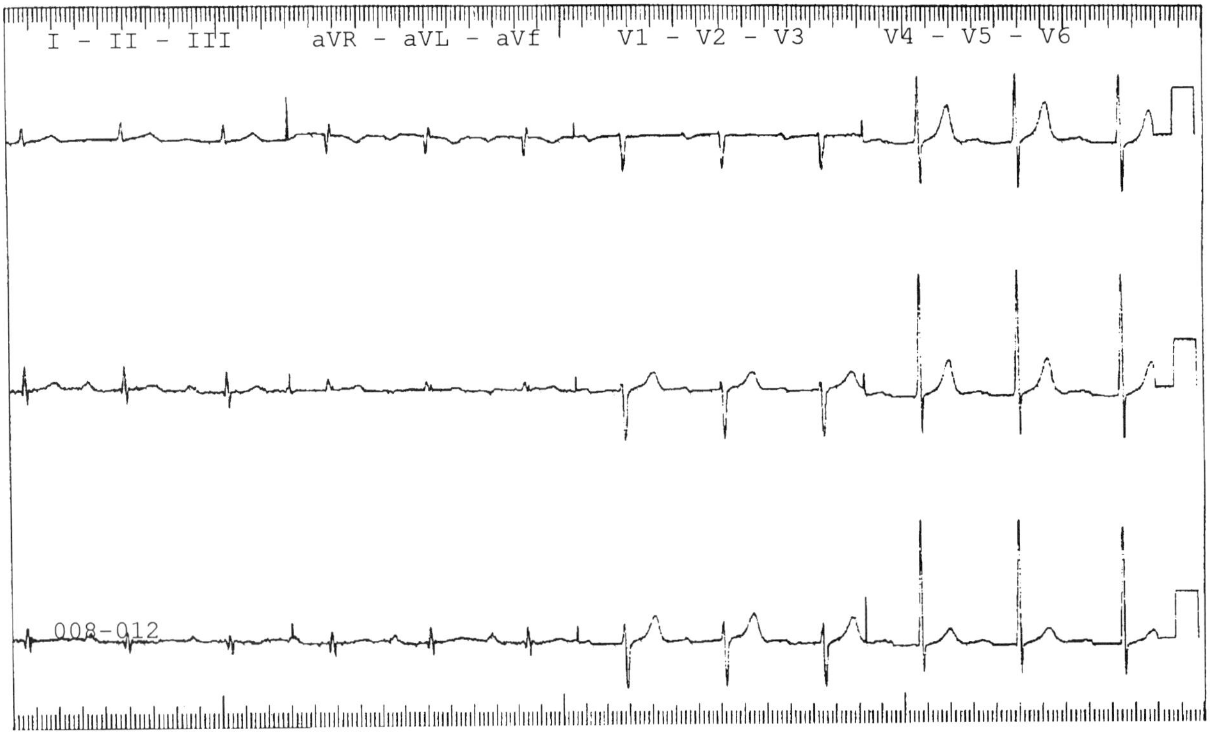

First Degree AV Block

70 70 32 08 40 sinus
+30 0:5 V3½ 25:0 normal
none
normal
±0 flat V1, positive V2-6

(1) Sinus mechanism, rate 70
(2) First degree AV block
(3) Otherwise WNL

The normal atrial wall conducts impulses at a rate of about 1000 mm/s; the AV node, about 20 mm/s. It takes about 0.20 s for an impulse to go from the sinus node to the beginning of ventricular depolarization, the PR interval. As with all intervals, this varies inversely with the rate, ranging between about 0.24 s for rates in the forties to 0.12 s at rates above 100. With impairment of AV conduction, it takes longer for an impulse to get through this electrophysiologic funnel (121), and PR is prolonged. P:QRS remains 1:1. This prolongation is called first degree AV block (150). With greater impairment of conduction, some atrial impulses fail to get through, second degree AV block (152). When no atrial impulses gets through, there is third degree, or complete, AV bock (153), and a distal focus must drive the ventricles.

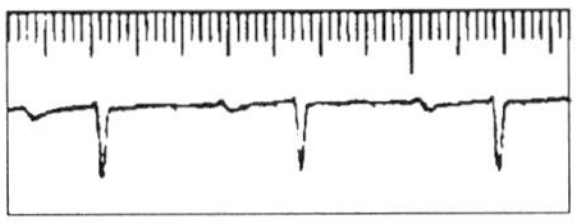
V1 from above

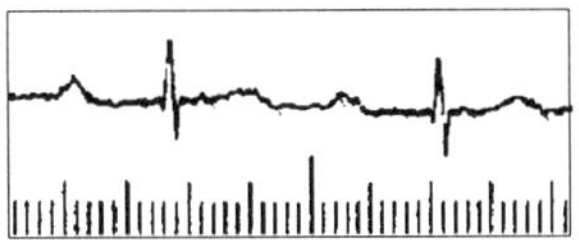
II from above

With the B point as its end, duration of PR depends on where P begins. It begins asymptotically, and PR cannot be measured usefully any closer than about 0.04 s.

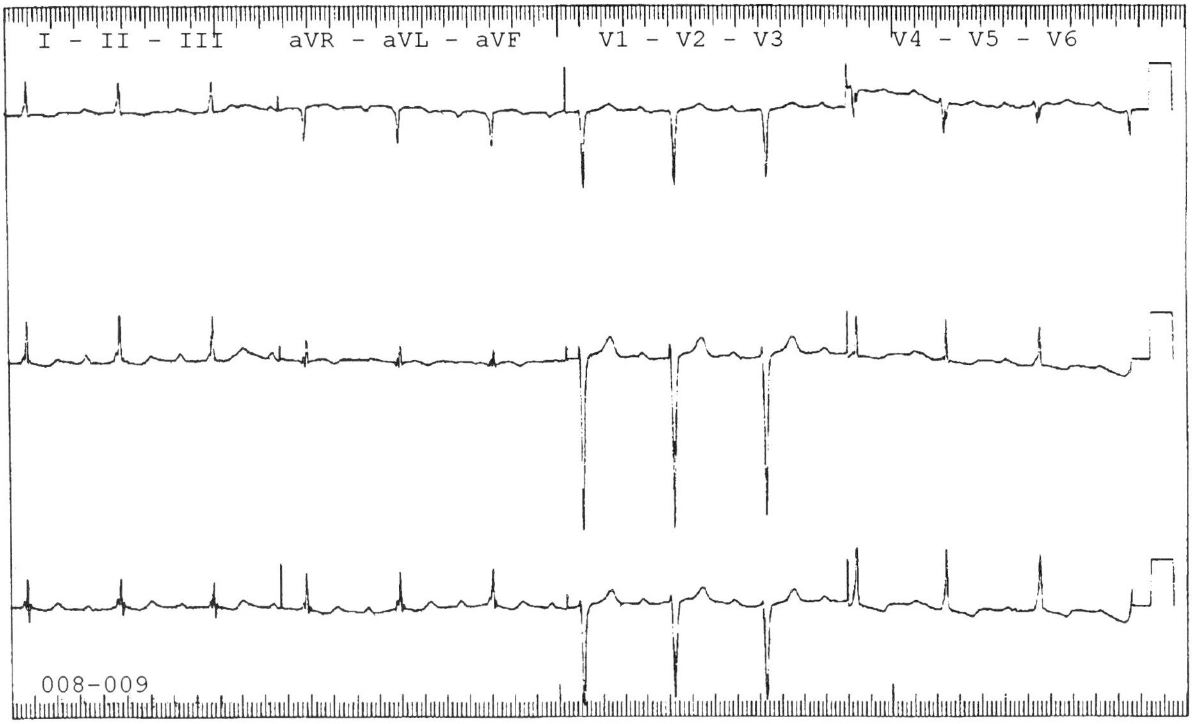

First Degree AV Block

ST-T abnormalities, nonspecific (LVO?)

```
75    75    28    08    36      sinus
+45   0:15    V4    12:0      normal
              none
          related to T
?+90 low   + V1-3, ±V4, neg V5-6

(1) Sinus mechanism, rate 75
(2) First degree AV block
(3) ST-T abnormalities, non-
    specific, suggestive of LVO
```

With the B point as a given for the end of PR, its duration is a function of where it begins (8). Because it begins gradually, at different places in different leads depending on the orientation of P (30), and P is often small, this is ill-defined. The computer applies the criteria programmed to identify these two points, measures the time between them, often to a thousandth of a second, and, when this exceeds the limit used by that program as normal, prints out "first degree AV block"...no judgment... nothing arbitrary... "right" by definition. At a human, clinically useful level, though, judgment is a big factor. The limits of the method must be respected; ±0.04 s is as close as PR should be called, and first degree AV block is a finding, not a disease.

There is no abnormality of P or QRS (structure). ST-T (function) is of normal duration (QT), amplitude, and contour, but the spatial orientation of its distal component, T, is nearly opposite that of QRS (80, 210). This is abnormal, and correlates better with an increase in demand for blood, left ventricular overload (187), than with diminution of supply, coronary insufficiency (207).

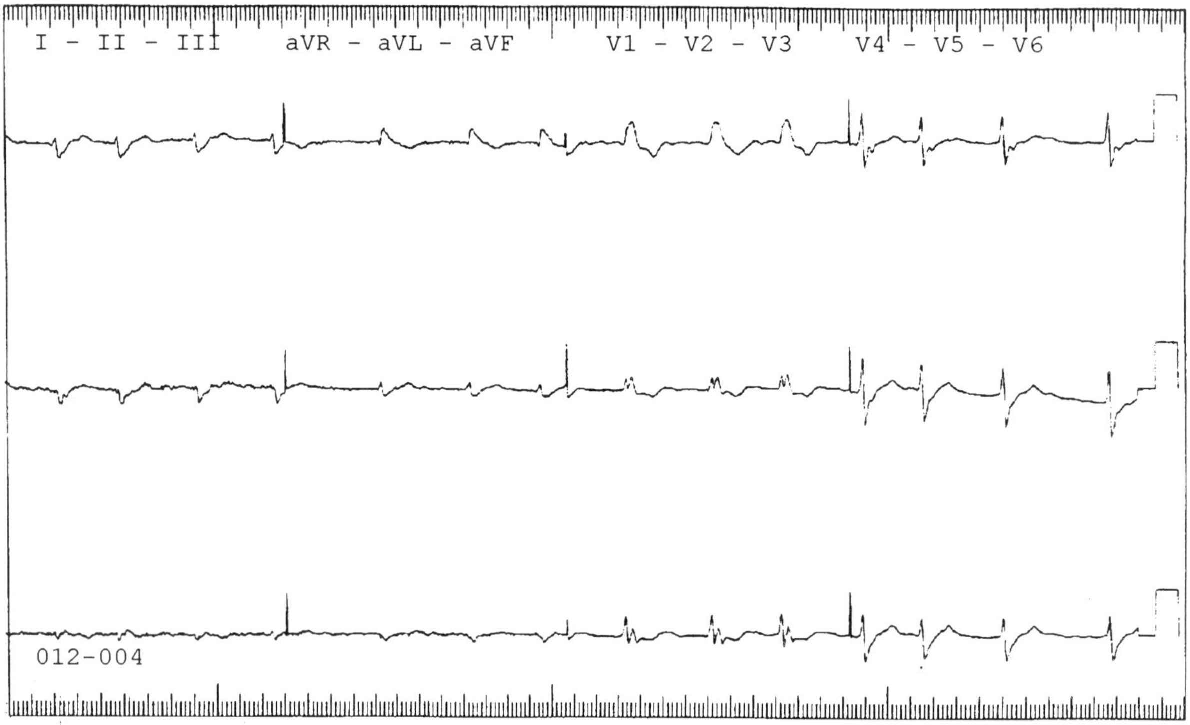

Atrial Fibrillation, Right Bundle Branch Block

```
--    85    --    16    36        AF
--    5:0    --     5:5      BSTDRA
              none
             normal
+30  neg V-2  ±V3-4      pos V5-6

(1) Atrial fibrillation,
    ventricular rate about 85
(2) Right bundle branch block
(3) Otherwise WNL
```

Undulation of the trace typical of atrial fibrillation is easy to see between ventricular complexes, especially in leads II, III, aVF, and V1 (19, 27, 131), and there is widening and slurring of the terminal part of QRS selectively, directed to the right (Lead I) and anteriorly (V1) (30), a pattern typical of right bundle branch block (159), an abnormality of structure. Note that this common diagnosis is objective; it translates the findings into a clinically useful name, but does not suggest an etiology.

All that is needed to complete the interpretation is an evaluation of the (electrophysiologic) function of the ventricular myocardium, the ST-T. Its duration, amplitude, and contour are easily normal, and so is its orientation, T is directed opposite the blocked part of QRS. The report is completed by saying that tracing is otherwise (i.e., what is left after mechanism and structure) within normal limits.

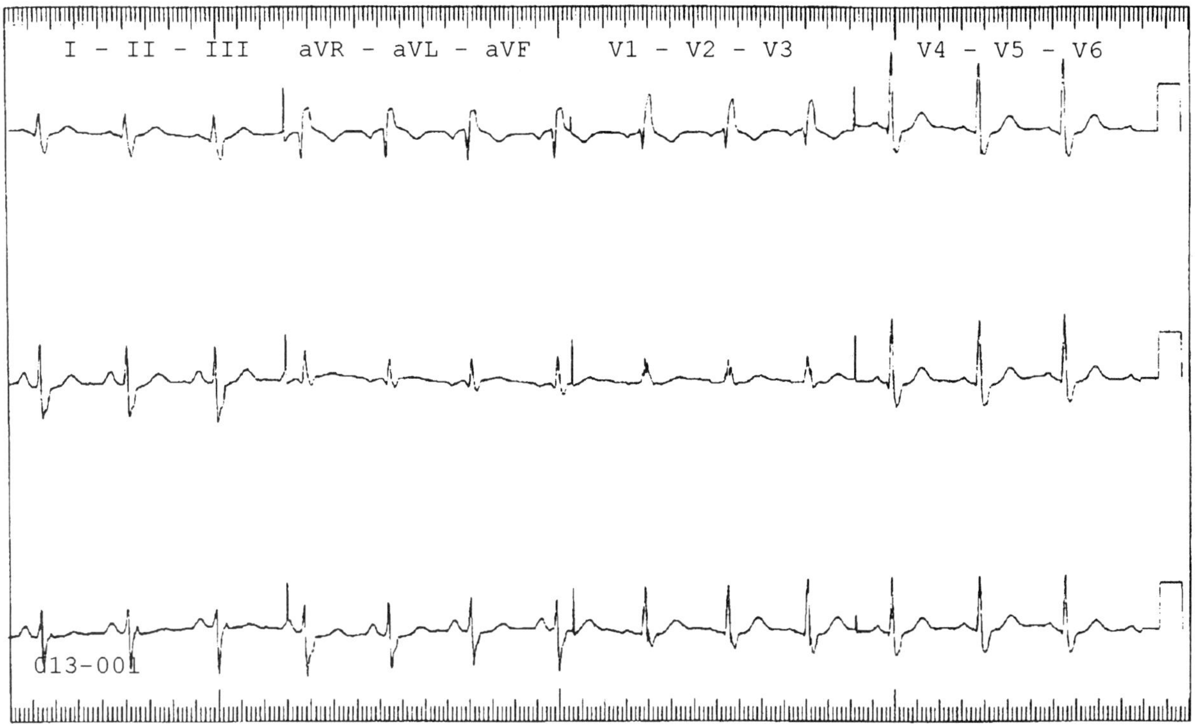

Right Atrial Enlargement, Right Bundle Branch Block

```
80    80    16    16    40     sinus
--    rSR 1:5:8   --    10:4   BSTDRA
                  none
                 normal
+45   neg V1    ±V2      pos V3-6
P: Prominent, peaked 2,3,F

(1) Sinus mech, rate 80
(2) Right atrial enlargement
(3) Right bundle branch block
(4) Otherwise WNL
```

The presence of P waves (27) shows that the atria are being depolarized in an organized fashion, and their orientation indicates their origin, the sinus node in this case. Their amplitude and contour, descriptors that cannot be separated completely, can point to enlargement of either or both atria. In this tracing, the relative prominence and symmetry of P2,3,F suggest right atrial enlargement (187), but not very strongly.

Right atrial enlargement almost always reflects loss of compliance of the right ventricle, and this is often secondary to increase in pulmonary arteriolar resistance, as with respiratory disease.

The most common basis for RBBB (159), but not the only one possible, is discrepancy between supply and demand for blood, "ischemia," and this may reflect change in either or both. The presence of RBBB invalidates one of the premises central to recognition of right ventricular enlargement, simultaneous radial depolarization of the ventricles, and to call both from the same tracing is beyond the limits of the method. The presence of either supports the idea that the P pattern means right atrial enlargement, and together they suggest pulmonary disease (232).

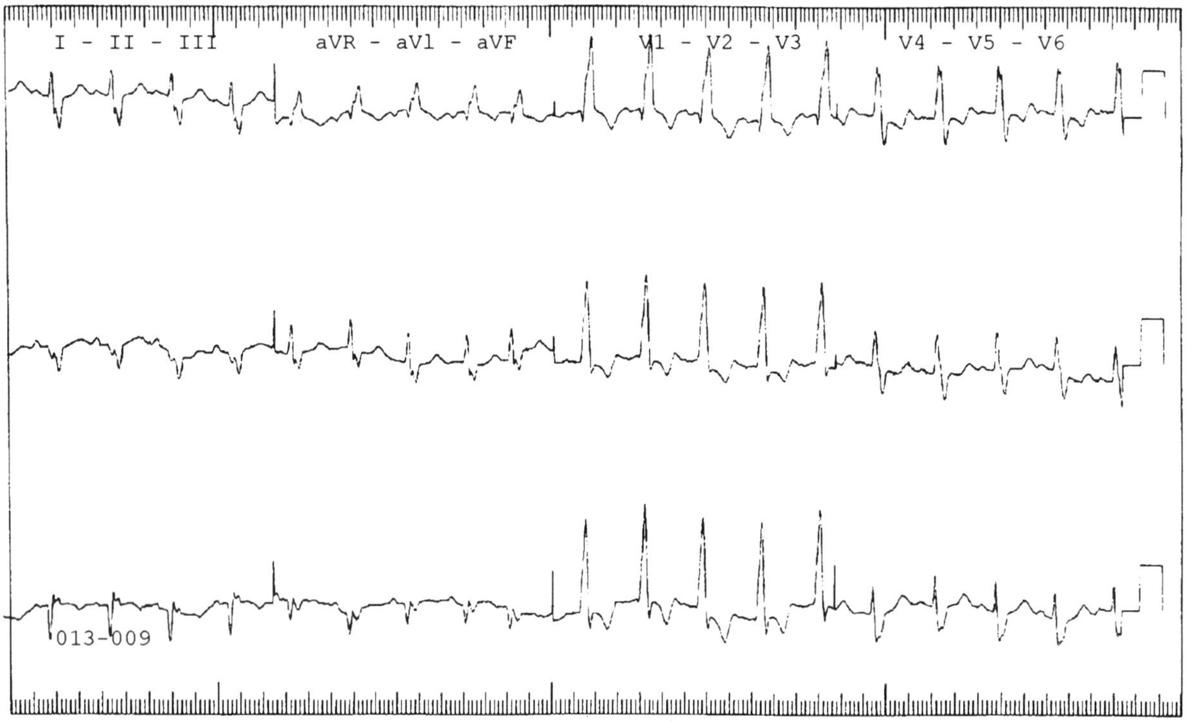

Right Bundle Branch Block, Old Inferior Myocardial Infarct

```
115    115    12  16    36    sinus
?-105   QR 2:15, V5, 6:8 (bstdra
                    QS2,F, Q3)
             none
         related to T
±0    neg V1-3    ±V4-5    pos V6

(1) Sinus mechanism, rate 115
(2) Right bundle branch block
(3) Old inferior myo infarct
```

Reasoning from things every student knows by the end of the first year of medical school, myocardial infarction would be expected to change the *initial* part of QRS (173), and this is exactly what happens. Because of the way the leads are deployed (68), this usually means an abnormal Q; not just a Q, an *abnormal* Q (174). The location assigned to infarcts indicates the position of the positive pole of the leads in which they are recognized, not the anatomic structures involved. The estimate of their age is based on the ST-T pattern (180).

The same knowledge of anatomy and physiology permits prediction of EKG changes as a result of right bundle branch block; broad, slurred *terminal* forces directed to the right and anteriorly (159). Left bundle branch block typically changes the whole QRS, and may preclude recognition of an infarct, but with right bundle branch block there is no conflict; both the infarct and the bundle branch block can be seen.

Note that RBBB names only the lesion; an infarct, both the lesion and an explanation for it.

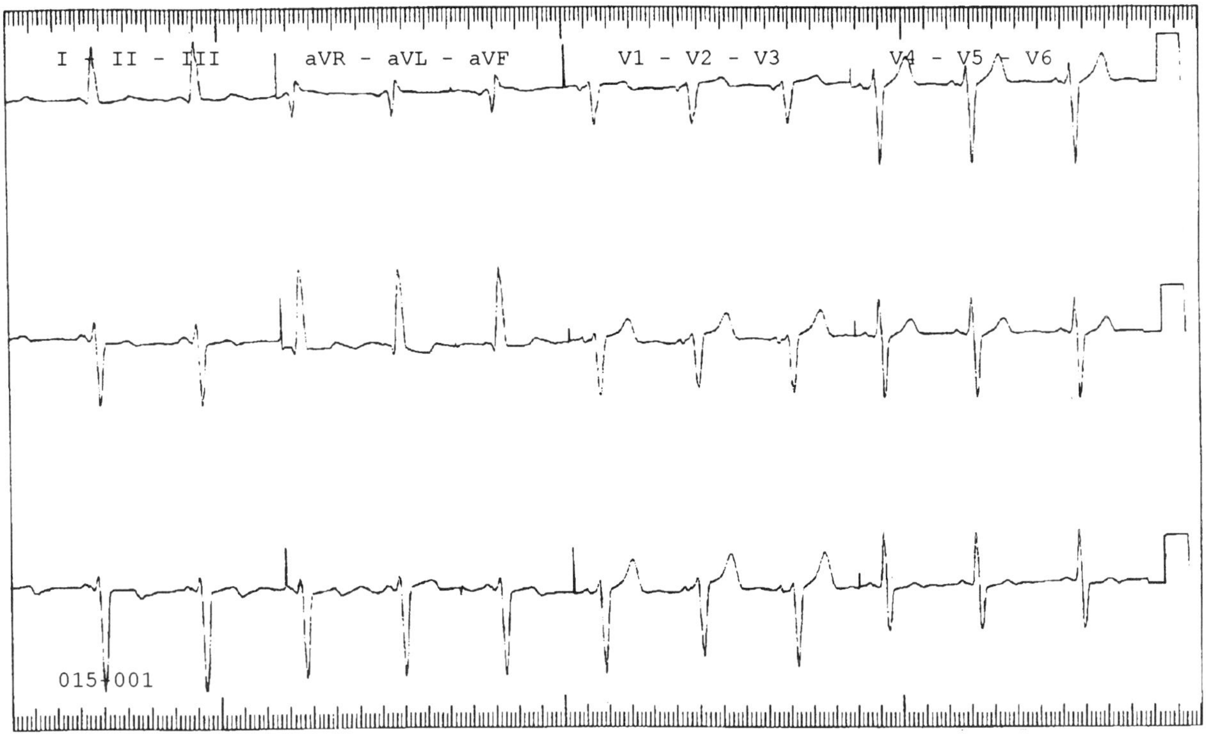

Left Anterior Fascicular Block

```
70    70    12    12    40      sinus
-60   1:6   V5½   10:8          normal
            none
          related to T
low    +15,  pos V1-6,   low V6

(1) Sinus mechanism, rate 70
(2) Left anterior fascicular
    block
(3) Otherwise prob WNL, at
    worst only small ST-T abns
```

QRS duration should be called no closer than 0.02 s; in this case, it may or may not be prolonged. The computer called it 0.126 s, defining it as abnormal, and attributed it to left bundle branch block. To differentiate between block of the whole bundle and only part of it is arbitrary, and that it is even possible assumes several nearly unprovable definitions (162). The reason left anterior fascicular block seems preferable here is that QRS contour is less distorted than typical of LBBB (160). The difference in clinical implication is probably small. The concept of LBBB is clinically secure, having been accepted for a long time as representing an anatomic reality, and its differential is small. The idea that block of only part of the bundle is a recognizable entity is newer, and EKG criteria for it are less clear, overlapping those for normal, right ventricular enlargement, and inferior myocardial infarct. Prolongation of IV conduction time may be present but is not a criterion for the diagnosis. Whether LBBB or LAHB, the implication is a lesion in the wall of the left ventricle without suggesting an explanation.

T voltage is low in V6, but the net QRS area is small there, too. If it is abnormal at all, the abnormality is small.

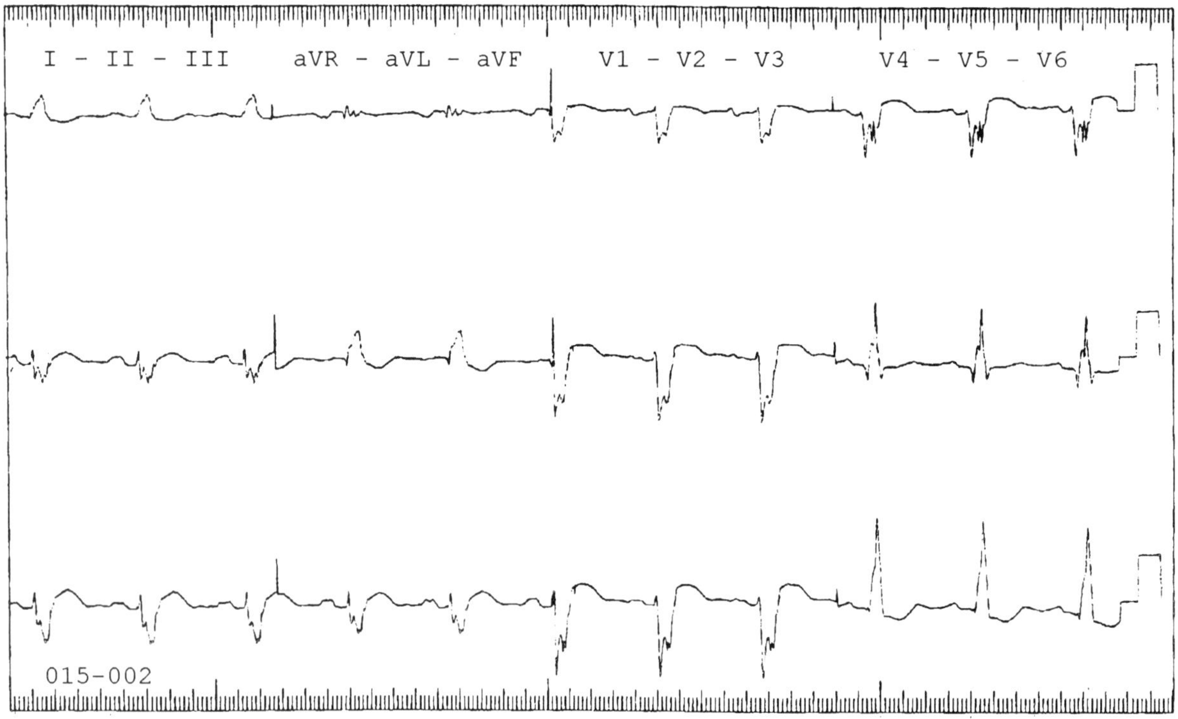

Left Bundle Branch Block, Anterior Myocardial Infarct

```
65    65    20    16    44     sinus
-60   1:6   V4½   20:1    diff slur
                         QSV4, QV5
      up 2,3,4,V2-4, down V6
          sagging/arched
+90    ±V1-5       negative V6 low

(1) Sinus mechanism, rate 65
(2) Left bundle branch block
(3) Anterior  myocardial  in-
    farct, probable, age indet
```

The effects of proximal (predivisional, complete) left bundle branch block, begin at the onset of QRS, changing the initial forces where evidence of the deep scar assumed to represent an infarct would be seen (174). This is the basis for the conventional wisdom that LBBB precludes the EKG diagnosis of an infarct. But sometimes it does not. In this tracing the pattern typical of LBBB, seen best in Lead I (160), offers an easy explanation for QRS prolongation, an objective finding that must be explained. The characteristics of initial QRS forces in the precordial leads, another feature that can be described objectively (174, 170), is typical of an infarct (184). A diagnosis of bundle branch block names a lesion, but not an explanation for it; an infarct, not only a lesion with universally defined anatomic characteristics, but also its etiology, a step that is really beyond the limits of the method but useful because of statistics and experience. An infarct may explain LBBB; both may be present. The ST-T pattern in this tracing suggests that the infarct, if there is one, is of recent origin, and this has to be noted. The clinical setting and stability of the findings are critical unknowns. An infarct requires action, LBBB does not. Other studies can be utilized.

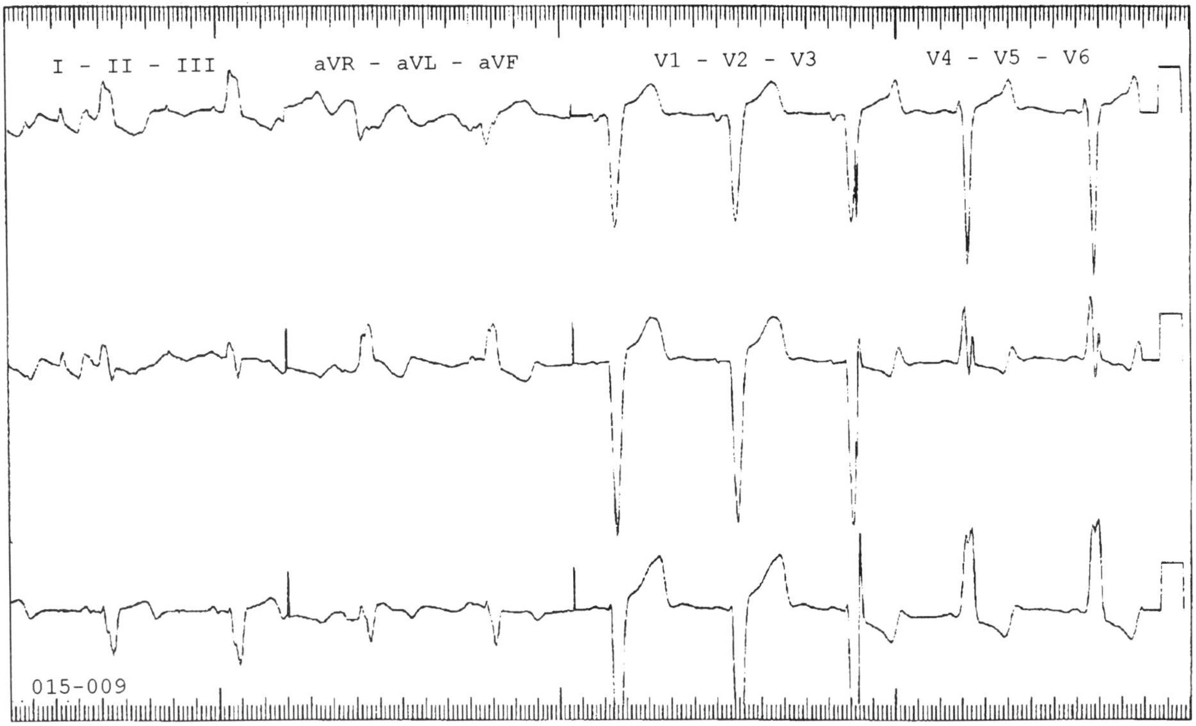

Left Bundle Branch Block, Typical

```
55    55    16    16    48      sinus
-30   0:25   V4½   20:0         DSLP
        down V6, up V1-3
          normal (see T)
+150   pos V1-4   ±V5   neg V6

(1) Sinus mechanism, rate 55
(2) Left bundle branch block
(3) Otherwise prob WNL, at
    worst only small ST-T ab-
    normalities
```

The pattern typical of left bundle branch block (160) is usually seen best in leads that view the heart from the left and/or below, I, aVL, and V6. QRS is wide, both upstroke and downstroke are nearly vertical, and the top is notched.

It is hard to know what to say about ST-T when there is bundle branch block. If function is normal, and the ST-T pattern simply reflects change in the route of depolarization due to bundle branch block, it will likely be normal in duration, amplitude, and contour, but directed opposite QRS. Intrinsic abnormality (duration, amplitude, contour) implies electrophysiologic abnormality.

Irregularity of the trace in Leads I and II, but not in III, points to an imperfect connection to the right arm, a component of I and II but not III, the "bipolar" leads. This kind of artifact is very common, and may obscure important information. Better training and supervision of technicians could eliminate it. It is easy to compensate for it with a bit of mental data averaging. When consistent throughout the recording, this kind of artifact affects all the other leads, too, but their "unipolar" configuration (88) makes it less noticeable. In this case, the problem occurred only during recording of I, II, and III, representing an isolated event.

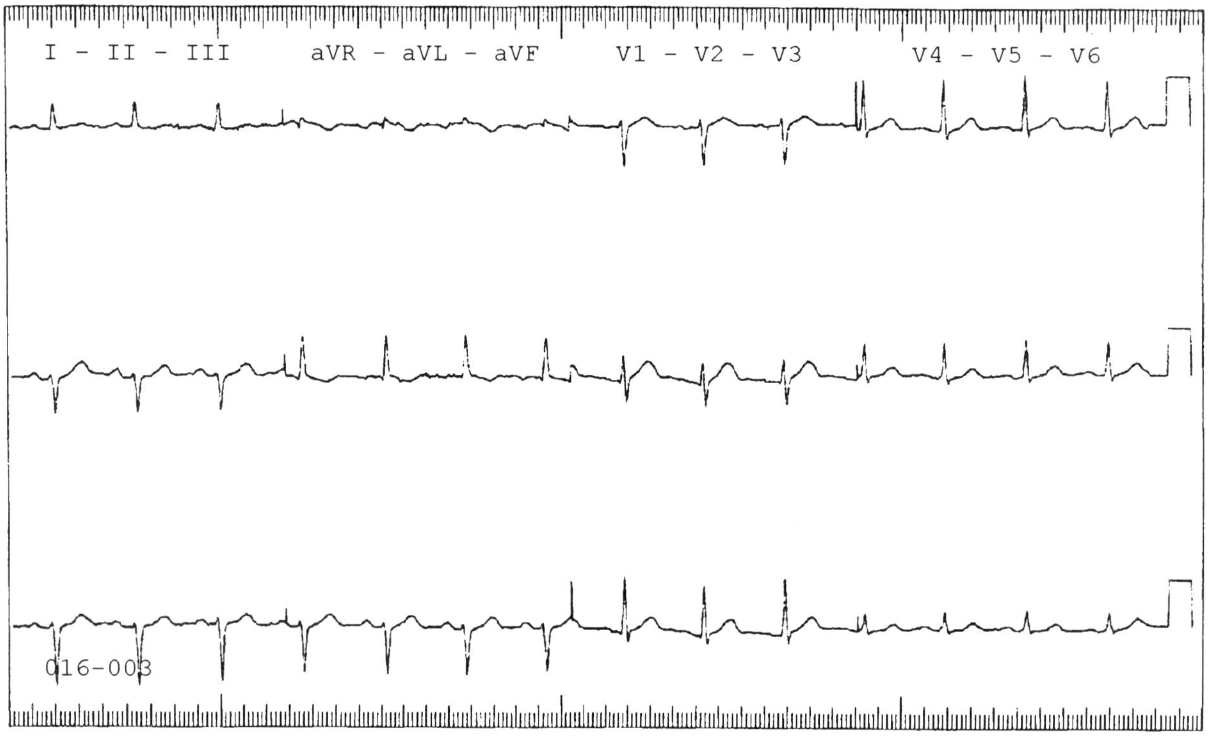

Left Anterior Fascicular Block

85 85 16 06 36 sinus
-60 1:8 V2 5:1 normal
none
normal
+90 positive V1-6 low V1

(1) Sinus mechanism, rate 85
(2) Left ant fascicular block
(3) Otherwise within nl limits

The orientation of MFQRS is a characteristic that can be expressed as a number and correlated usefully with other features and the clinical picture. This is known as the electrical axis, or just the axis, and is represented as an arrow extending outward from the center of the system. Its position is estimated on the basis of the net area enclosed by the complex (34), and usually falls between –30% and +105%. Values counterclockwise to –30% became known as left axis deviation; clockwise to +105%, right. The area of the curves is very difficult to calculate, though, and, except when there is widening of the distal part, but not the proximal (as in RBBB, and, less obviously, left anterior fascicular block), their amplitude alone suffices. However defined, the possible explanations for deviation are numerous (226). It is generally accepted as reasonable that, in the absence of other explanations, a mean frontal QRS between about –60% and –90%, when initial QRS contour is normal, represents LAFB. The clinical importance of the diagnosis by itself is usually small. Differential includes, especially, inferior infarction, right ventricular enlargement, and pulmonary emphysema (163). (See also EKGs 36, 44, 65, 74, and 98 for further discussion and examples.)

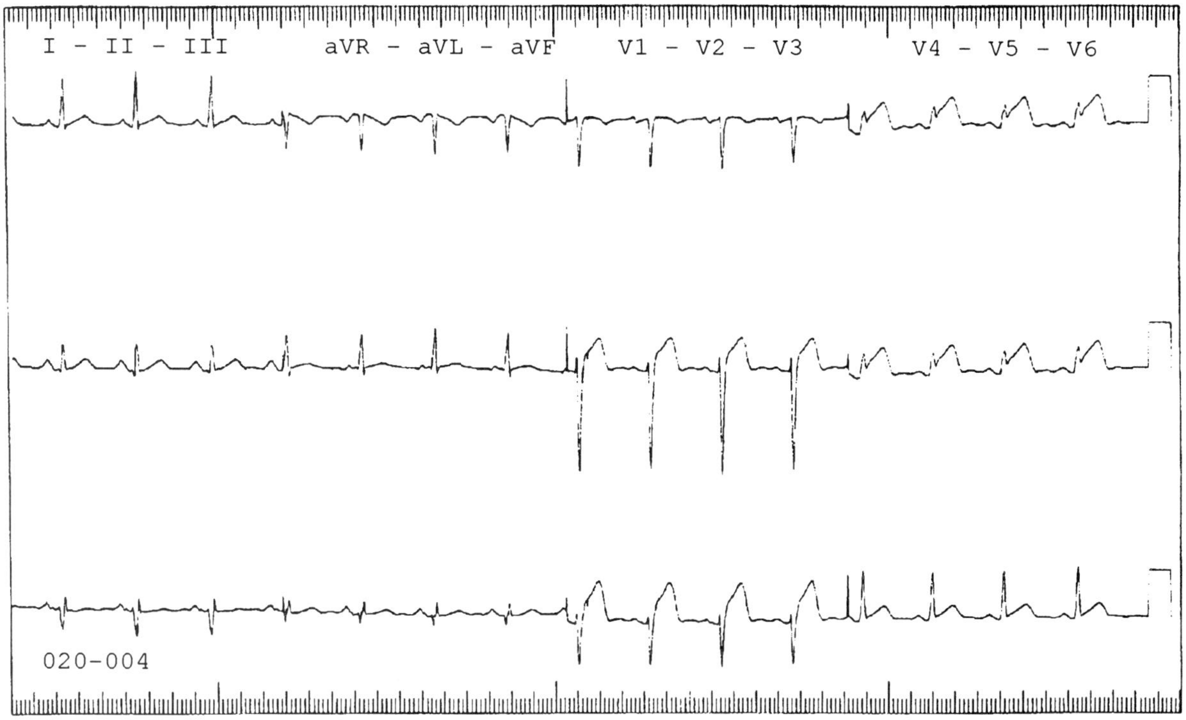

ST Elevation (Myocardial Injury)

```
95    95    16    08    32      sinus
±0    0:10    V3½    10:0    normal
          up V2-6
        straightened
+45   negative V1   positive V2-6

(1) Sinus mechanism, rate 95
(2) ST T abnormalities typical
    of anterior myo injury
```

The computer readout for this tracing says anterior infarct...with no caveats.

The anterior ST elevation implies subepicardial injury, and offers strong support for a clinical suspicion of a new infarct, but there is no identifiable evidence of the anatomic lesion itself (173); i.e., of deep myocardial scarring. That would show in the initial part of QRS. See *myocardial infarct* in the index for examples.

ST displacement this marked, and in a direction implying subepicardial location, implies injury to a relatively large mass of muscle. It is probably explained best as outward extension, toward the point of coronary narrowing, of the process first manifest deep in the myocardium at the distal end of the blood supply (208). Compare it to the relatively small displacement brought about by injury from outside the epicardium, pericarditis, involving only the tissue immediately beneath it. (EKGs 54, 86, and 115). EKGs 41 and 42 show other examples of injury similar to this one.

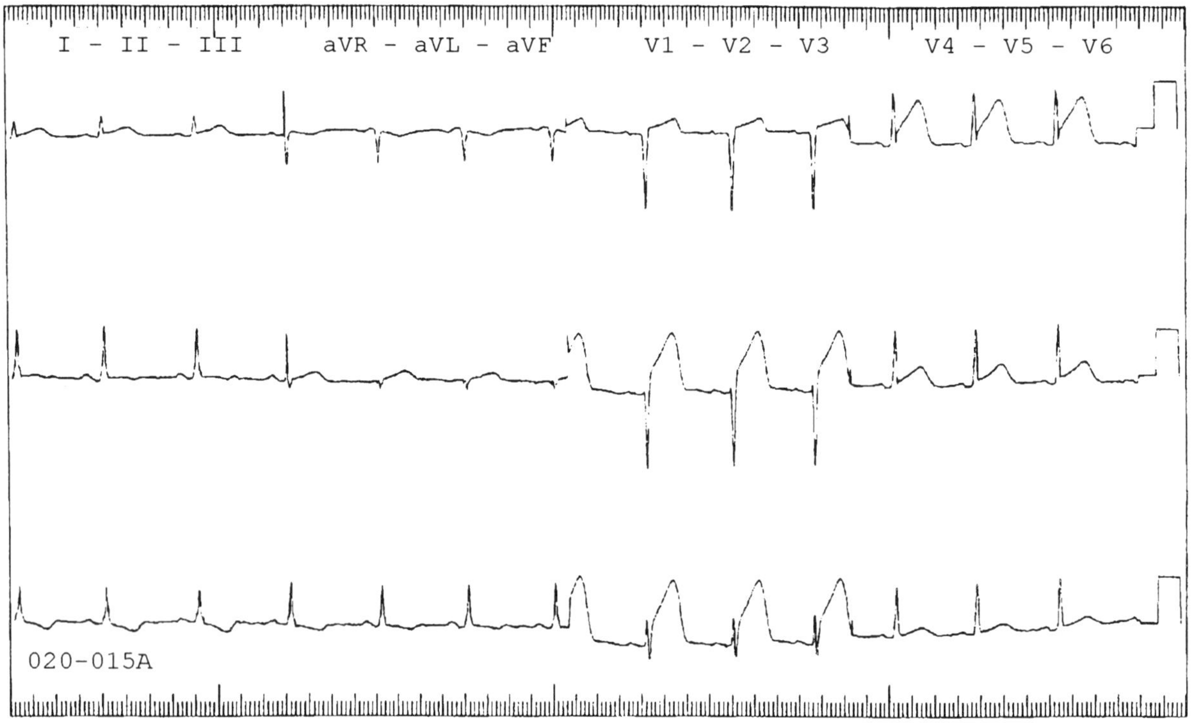

ST Elevation (Myocardial Injury)

```
80    80    16    08    40     sinus
+75   0:15    V3    10:0     normal
              up V2-5
           straightened
-30       pos V1-6,   tall V2-4

(1) Sinus mechanism, rate 60
(2) ST-T abnormalities typical
    of ant myo injury, as with
    at least cor insufficiency

--probably an early phase of an
  infarct
```

This ST-T pattern is typical of anterior injury, probably transmural, and is seen often very early in myocardial infarction, the "hyperacute" phase. EKG 42 shows a later stage of this same lesion.

ST contour is one of the most difficult features of the tracing to describe, and there is no standard, no right or wrong vocabulary for it. In this tracing, J is elevated in anterior leads, and the line connecting it with the well-defined peak of a tall T, the ST segment, is nearly straight. The back side of this process, ST depression, does not show, but the EKG documents the motion of point. When that point is apart from its resting position, the B point, toward one part of the body, it is away from some other part, but the volume conductor (thorax and abdomen) is not a sphere, and the leads are not deployed diametrically opposite each other. Both views may be seen when the forces of injury are directed caudad and dorsad (ST up in aVF and down in V3-4), as with many acute inferior infarcts (EKG 145), or cephalad and anterior (ST up in anterior leads and down in inferior ones), as with some anterior infarcts (EKG 62) (47, 202).

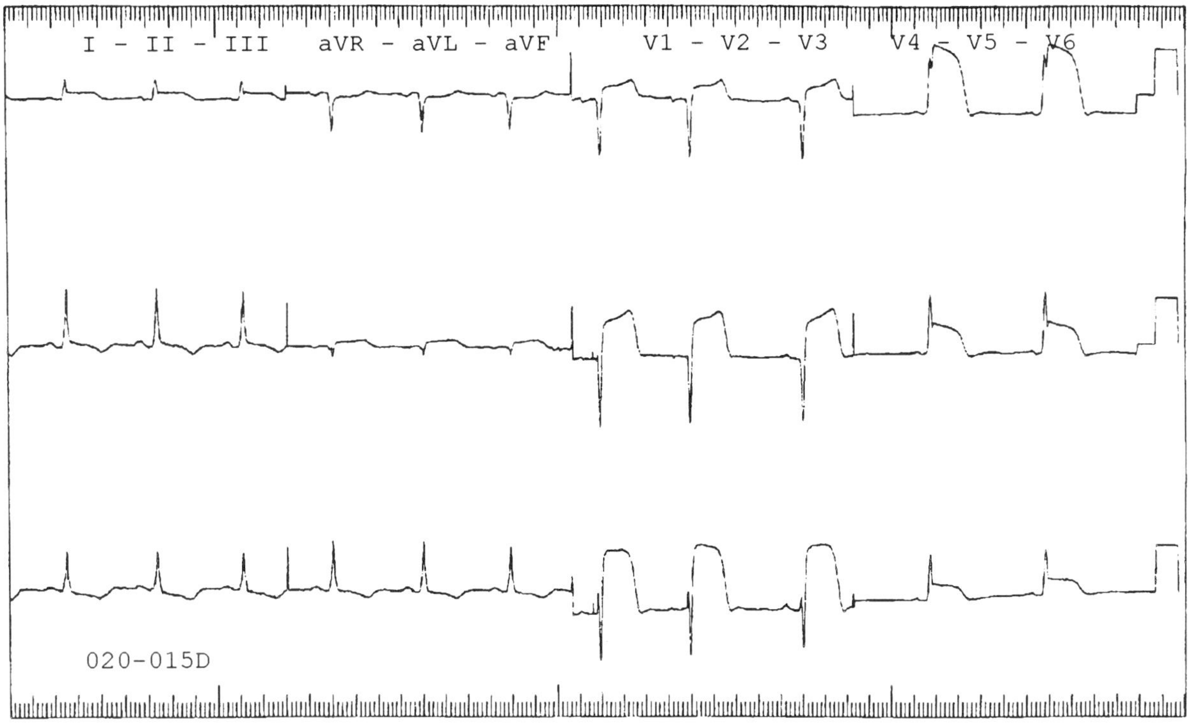

Anterior Myocardial Injury

```
70    70    16    08    40      sinus

+75   0:12    V3½    10:0      QSV2
      up I, V1 6, sl dn aVR
         flattened/arched
-90   pos V1-2,     insep ST V3-6

(1) Sinus mechanism, rate 70
(2) ST-T abns typical of at
    least ant myo injury
(3) Acute ant myo infarct, prob
```

There is no single "right" way to describe this pattern. Its important features are marked ST displacement ventrad, almost perpendicular to the frontal plane. Its contour in those leads where displacement is marked can be described as arched and/or flattened. The judgment that this is due to transmural injury, as with coronary insufficiency, instead of localized subepicardial injury, as with pericarditis (q.v.), is based on the amplitude of ST displacement (compared to the amplitude of QRS), presumably evidence of involvement of a larger mass of muscle than the thin layer immediately subjacent to the epicardium with pericarditis. With coronary insufficiency, the first tissue to suffer is deep, and the area involved extends outward, toward the lesion in the coronary artery, as the insufficiency progresses (208).

The evidence for infarction, the anatomic lesion itself, is the prominent Q in V2. It is clean. and not very wide, and the clinical setting is an important unknown, but considering the ST-T pattern of injury, and the change since the tracing of a little over an hour ago (EKG 41), the picture as a whole leaves little doubt that there is a new infarct.

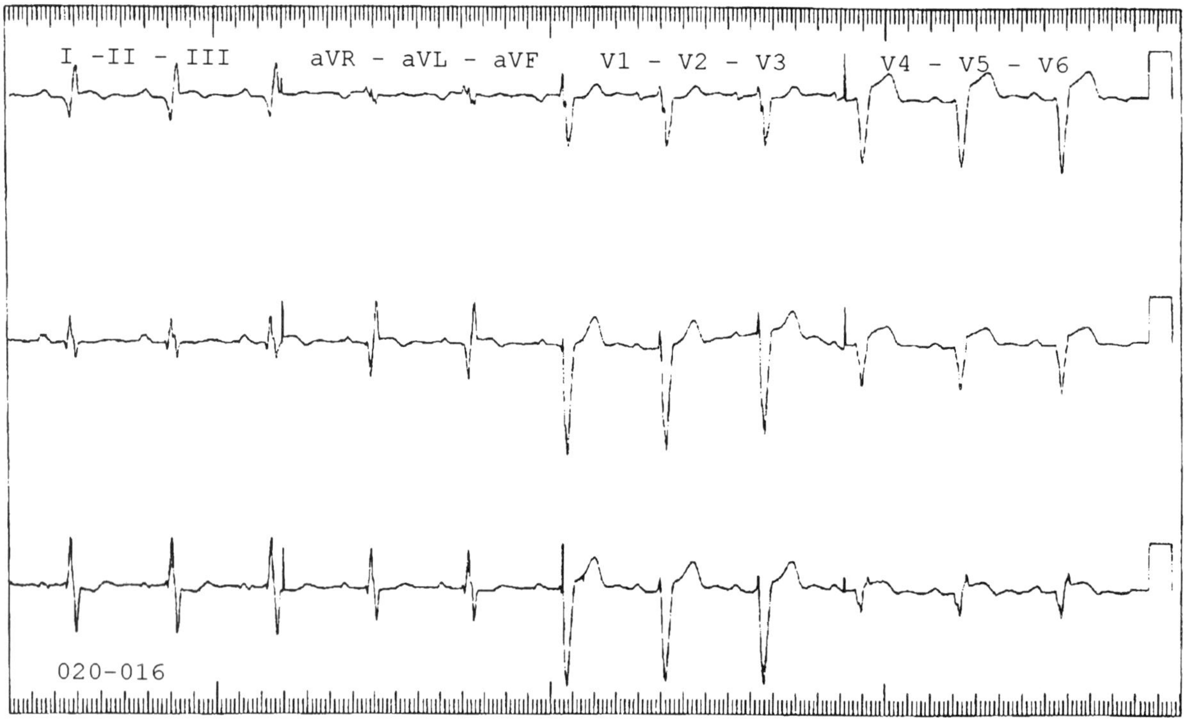

Anterolateral Myocardial Infarct

```
70    70    20    12    40     sinus
??   3:10   V6   QRV6  5:2   Q1,L,V6
        up I,  aVL,  V4-6
         flattened/arched
low     pos V1-5,    insep ST V6

(1) Sinus mechanism, rate 70
(2) Anterolateral myocardial
    infarct, age indeterminate
```

The *sine qua non* for the electrocardiographic diagnosis of an infarct is abnormality of the initial part of QRS (173). The position of the positive pole of the leads in which this is recognized names its location (177), and ST-T evidence of injury, or its absence, determines whether it is called new or old (180). The first of these criteria is satisfied in this tracing by the broad, ragged Q in I, aVL, and V6, and the QS in V4-5 following an rS in V1-3; the second, by the view from the front (V4-5), and side (I, aVL, and V6). Little, if any, ventricular myocardium depolarizes toward the right; "lateral" means left lateral.

Injury is transient and, assuming that it is a result of the same thing that caused the infarct, the infarct must have occurred recently, usually somewhere between minutes and a day or two. In this case, evidence of injury (202) is clear, but the age of an infarct is always subject to interpretation. A new one may not look new, and ST displacement characteristic of a new one, but persistent, may mean ventricular aneurysm (185).

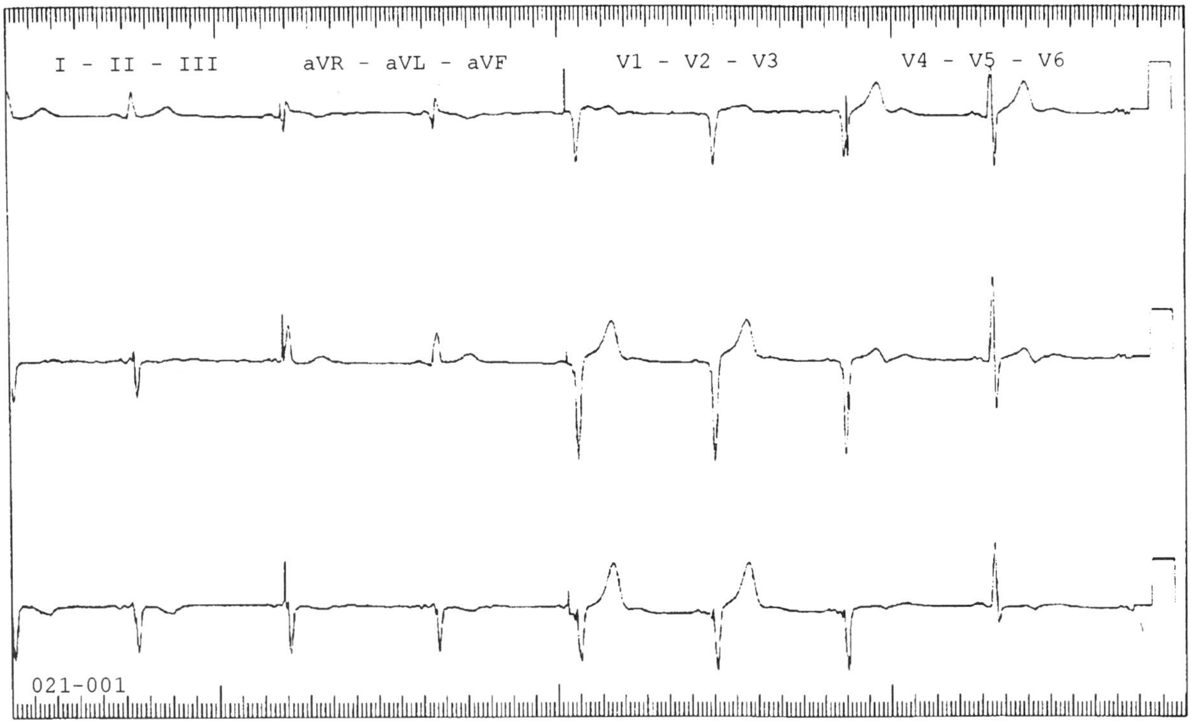

Left Anterior Fascicular Block, Old Anterior Myocardial Infarct

```
50    50    ?12    10    44    Sinus
-60   0:10  V4    15:3   early slur
                           QS V2-3
       slightly up V2-V4
         related to T
-30   ±V1   positive V2-5      ±V6

(1) Sinus mechanism, rate 50
(2) Left ant fascicular block
(3) Old anterior myo infarct
```

The evidence for left anterior fascicular block (or hemiblock) is a marked counter-clockwise direction of QRS in the frontal plane (about –45% to –90%), with normal initial QRS contour in those leads (163). The principal alternative to be considered as an explanation for this "left axis deviation" is an inferior infarct. The two lesions may coexist, but cannot both be identified in the same tracing. Either may explain "left axis deviation," but an infarct deforms initial QRS forces, while they are normal in uncomplicated LAFB (164). Remember that the tracing shows the course, in time and space, of only one point (70, 121), and there is only one QRS. All leads show the same events, but in different projections. Evidence for an anterior infarct is clear, notching of initial QRS in views (leads) from the front of the body. Note that the critical finding, abnormality of initial QRS forces, is in a QS in this case, not a Q; there must be an R to distinguish between a Q and an S. Calling it very close, there is a tiny, clean Q in V3, but it does not initiate a predominantly positive QRS, and it disappears in leads farther to the left (175). The lesion is assumed to be old because nothing looks new, but the clinical setting, and stability of the findings, are not known. The location of the infarct suggests an explanation for the fascicular block.

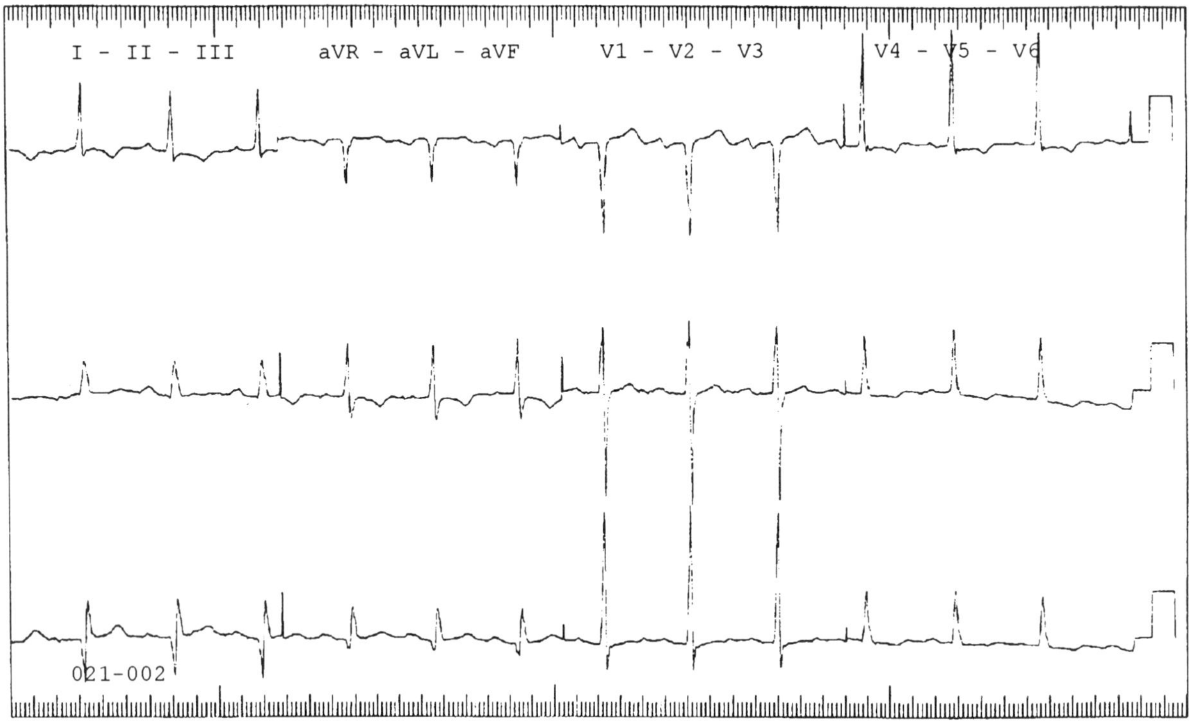

Old Inferior Myocardial Infarct

```
80    80    24    08    40      sinus
+30   0:20    V2    10:0        Q3,F
                none
           related to T
+150   +V1-2, ±V3, neg V4-5, ±V6

(1) Sinus mechanism, rate 80
    with borderline AV conduc-
    tion time
(2) Old inferior myo infarct
```

PR is about 0.24 s. The computer called it 0.228, a value greater than the traditional 0.20 for the upper limit of normal, and therefore first degree AV block (27, 150), but the implication of such precision is an illusion. To call PR closer than 0.04 s is beyond the limit of clinical usefulness, and if first degree AV block is perceived as disease, instead of a finding, the patient is put at inappropriate risk.

The evidence for an infarct is mostly in the breadth of the Q in II, III, and aVF (174) with some notching in aVF. The absence of abnormal ST displacement to imply injury (202) suggests that the lesion is not of recent origin, i.e., old (180).

T is a little deeper in V4-5 than in V6, suggesting coronary insufficiency (211, 212), but, in this case, not enough to make much of by itself, an observation that might be added to the interpretation. The clinical setting, and stability of the pattern, are potentially important factors, known to the primary physician who may have access to previous tracings, and can decide whether to order subsequent ones.

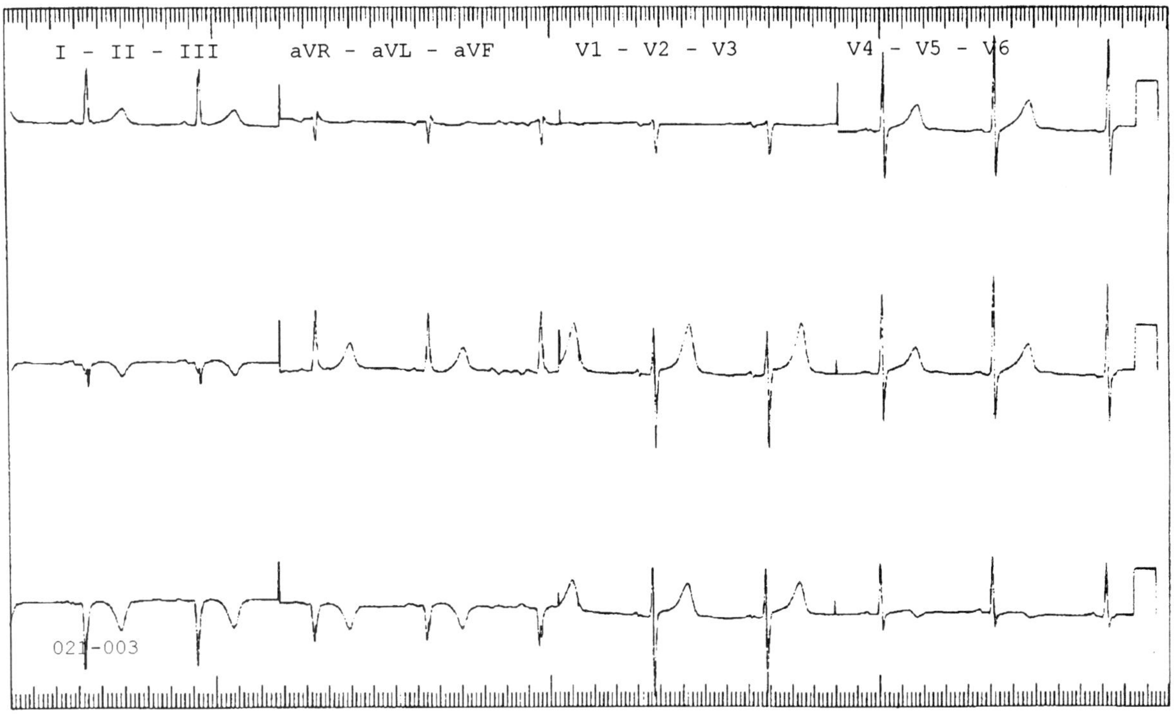

Inferior Myocardial Infarct, Age Indeterminate

```
60    60    16    08    40       sinus
-45   1:5   V3½   10:2         QS2,3,F
              none
             arched
-60   +V1   pos V2-5    neg V6 low

(1) Sinus mechanism, rate 60
(2) Inf myo infarct, age indet
```

First, a caveat that can be very important: Remember that EKG evidence for a myocardial infarct can approach 100% accuracy as confirmation of a clinical impression (180), and can be very strong evidence for one even when the clinical picture does not suggest it, but never establishes the diagnosis by itself. The tracing shows dead (electrically inactive) tissue in the presence of living tissue, but not what caused it to die. Similarly, an infarct can never be eliminated from consideration, "ruled out," by EKG. That said, the practice of reporting tracings as showing infarcts is justified because there are so few other lesions that can produce the whole picture, and the report assumes that the physician to whom it is addressed knows this and knows the patient. It is an interesting paradox of computer readouts that, though they commonly include warnings such as "possible" and "consistent with", they sometimes make the unqualified statement that the tracing shows an infarct when it does not. The evidence for one in this tracing, QS in II, III, and aVF, especially the notch early in QS II, is strong. There is no ST displacement to imply a recent origin. The symmetry of the negative Ts in II, III, and aVF (210) may have that significance, or it may mean coronary insufficiency in a patient with an old infarct, or may be a stable part of an old lesion.

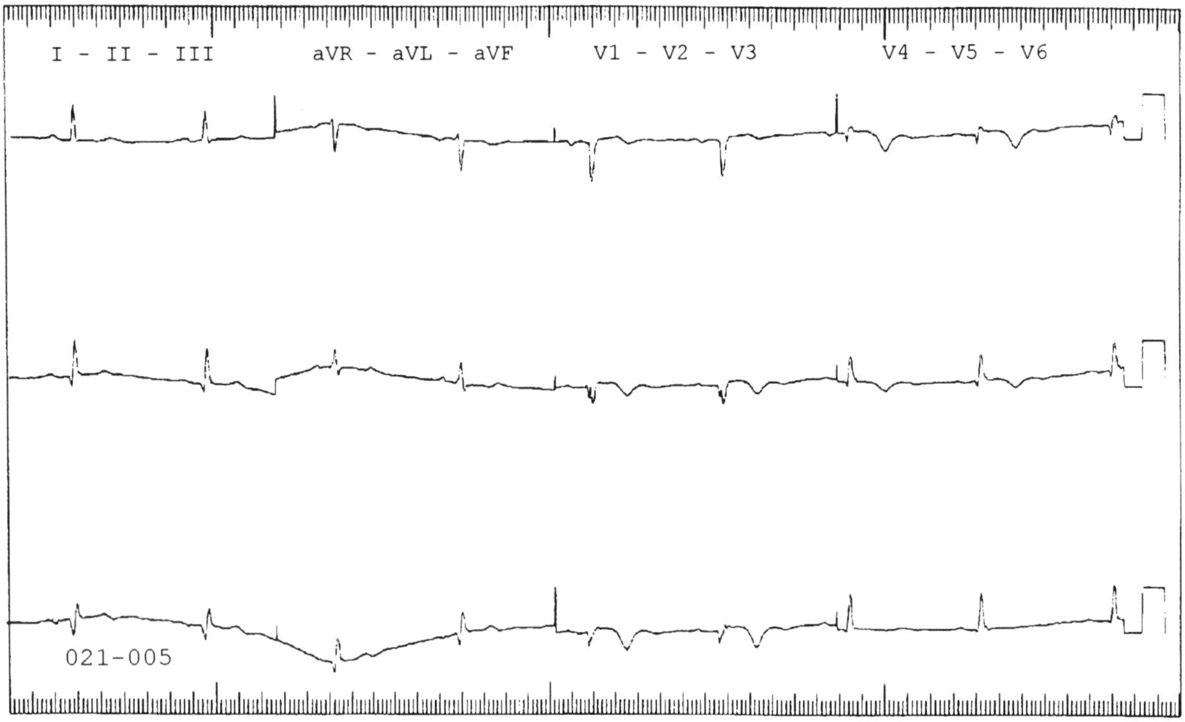

Anterior Myocardial Infarct, Probably New, Suggests Old Inferior Myocardial Infarct

50 50 20 08 40 sinus
+30 0:8 V4 8:0 QSV2-3,QV4
Q2,3,F
slightly up V2-4
arched
low neg V1-5 ±V6

(1) Sinus mechanism, rate 50
(2) Ant myo infarct, prob new
(3) Suggests old inferior mci

An infarct is a wedge-shaped section of dead tissue at the distal end of a branch of an artery, in the presence of living tissue. It results from inadequacy of its blood supply. Coronary arteries originate superficially and ramify deep, while excitation is in the opposite direction (174). Evidence of an infarct, when identifiable, is in the initial part of QRS; how long it has been there is suggested by the presence or absence, in ST-T, of evidence of injury (180).

In this tracing, an anterior lesion is clear (175), QS V1-3 with early notch, and prominent QV4-5 followed by completely positive QRSV6, but the ST-T pattern, elevated STV2-4 arched into a negative and symmetrical T, is only suggestive of injury (47,180).

The evidence for an inferior scar (175), Q II, III, AVF, is less. In lead III, Q is as large as R, but sharp and clean, not quite so prominent in aVF, and very small in lead II. Nothing at all looks new in this area.

An anterior infarct shows mostly in the horizontal plane, an inferior one in the frontal. Both may be seen in a single tracing.

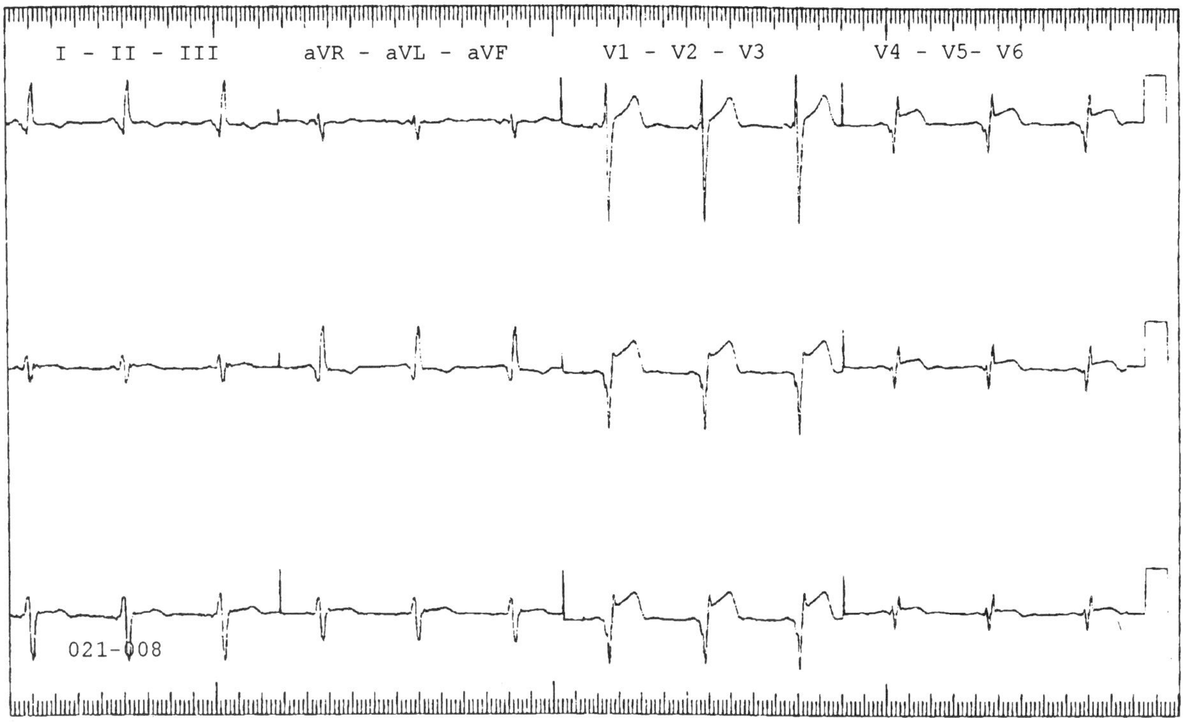

Acute Anterior Myocardial Infarct (vs Pre-Excitation??)

70 70 ?? ?12 40 sinus
-30 10;20, V4-6, RSR 1:3:2
QV2-5
up V2-6
related to T
low +120 positive V1-4 ±V6

(1) Sinus mechanism, rate 70
(2) Acute anterior myo infarct, probably

--Ventricular pre-excitation is a less likely explanation for the early QRS contour.

The mechanism is sinus. PR is short. That is not abnormal by itself (21, 154), no lower limit for its duration can be set, but combined with abnormality of initial QRS contour, it raises the question of ventricular preexcitation. The only other common lesion that changes selectively the forces at the beginning of ventricular depolarization is myocardial infarction (182). The marked anterior displacement of ST is strong evidence for myocardial injury, though its contour is not rounded enough to be quite typical, and injury is not part of ventricular preexcitation. All things considered, the combination of the ST-T and QRS pictures makes a report of acute infarction appropriate, at least at the level of probability.

Myocardial infarction and ventricular preexcitation are not mutually exclusive, but cannot both be diagnosed from a single tracing.

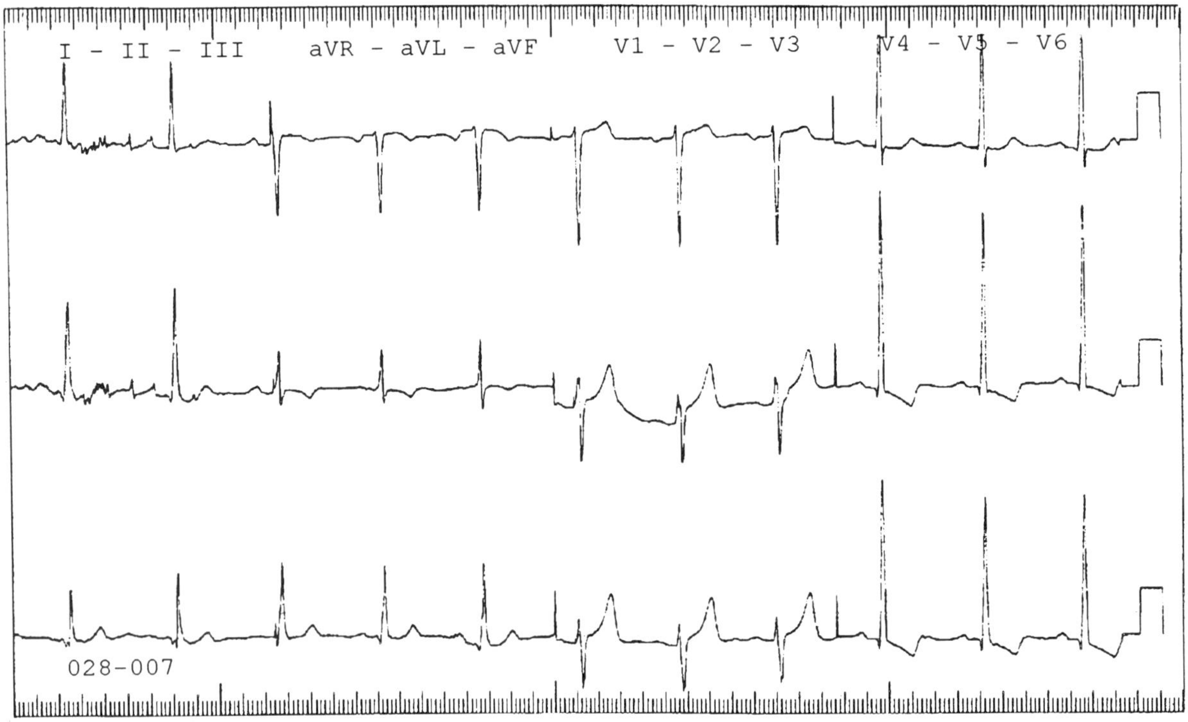

Left Ventricular Overload, Left Ventricular Hypertrophy, Inconstancy of QRS Amplitude

```
65    65    20    08    40     sinus
+45..3:20, V2½, 40:0(V5) normal
              none
             normal
+90   pos V1-3,  ±V4    neg V5-6

(1) Sinus mechanism, rate 65
(2) ST-T abns, probably left
    left ventricular overload
(3) Left ventricular hyper-
    trophy, probable
```

This tracing offers a good opportunity to separate evidence of structure from that of function, and to draw attention to the limits of the method.

The mechanism is sinus and uncomplicated. There is no abnormality of P to suggest atrial abnormality. QRS orientation, duration, and contour are normal. Its voltage is high by at least one criterion (192), but note that the value depends on which beat is read; R is 43 mm tall in the first beat in V5, 38 in the second. QRS voltage is the only useful EKG measure of left ventricular hypertrophy, but weak at best. Several sets of EKG numbers are available for this purpose, but the only way any EKG criterion can be validated is by correlation with clinical reality, and not many investigators have used the same definition for hypertrophy.

ST-T amplitude, duration, and contour are normal, but T is almost 180° from QRS in space, a pattern that correlates well with left ventricular overload (strain) (189). Together, the evidence of a functional lesion of the left ventricle, strain, and its consequence, hypertrophy, point strongly to that chamber as the seat of disproportionate burden.

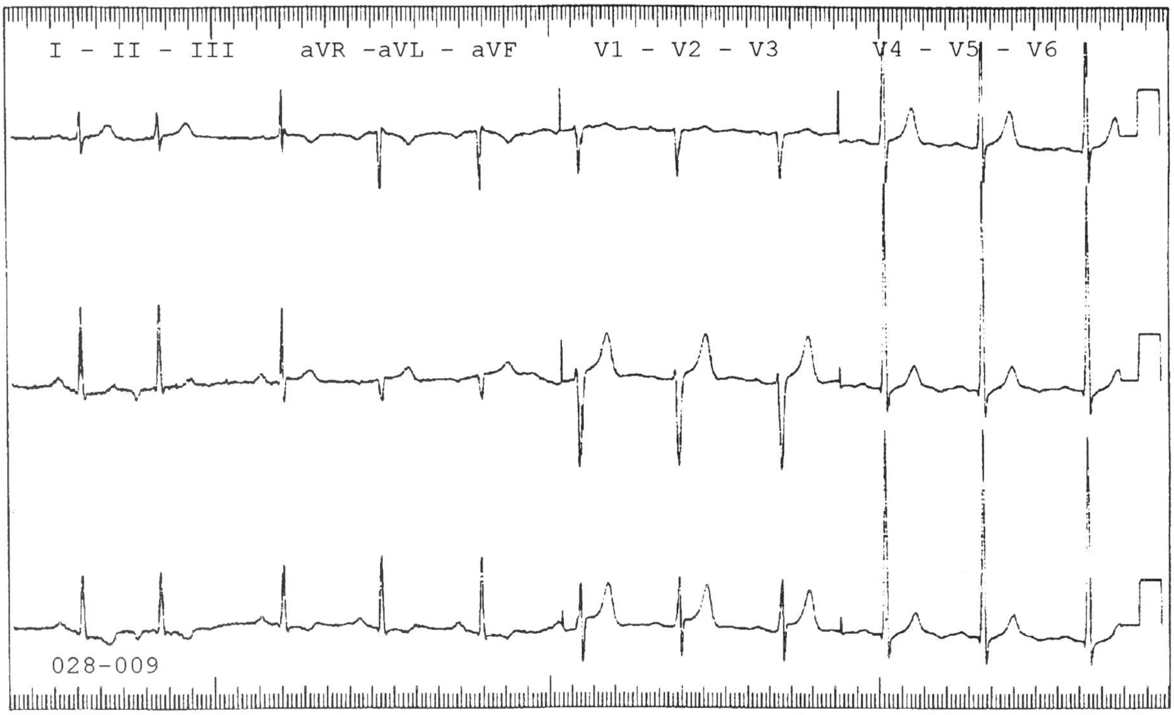

Left Ventricular Hypertrophy

Other EKG criteria for left ventricular hypertrophy are available, but that of Sokolow and Lyons (192) has been around a long time and has a lot of credibility; the sum of SV1 and RV5 (or, if it is taller, RV6) exceeds 3.5 Mv. The limit of the method is about 0.5 Mv, and there are many other explanations for high voltage (228). Voltage can vary from beat to beat and day to day (see EKG 51), but the value here is great enough to justify a presumptive diagnosis. If the patient is very thin, scoliotic, has had a pneumonectomy, has normal blood pressure and no murmurs, the tracing may be normal. An EKG diagnosis of left ventricular hypertrophy, by itself, much less just a computer readout, has little value, but can put the patient at risk for unpleasant consequences if this is not recognized.

65 65 20 08 36 sinus
+75 0:10 V2½ 45:3 normal
none
normal
±0 ± V1 positive V2-6

(1) Sinus mechanism, rate 65, with one PAC
(2) Left ventricular hypertrophy
(3) Otherwise WNL

ST-T here is normal in duration, amplitude, and contour. Its spatial relation to QRS is borderline. It may represent left ventricular overload (186, 189), but, given the limits of the method, especially for estimating the T axis, it is not clearly abnormal at all.

The PAC is classic; early, P inscribed retrograde, QRS-T unchanged.

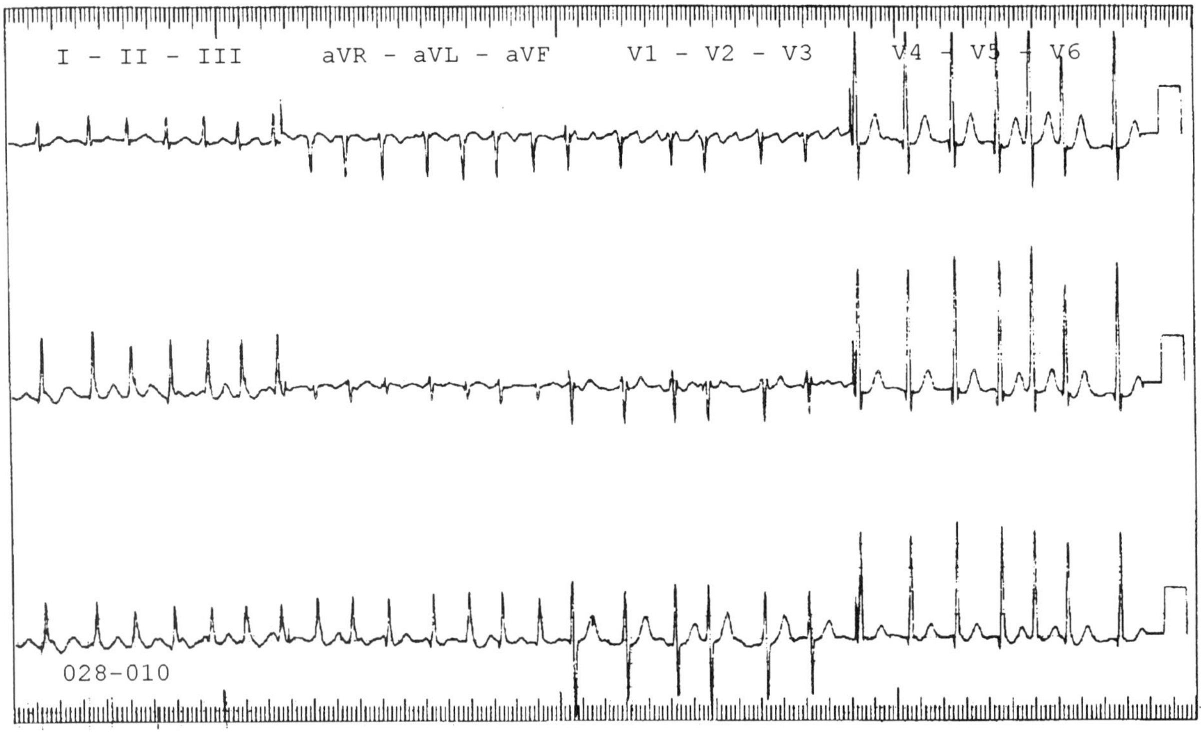

QRS Amplitude is not Constant, Atrial Flutter

300	165	--	08	32	see below
+60	0:6	V3		20:0	normal

none
normal
+60 ±V1-2 positive V3-6

(1) Atrial flutter, 300/165
(2) Otherwise WNL

The QRS is the most stable part of the ventricular complex (43), but it is not an absolute; its amplitude, more than its orientation, duration, and contour, is subject to wide variation, even from beat to beat, and can be influenced by many factors (228). The sum of SV1 and RV5 in this tracing can be read as anywhere from 30 mm to 40 mm, depending on which beat is considered, and what limits of measurement are accepted. Note the difference of eight mm in consecutive beats in V5. The importance of recognizing this is that QRS voltage is the only useful EKG evidence of left ventricular hypertrophy no matter whose figures are used (192), and the anatomic reality needed to validate them is hard to define, but left ventricular hypertrophy is one of the most frequent of all computer readouts produced by all programs. If the limitations of the method are not understood, this can have unfortunate consequences.

The mechanism in this tracing is atrial flutter (129). Irregularity of ventricular rhythm is implicit in the figures for atrial and ventricular rates. The ST-T pattern is normal, even in places where the ventricular rate is as great as 200, suggesting normal electrophysiologic function.

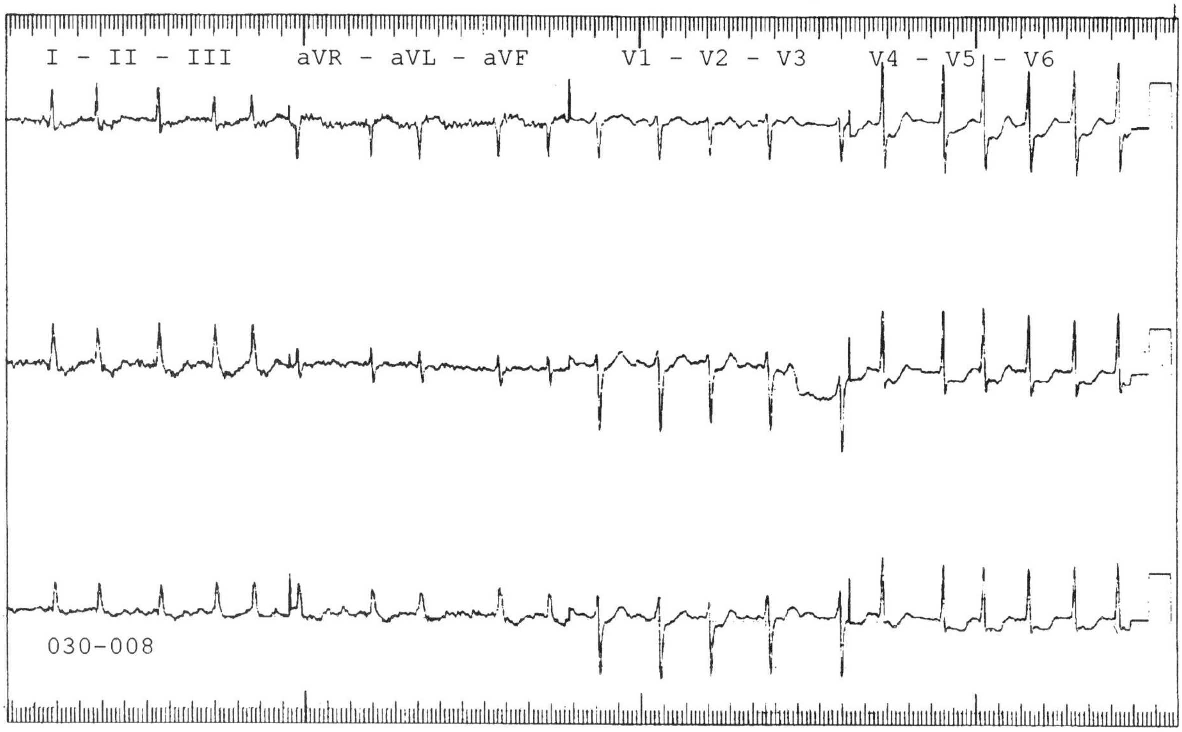

Atrial Fibrillation, Subendocardial Injury

```
--    125   -- 08   32    see below
+60   1:8    V3½    12:2    normal
             down V3-6
             flattened
low   ±V1,   pos V2-3 low, ±V5-6

(1) Atrial fibrillation, ven-
    tricular rate about 125
(2) ST-T abnormalities,
    typical of subendocardial
    injury as with coronary
    insufficiency
```

This is a good example of atrial fibrillation; the trace is not the same between any two consecutive QRSs in a given lead. The rate and strength of atrial impulses entering the AV junction are inconstant, and so is their penetration of the system. They do not all get through; second degree AV block is implicit in the diagnosis and need not be mentioned. Exceptions include third degree AV block, acceleration of a junctional pacemaker, and rarely, when there is also ventricular pre-excitation, ventricular fibrillation (EKG 150).

In this tracing, ST orientation (displacement), is discordant; i.e., directed opposite the dominant QRS, and of moderate amplitude; its contour, flattened/sagging. These characteristics are typical of subendocardial injury, and coronary insufficiency is the usual explanation for them (207). In this distribution, the lesion is probably in the left anterior descending artery. Did the rapid ventricular rate precipitate the insufficiency? The other way around? QRS is normal.

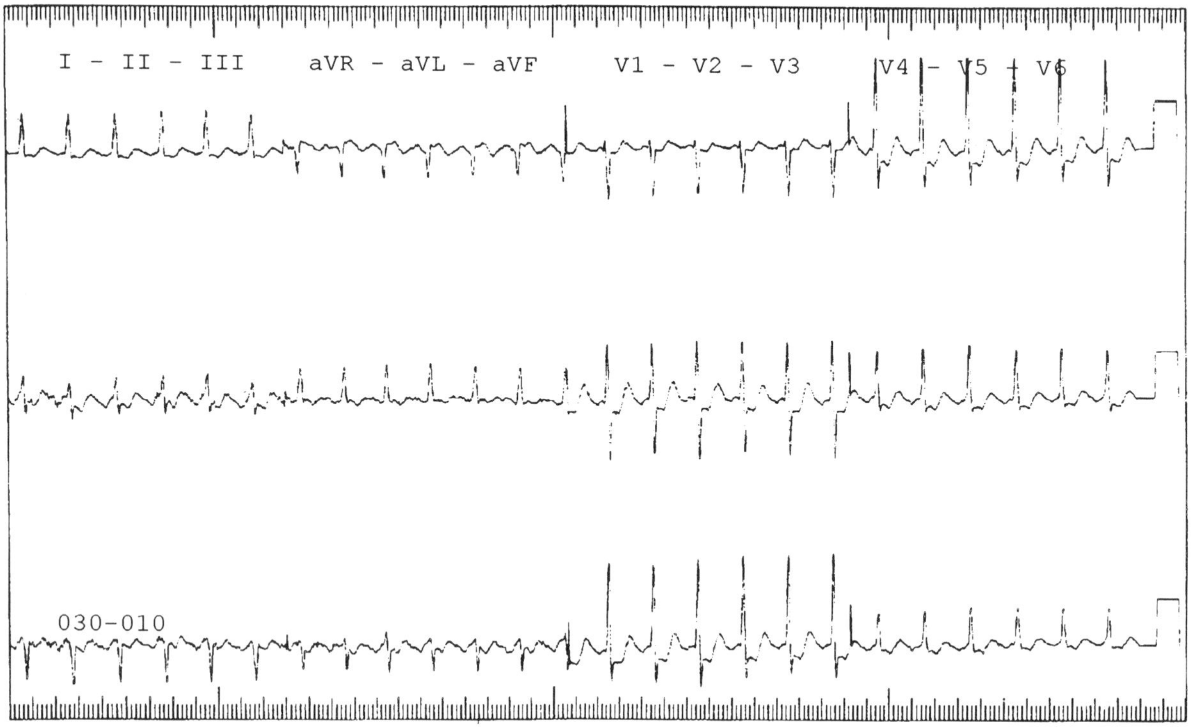

Atrial Flutter, Subendocardial Injury

```
300   150   --    08   32   see below
-15   1:10      V2      8:0     normal
       down V2-5, sl up aVR
         sagging/flattened
low    ±V1      +V2-6       low V6

(1) Atrial flutter, 300/150
(2) ST-T abnormalities, typical
    of subendocardial injury as
    with coronary insufficiency
```

The mechanism is atrial flutter (120). In some cases, as in this one, the "extra" P is continuous with QRS and may be interpreted as a Q, an S, or as prolongation of QRS. Here, though, it follows the previous QRS far enough that neither of these is likely to be a problem. It appears early in ST and is seen best in aVF.

Abnormal ST displacement means myocardial injury (202), and when injury involves the deep layers of the myocardium selectively, the displacement is discordant, approximately opposite QRS, toward the injured area. Its contour is sagging, flattened, or arched depending on the view. In this case, the pattern is typical, and the lesion is presumably in the territory of the left anterior descending artery.

It is clear what the tracing shows, but the etiologic relation between the rapid ventricular rate and coronary insufficiency, in either direction, if any, is speculative. The clinical history is an important unknown.

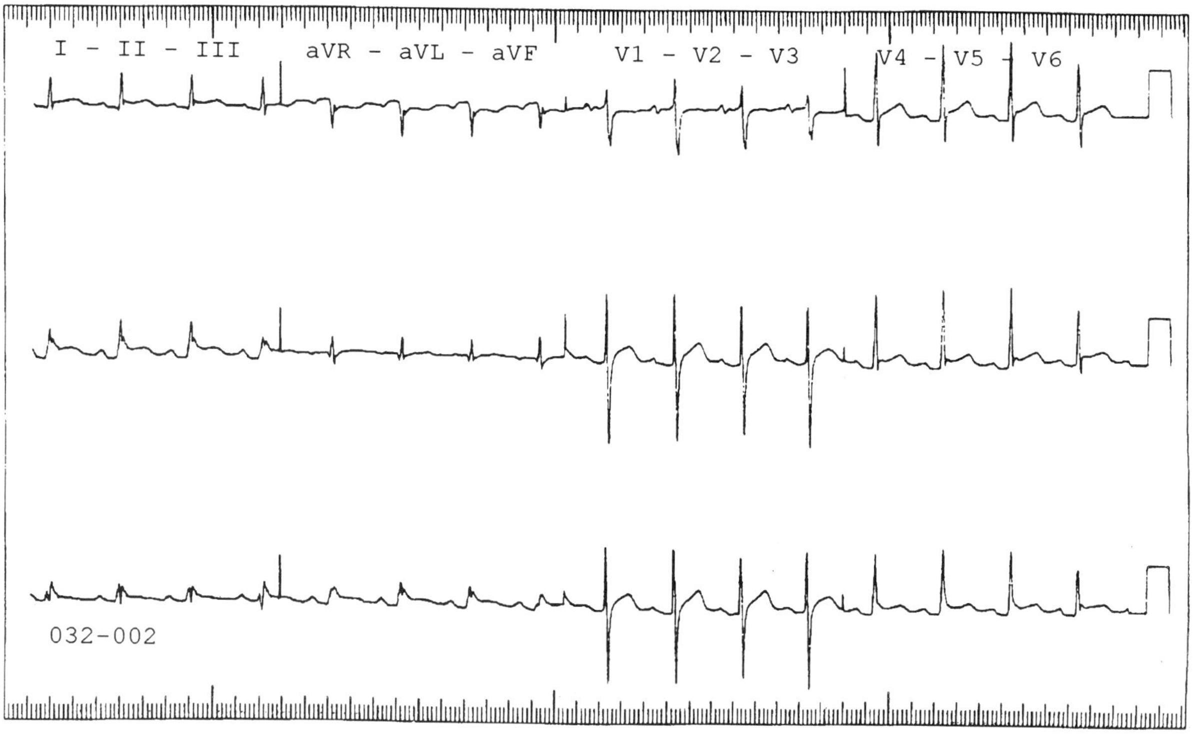

Subepicardial Injury, Pericarditis

100 100 20 08 36 sinus
+45 6:8 V2-3 12:0 normal
up 1,2,F,V2-6, dn aVR
related to T
low ±V1 positive V2-6

(1) Sinus mechanism, rate 100
(2) ST-T abns, typical of subepicardial injury as with pericarditis

Myocardial injury, when identifiable, produces abnormal ST displacement and contour (47), and its location in the myocardium, whether superficial or deep, can often be localized (202). When only a thin layer subjacent to the epicardium is involved, as with pericarditis, the displacement is small, nearly concordant with QRS, ST is flat, and T voltage is low. When superficial layers are involved by extension outward from the endocardium, as with acute myocardial infarction, displacement is typically much more marked, and ST is arched (180, 208), probably indicating involvement of a greater mass of muscle.

Remember to distinguish between pericarditis and pericardial effusion (228). They are not mutually exclusive, but are not the same thing. Voltage may, or may not, be low with effusion, but is not affected by inflammation.

The back side of ST displacement, depression, can be seen here (in aVR), but this is not always the case. Such "reciprocal" patterns are more likely with coronary insufficiency and myocardial infarction. See the Index for examples.

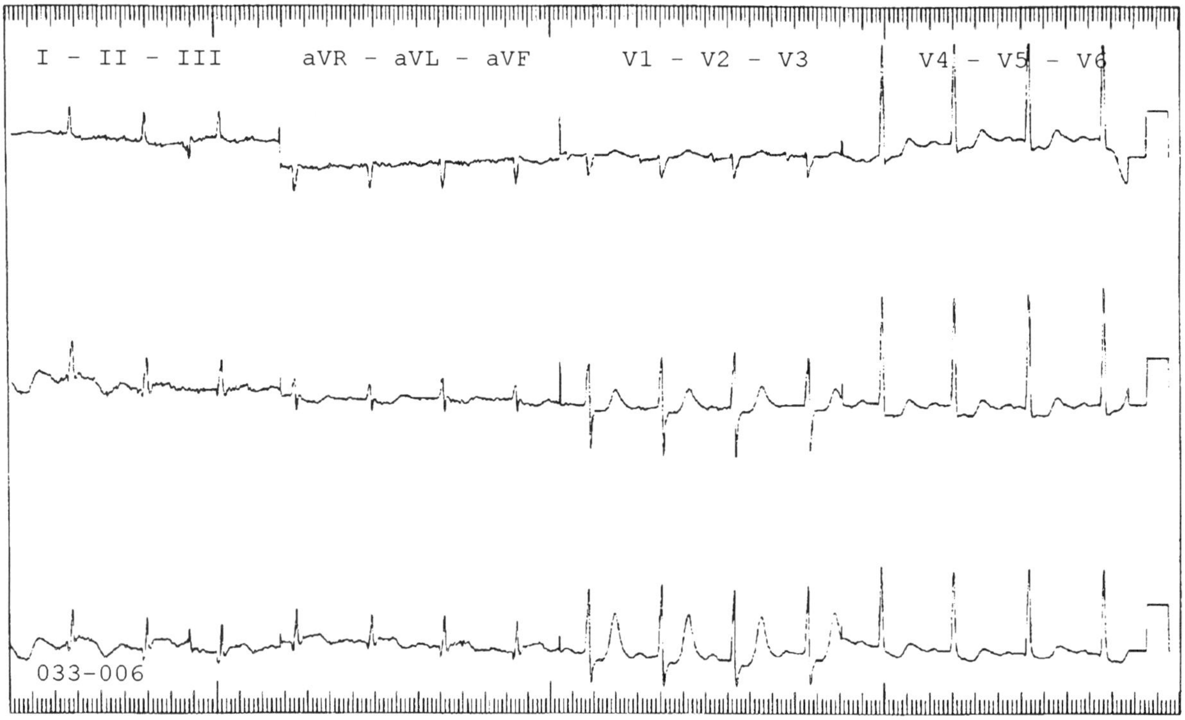

Subendocardial Injury, Coronary Insufficiency

```
90     90     16     08     36     sinus
+45     1:5     V2     18:0     Q2,3,F
     down V2-6      sl up 2,3,F
              flattened
Low     ±V1     +V2-6          low V4-6

(1) Sinus mechanism, rate 90
(2) ST-T abnormalities typical
    of coronary insufficiency
(3) Suggests inf mci, age indet
```

Myocardial injury is characterized by ST displacement, whether elevation or depression depends on the lead in which it is found. Both sides of the lesion, the boundary of potential difference (78, 203), can be seen in some instances, elevation in some leads and depression in others (202). Often findings are not described in detail and attention is called to the abnormality by saying only that the tracing shows elevation or depression. In this tracing, the injury force is directed dorsad, almost perpendicular to the frontal plane, and its only identifiable manifestation is ST depression in precordial leads. The picture is typical of subendocardial injury, as with coronary insufficiency. When depression extends as far to the left as V6, elevation in aVR is often present.

P is hardly identifiable in the frontal leads, but easy to see in V1 where its biphasic contour implies a sinus origin.

The glitch in the baseline between the second and third beats, seen in leads I and III but not II, came from the connection to the left arm (86, 102).

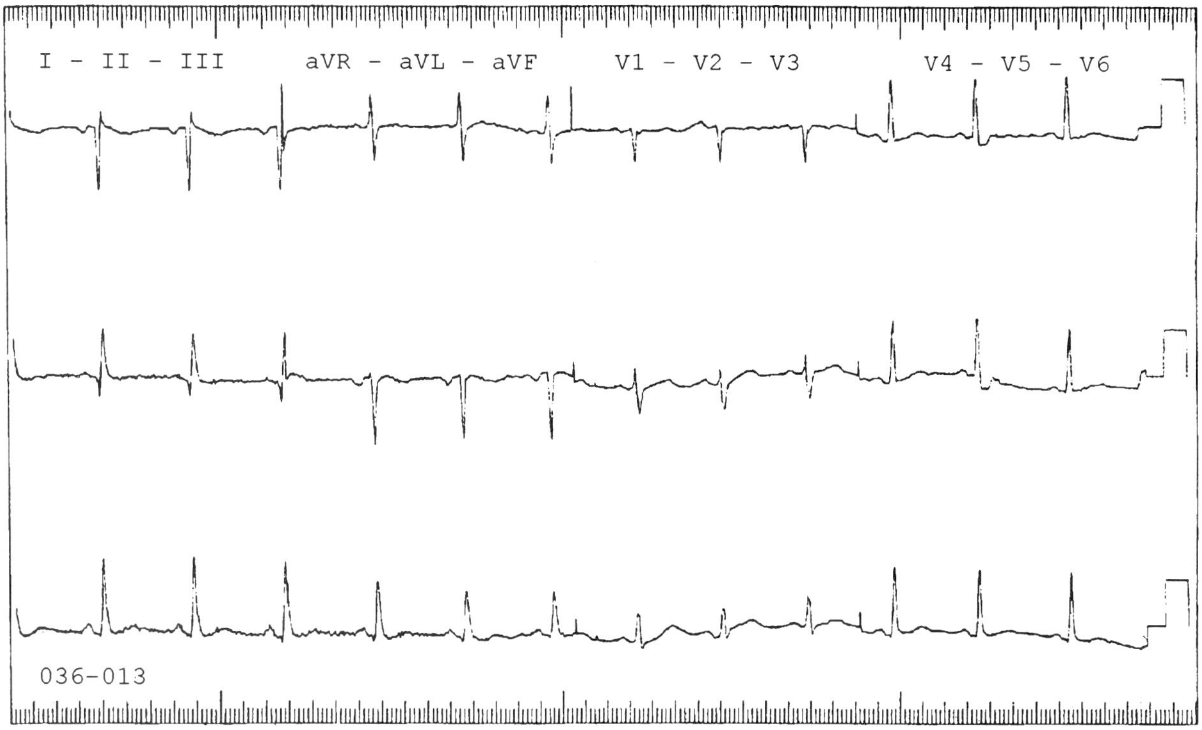

Crossed Arm Leads, Nonspecific ST-T Abnormalities

Crossed (transposed) arm leads, the most common of all technical errors, is easy to identify in most instances. Technicians will often recognize it as "it's upside down in Lead I"; P and QRS are negative. It cannot be differentiated from dextrocardia, "crossed heart," in the frontal leads alone, but is clear when the precordial leads are taken into account. With crossed arm leads, all three corners of Einthoven's triangle are still represented, and V leads are not affected (88, 97, 107). The tracing is complete but mislabeled. Interpretation is like reading print on a page seen upside down; all that is needed is that the problem be recognized. Correction is easy: the lead labeled I is I, but upside down, II is III, III is II, etc. (107)

Depending on the characteristics of the heart, crossed arm leads may not make much difference, but may lead to a report of lateral myocardial infarct. Computer programs often recognize the problem but do not correct for it.

```
80    80    16    08    40    sinus
+60   0:5   V2½   15:0        normal
            none
         related to T
+30 low    ±V1,  +V2-3.  ±V4-6

(1) Sinus mechanism, rate 80
(2) Nonspecific ST-T abn

--Just low T voltage, not far
  from normal
--Interpretation corrects for
  crossed arm leads.
```

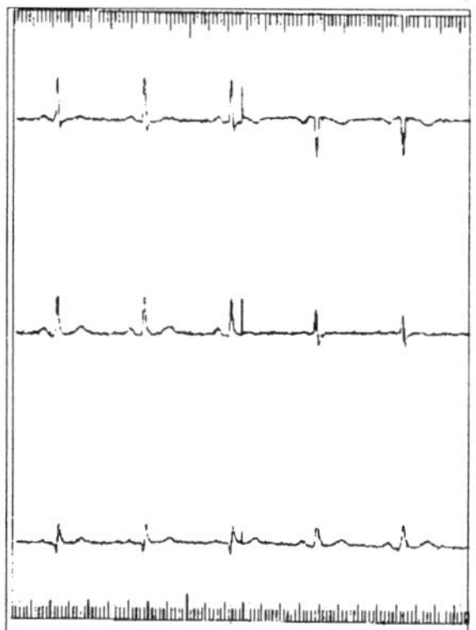
Frontal leads EKG #56 recorded correctly

EKG 57

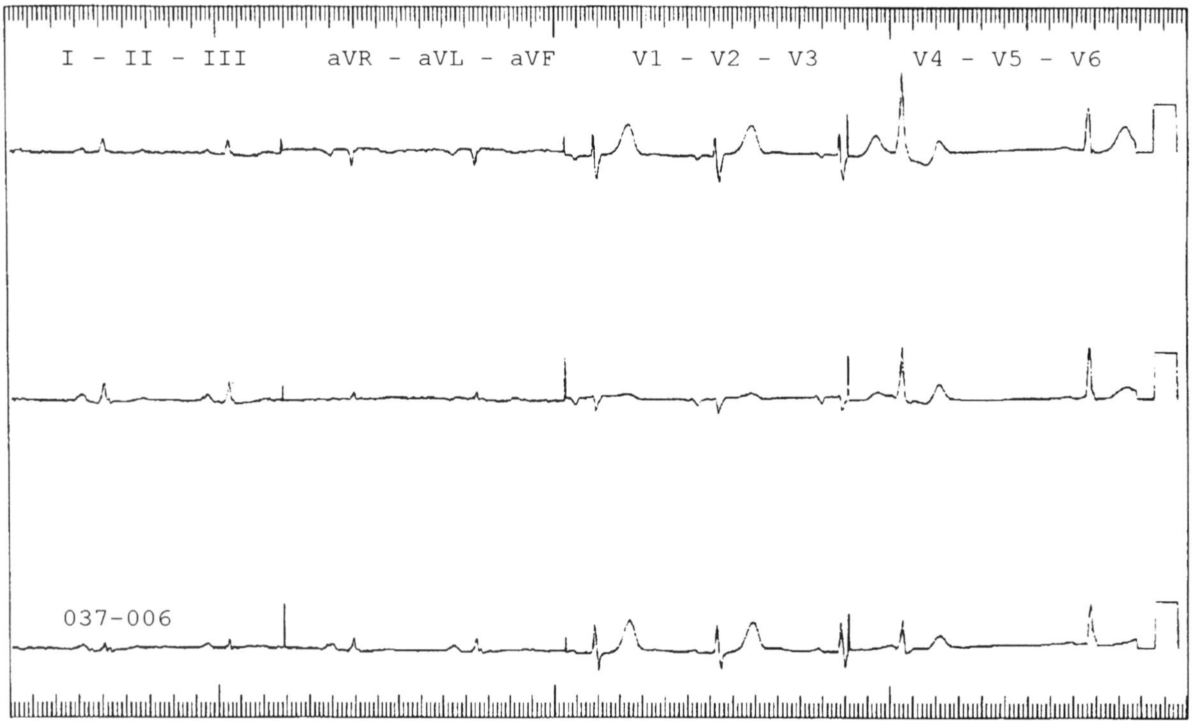

Artifact Called Infarct, V1 and V2 are Transposed

```
55     55     20     08    44        sinus
low  +45    0:3    V2½   8:0       normal
                 none
          sagging/flattened
low          pos V1-6          low V1

(1) Sinus mechanism, rate 55
(2) ST-T abnormalities, non-
    specific

--Interpretation corrects for
  transposition of V1 and V2.
```

Any patient having an electrocardiogram accepts a certain risk; as with any other study, findings have to be interpreted, and mistakes may be made. This was emphasized by Dr. Frank Wilson, one of the founders of the method (4), and has become a larger problem with time. The risk is much greater if the doctor relies too heavily on the technician's ability to count intercostal spaces and identify the midclavicular and anterior axillary lines for accurate placement of electrodes (93). It is even greater if the role of the computer is not kept in perspective (183, 225). The readout for this tracing included an anterior infarct...no caveats. This would be appropriate if the leads were labeled correctly, but they are not. The P wave is the key to recognizing transposition of precordial leads. As labeled, PV2 is deeper than PV1 (107), and TV2 is smaller than TV1 or TV3, a "break in the trend of the T wave." Both suggest that V2 was recorded to the right of V1. Assuming this, progression of QRS is normal, and nothing looks like an infarct. The tracing is not quite normal, but not far from it, especially for a seventy-five year old with no previous tracings, and whose clinical status is not known. First, do no harm. Transposition of precordial leads is one of the most common technical errors.

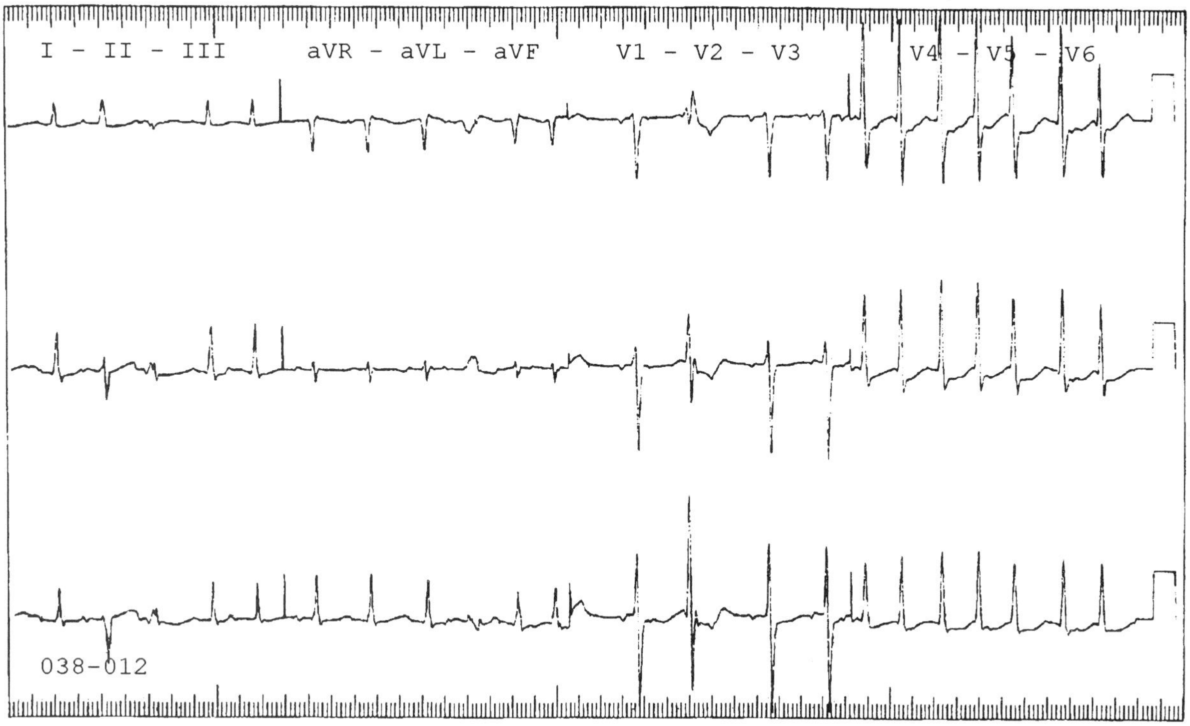

Inconstancy of QRS Voltage (Amplitude)

```
115    115    12    08    --   sinus
+60    1:12   V3    12:1       normal
              down V4-6
           sagging/flattened
low         isoelectric V1-6

(1) Sinus mechanism, rate 115,
    with normal AV conduction
(2) Frequent PAC's, some with
    aberration
(3) ST-T abnormalities suggest-
    ive of coronary insufficien-
    cy, but small
```

The computer called the mechanism in this tracing atrial fibrillation, but it is not; there are P waves (27, 70) (seen best in V1), and P waves and *f* waves are mutually exclusive. On physical examination, atrial fibrillation would probably be assumed because of the irregular irregularity of ventricular rhythm, but in the electrocardiogram atrial activity is observed directly.

There are frequent PACs, some in runs (or salvos, or paroxysms) at rates of nearly 200. These are associated with depression of ST typical of subendocardial injury as with coronary insufficiency (202), probably as a result of shortening of diastole as well as a possible increase in need for oxygen. In effect, the same sort of thing that happens in a positive response to an exercise test (219).

The wide QRS's may be PVCs, but also may represent ventricular aberration (169). And note the wide variation in QRS amplitude. To assume that high QRS voltage by itself, by whatever standard, represents left ventricular hypertrophy is a potentially serious mistake (38, 192).

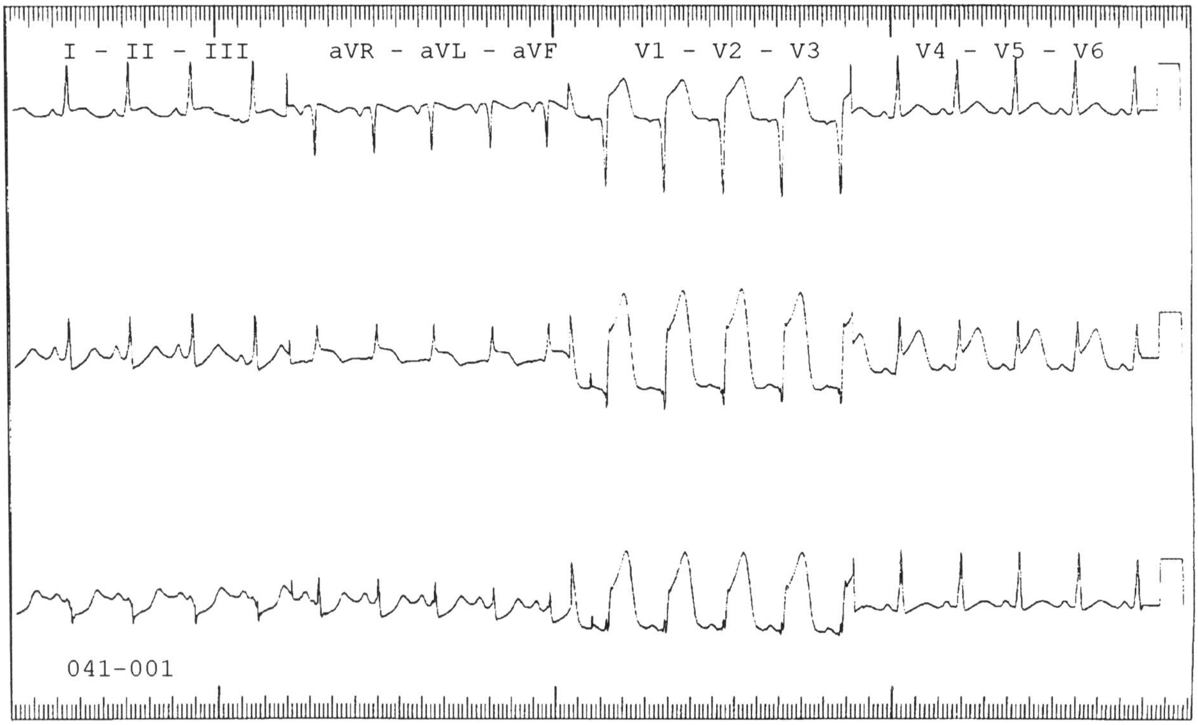

Acute Anterior Myocardial Infarct

"Reciprocal" ST displacement

115	115	12	08	36	sinus
±0	QR	15:5	V1½	10:0	QV1-2

down 2,3,F, up 1,L,V1-3
straightened
+60 positive V1-6, low V6
P: prominent, peaked, 2,3,F

(1) Sinus mechanism, rate 115
(2) Right atrial enlargement
(3) Acute anterior myo infarct

This tracing demonstrates nicely the value of recognizing that an EKG documents the course in time and space of a single point (70, 121). The marked ST displacement means myocardial injury (47, 202), and implies that the anterior infarct (prominent QV1-2) (174, 177) is of recent origin (180). In most anterior infarcts, evidence of injury is directed anteriorly and to the left, with very little cephalad component, i.e., there is ST elevation in chest leads and/or I and aVL, but very little displacement in II, III, or aVF. In this one, there is a strong cephalad component, and both sides of the boundary of potential difference show nicely; ST is down in inferior leads at as well as up in those whose positive poles are anterior and to the left (78, 203). This is commonly called "reciprocal" displacement, but that must not be taken to mean that one side of the picture is in response to the other; they are two views of the same thing. With inferior lesions, it is common to see both sides, ST depression in midprecordial leads and elevation in inferior ones (EKGs 144 and 145).

The evidence for infarction is less clear, but the Q in V1-2 followed by notching of initial QRS in V3 and an initial R in V4 leaves little doubt...especially when the ST-T pattern is included.

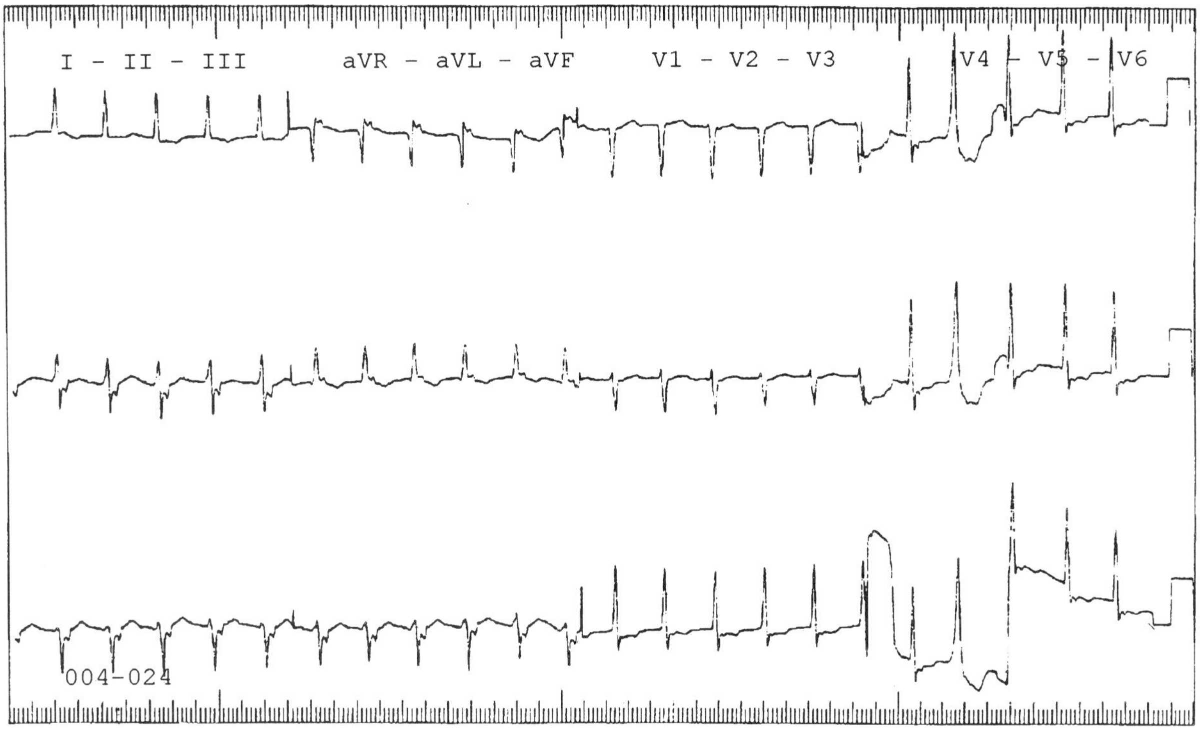

Low Junctional Mechanism, Rate 135; ST-T Abnormalities, Probably Coronary Insufficiency

P is negative in aVF, indicating retrograde depolarization of the atria, and QRS is not wide, identifying depolarization of the ventricles from a supraventricular focus. P follows QRS. The implication is that both are activated from a focus above the bifurcation of the Bundle of His, presumably closer to the ventricles than the atria since the impulse reaches the ventricles first; thus, "low junctional," probably the His bundle (126, 133).

This could be reported as just "junctional tachycardia" (120), and "tachy" it is, but to specify the rate is better than simply saying that it is fast. The doctor who ordered the tracing already knows the rate and rhythm, but not the locus of the pacemaker.

The instability of the trace in V4,5,6 is explained by motion at the skin/electrode interface (103). The ST-T pattern, low T voltage and flattened depression of ST in V3-6, is typical of subendocardial injury as with coronary insufficiency, but the abnormality is small.

135 135 -- 06 -- see below
-30 0:10 V2½ 15:3 normal
slightly down V3-6
related to T
low positive V1 low ±V2-6
P: follows QRS negative 2,3,F

(1) Low junctional mechanism, rate 135
(2) ST-T abnormalities, prob cor insuf, but small

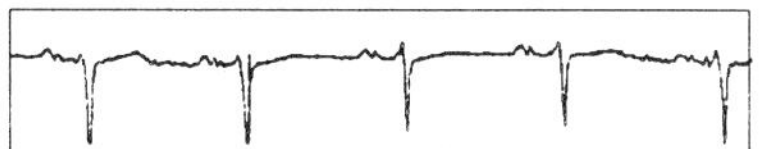
Leads III and aVF from the same patient in sinus mech

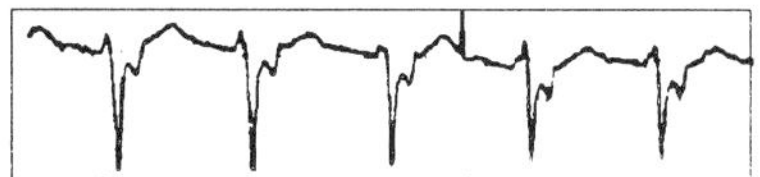
Leads III and aVF from above

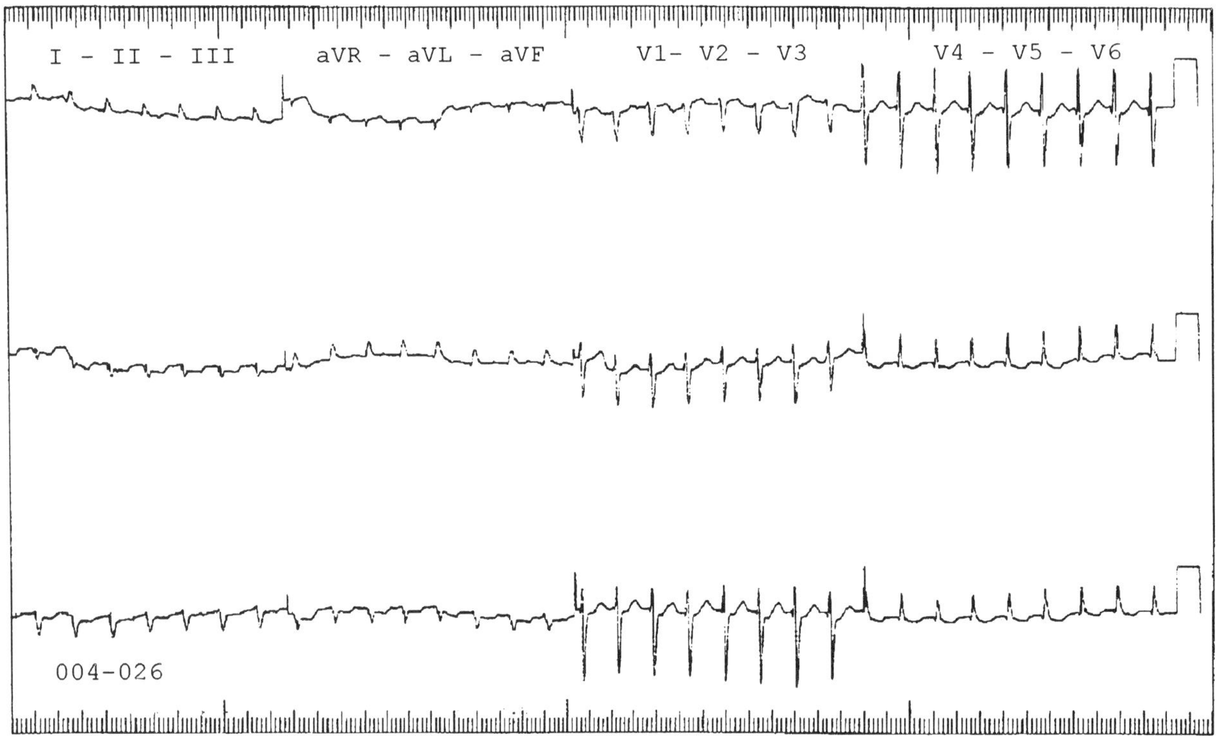

Supraventricular Tachycardia ("SVT")

```
--   195   --   06  24    see below
low  -45?  1:5  V4½  5:0  normal
        slightly down V4
          related to T
low     ±V1    pos V3-4 low   ±V6

(1) Ectopic supraventricular
    mechanism, rate 195, with
    regular rhythm, probably of
    junctional origin.  Atrial
    activity is not identifi-
    able
(2) ST-T abnormalities, non-
    specific
```

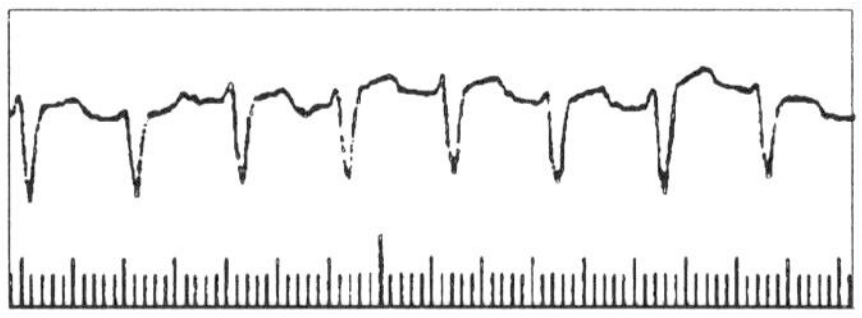

V1 from above

This is, probably, what is understood by most doctors when they hear "SVT" (133), and the only thing wrong with that term is that it is not as specific as it can be (242). Supraventricular, yes (QRS is not wide), and "tachy," yes (everyone would agree that 195 is fast), but it refers to the ventricles only. What about the atria? Their rate may not be the same...and it makes a difference. Supraventricular mechanisms may be of sinus, atrial, or junctional origin. The regularity of ventricular rhythm here is strongly against atrial fibrillation, the rate almost rules out sinus, and the combination of the two is against atrial flutter because, QRS rhythm being regular, atrial rate would have to be a multiple of 195, well beyond the rate at which most atria can function in an organized, repetitive fashion. This leaves the AV junction as the probable source. Speculation as to the means by which the mechanism is sustained may be appropriate in a supplemental comment, but not in a statement of what is in the tracing.

T voltage is low, a minimal abnormality, especially for this rate.

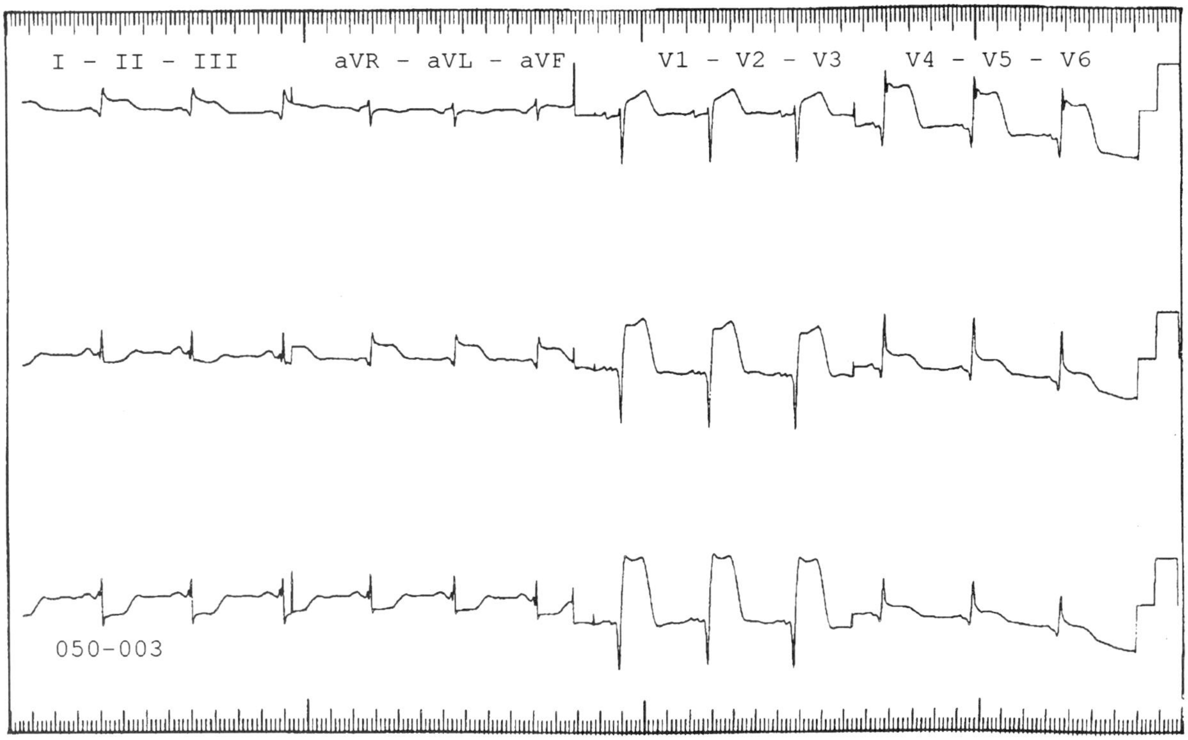

Acute Anterior Myocardial Infarct

```
75    75    16  08    40     sinus
+15   1:10   V2  prominent QV2-6
  up I,L, V1-6,  down II,III,F
            flattened
low    pos V1-2, insep ST V3-6

(1) Sinus mechanism, rate 75
(2) Acute anterior myo infarct
```

An estimate of the age of an infarct is based on the presence or absence of evidence of injury, abnormal ST displacement (202). Injury is transient, and, if one assumes that it is a result of the same process that caused the infarct, its presence implies that the event must have occurred recently, but "recent," is not precise, and there are exceptions in both directions. In the classic, and common, example, displacement is opposite the deformity of the initial part of QRS that is evidence of the anatomic lesion. This means elevation in anterior leads with an anterior infarct, as here. The same force produces ST depression in leads whose positive poles are on the other side of the boundary of potential difference, and, depending on the location of the lesion, this may, or may not, be visible in the routine tracing The injury associated with most anterior lesions is nearly perpendicular to the frontal plane, and, because there are no leads made from the back, ST depression is not likely to be seen. In this one, however, the "injury current" has enough cephalad component to be clear from inferior leads. With inferior infarcts, both sides are seen commonly, elevated ST 2,3,F, and depressed ST V4 (EKG 144, 145). The contour of ST in these lesions is likely to be more curved than here; arched where elevated, sagging where depressed.

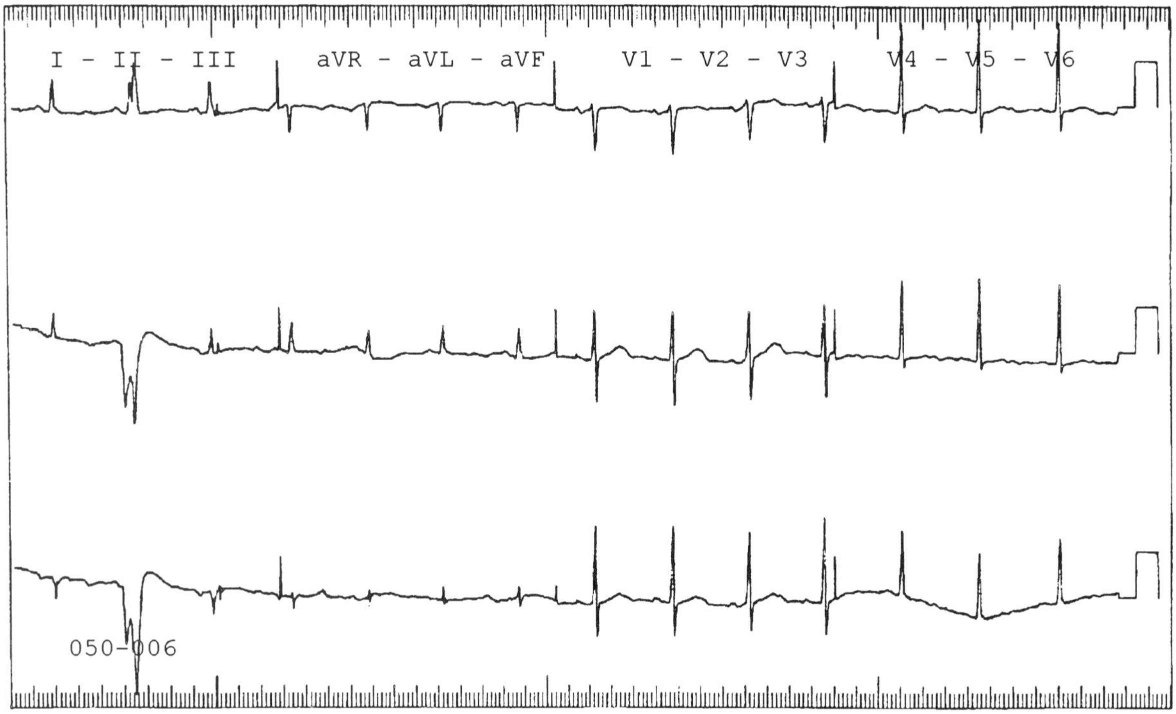

ST-T Abnormalities, Nonspecific

The second QRS is wide, and its contour is different from that in the other beats in the same lead. It may be a PVC, not related to the P that precedes it (seen best in Lead I), an "end-diastolic PVC" (143), or a fusion beat, combining information from two wave fronts, one ectopic and one conducted (169). Another explanation, but less likely, is that it is an artifact that happens to coincide with a QRS. It is much more prominent in leads II and III than I, suggesting origin in the connection to the left leg, but the fact that it shows in Lead I at all is against that. A random contraction of a striated muscle may be a factor. Almost any finding may have more than one explanation, and not all artifacts can be explained, but to attribute a finding to an artifact without coming as close to an explanation as possible is not very helpful.

```
100    100    16    06    40   Sinus
±0    1:18    V2   15:0       normal
                none
            related to T
low      ±V1    +V2-4 low    ±V5-6

(1) Sinus mechanism, rate 100
(2) ST-T abnormalities, non-
    specific

--Just low T voltage, not far
  from normal
```

There is no abnormality of P or QRS, and ST is not displaced. The only abnormality is low T voltage, a minimal departure from normal, and completely nonspecific (213).

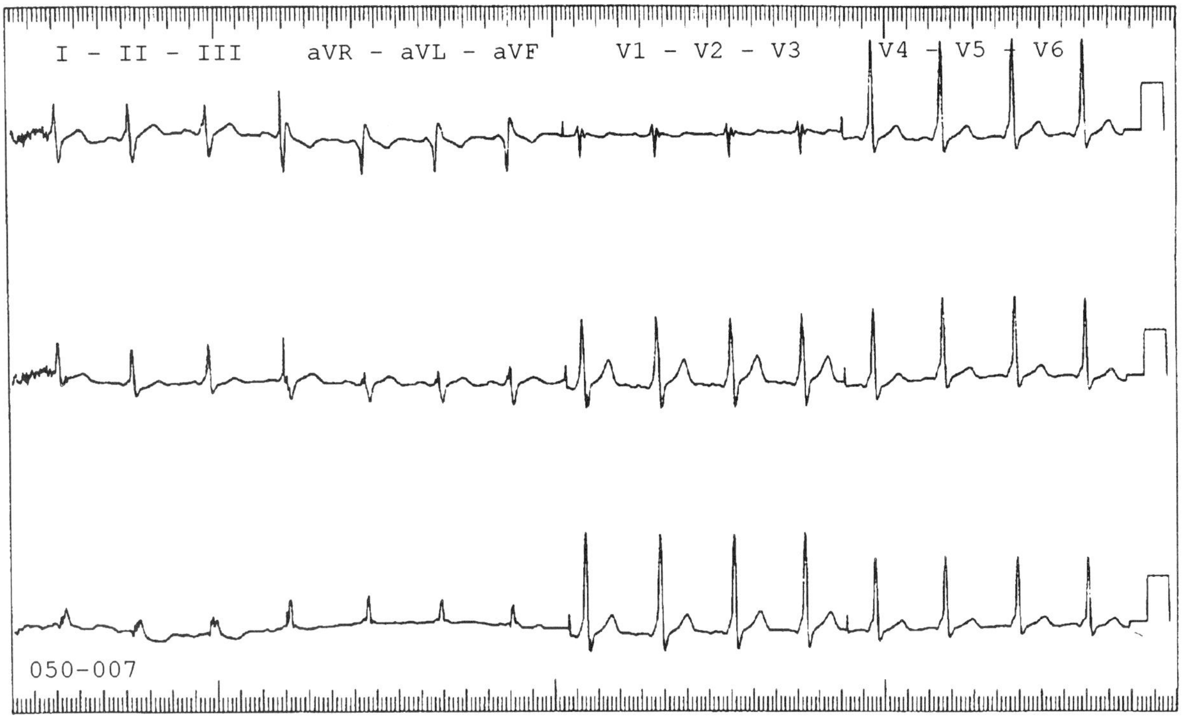

Ventricular Pre-excitation (WPW Syndrome)

```
90    90    12    16    40    sinus
+90   rSr  2:5:1  V1   15:2  early
           none               slur
         normal
±0     ±V1    positive V2-6

(1) Sinus mechanism, rate 90
(2) Ventricular pre-excitation
(3) Otherwise within nl limits
```

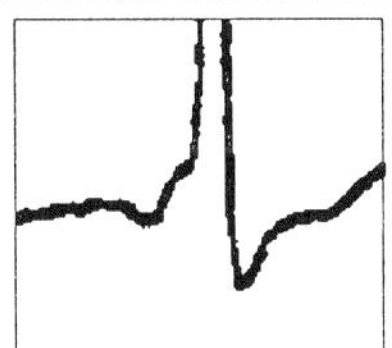
V6 from above, "delta"wave

The clinical syndrome described by Drs. Wolff, Parkinson, and White in 1930 (155) consists of paroxysms of rapid heart action in young people whose EKGs show a short PR and a wide QRS with distortion of its initial contour. The EKG was thought to represent an unusual form of bundle branch block. It was much later that the congenital anomaly described by Kent was recognized as the basis for both the clinical and electrocardiographic picture, and later still that the EKG picture alone was called "the WPW syndrome" and the distortion of QRS a "delta wave." See EKG 17.

No absolute value can be given for either the lower limit of normal for PR or the upper limit for QRS; both are subject to judgment, but when both are present, and the initial slope of QRS is abnormal, pre-excitation can be diagnosed with confidence.

The only other common explanation for abnormality of initial QRS forces selectively is myocardial infarction. Both may be present, but both cannot be recognized in a single tracing (182).

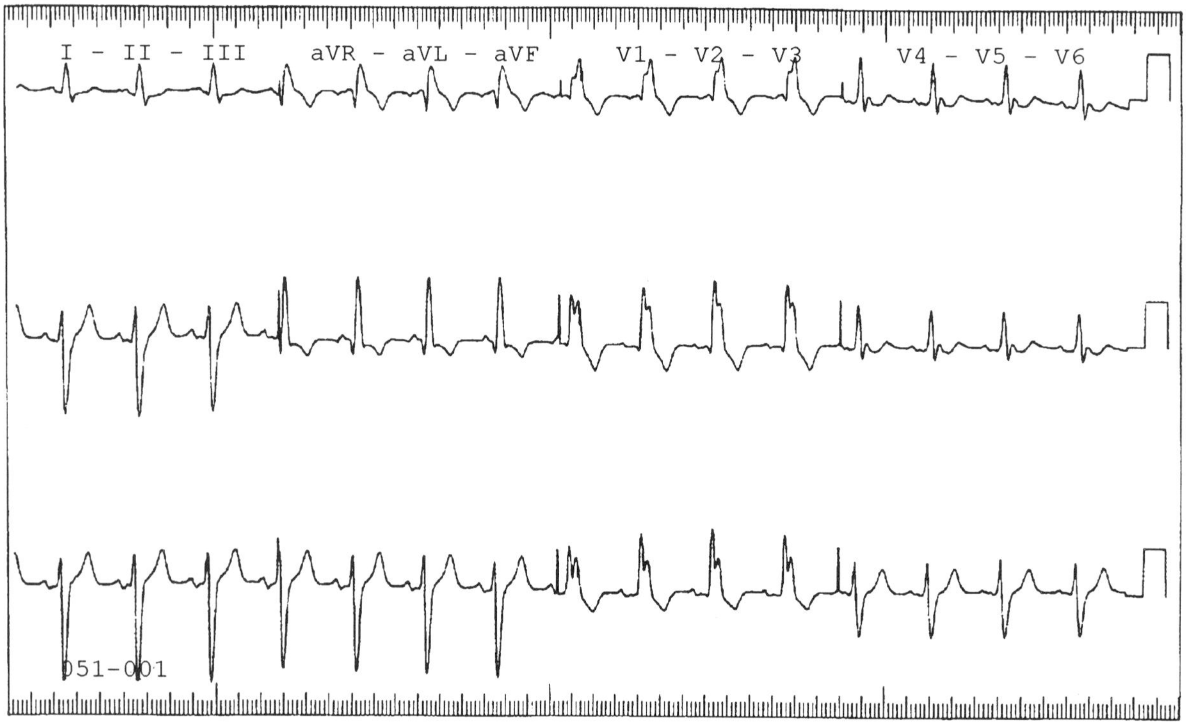

Right Bundle Branch Block, (and Left Anterior Fascicular Block?)

```
95     95    12    16    36      sinus
?-75  qR1:8   --    8:10      BSTDRA
               none
          related to T
+75   neg V1-3,  ±V4-5,   pos V6

(1) Sinus mechanism, rate 95
(2) Right bundle branch block
(3) Left anterior fascicular
    block, probably
(4) Otherwise WNL
```

The diagnosis of block of the right branch of the Bundle of His is rarely subject to anatomic or physiologic proof, but is based on findings that are easily predictable from things every medical student learns in the first year of school (154). The concept is supported by many years of experience, and its clinical value is uncontroversial. The example here is (almost) classic: broad, slurred terminal QRS forces directed to the right and, especially, anterior. The initial part of QRS is unaffected.

Left anterior fascicular block, given that there is such an electrocardiographic entity, also affects the terminal forces selectively (164). Their direction to the left and cephalad ("left axis deviation") is a criterion, but left axis deviation is defined in many ways, and refers to the whole complex, not just the terminal part. It is reasonable to assume that the lesions may coexist, but criteria for "bifascicular block" are difficult to explain and defend (16), and the concept is less popular than in the past. This tracing comes as close as possible; there is almost no rightward QRS component.

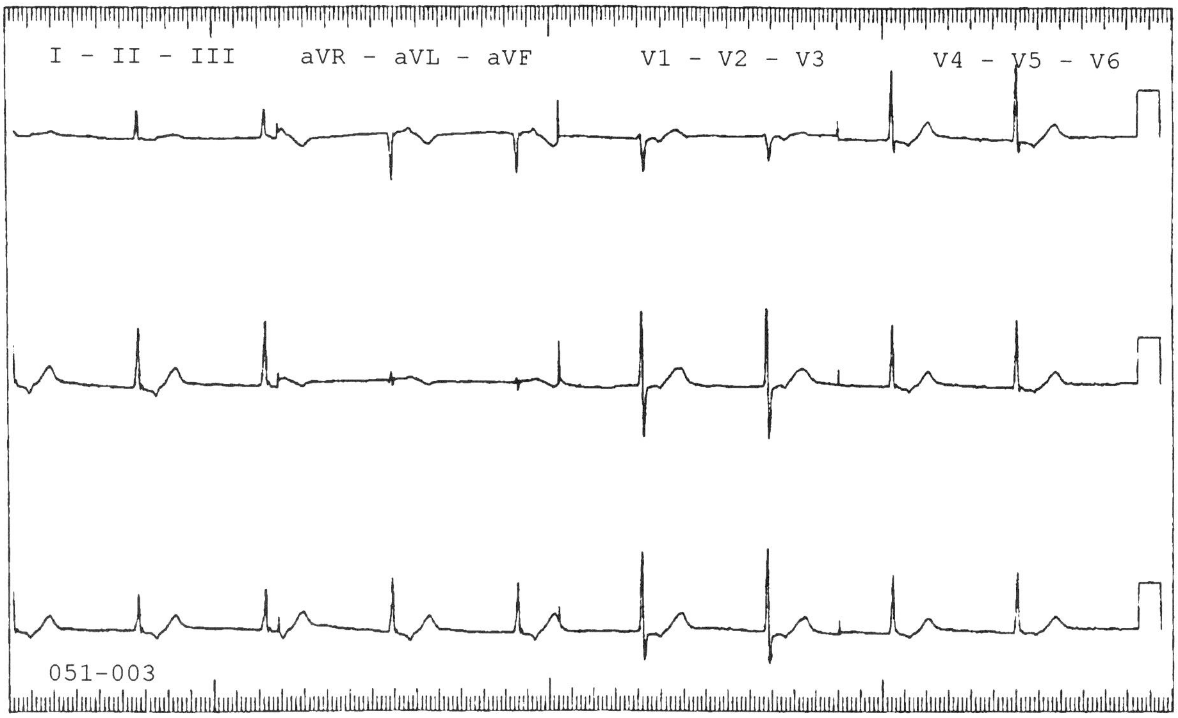

Low Junctional Mechanism

Some would call this just junctional (19, 125, 243), saying that whether low, mid, or high is not important. The negative P in II, III, and aVF is clear, though, and it follows the supraventricular QRS. This implies an origin closer to the ventricles than the atria, probably the His Bundle; i.e., low junctional (formerly known as low nodal). The significance to the patient in the difference between low, mid, and high, if any, is a separate question.

Any pacemaker other than the sinus node is ectopic (121), and ectopic mechanisms are either usurping or default (122). The EKG shows the locus of the pacemaker, and its rate and rhythm, but whether it is "accelerated" (usurping, abnormal) (134) or compensatory (default, normal) is a clinical judgment.

The term "ectopic" as applied to a mechanism originating in an atrium is redundant, but is in common use, and seems to imply automaticity as the means by which activity of a focus is maintained, as distinct from reentry.

55 55 -- 08 44 see below
+60 1:5 V1½ 10:0 normal
none
normal
+75 positive V1-6, low V1

P: follows QRS and is negative in leads II, III, and aVF

(1) Low junc mech, rate 55
(2) Otherwise WNL

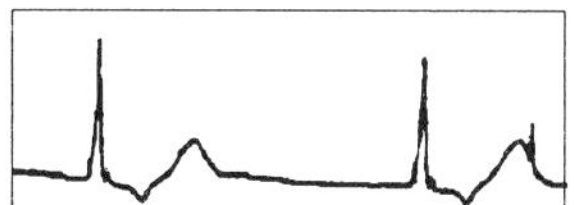

Last two beats in aVF from above. The spike in the second T is a lead change.

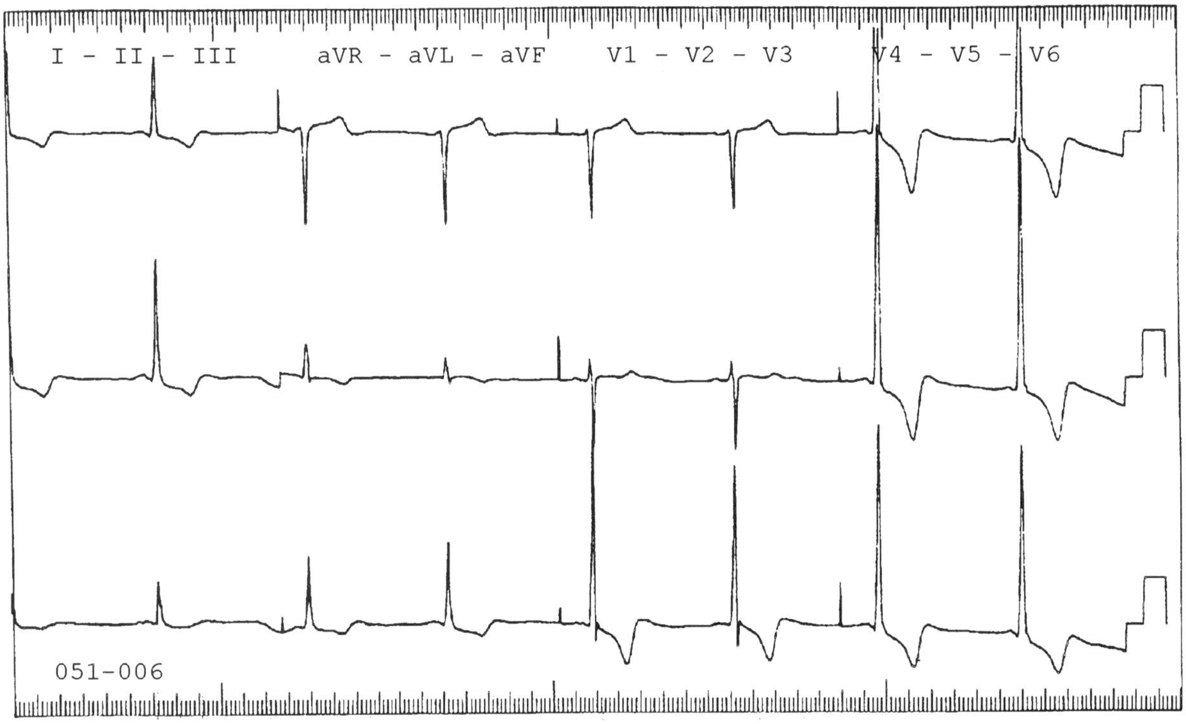

Left Ventricular Hypertrophy, Left Ventricular Overload (Strain)

Discrepancy between supply and demand for oxygen in the wall of the left ventricle results from either exaggeration of demand (left ventricular overload) and/or impairment of supply (coronary insufficiency). With LVO, as in this tracing, the distinguishing feature is a wide QRS-T angle (53, 189). ST-T contour is normal, and this can be demonstrated by projection of the curve from the peak of T back through the QRS. It will come out at the B point, where both QRS and ST began. ST depression, defined by the level of J with relation to the baseline, is minimal if there is any at all (45). Coronary insufficiency produces flattening *and* depression of ST. See insets and "A tutorial: Examination of one heartbeat" in Chapter 3. These two patterns overlap widely, and may coexist. They are both likely to be called simply "ischemia" (136), but can often be distinguished from each other. The difference between form and function, between hypertrophy and strain is real. Hypertrophy follows strain, not vice versa; ST-T abnormality is not secondary to hypertrophy. See EKGs 26 and 50.

```
45    45    16    08    44     sinus
+45    1:15    V2½  40:0    normal
       minimally down V4-6
            related to T
+135   pos V1,   ±V2,   neg V3-6

(1) Sinus mechanism, rate 45
(2) Left vent hypertrophy
(3) ST-T abns, prob LVO and
    suggestive of cor insuf
```

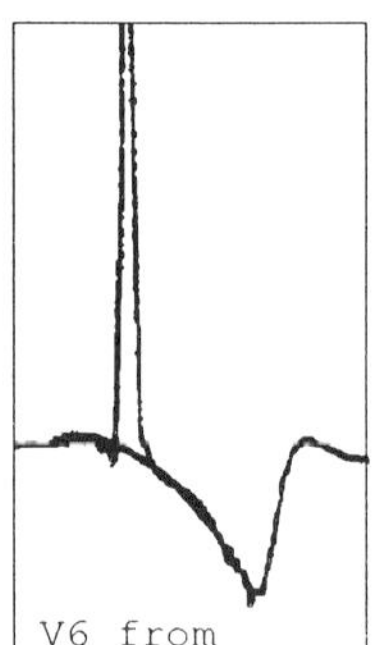

V6 from tracing above

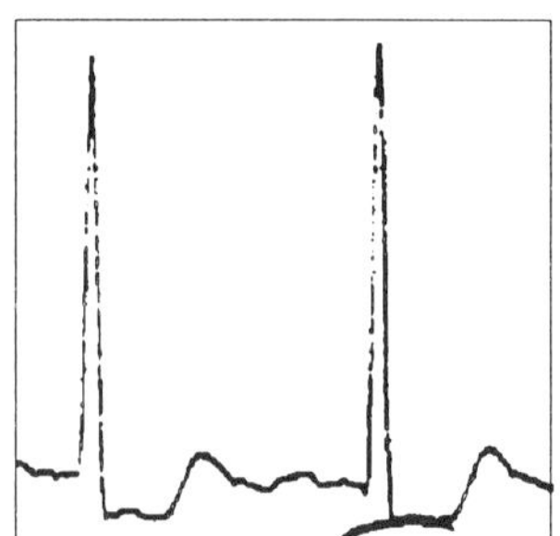

V5 from EKG #55

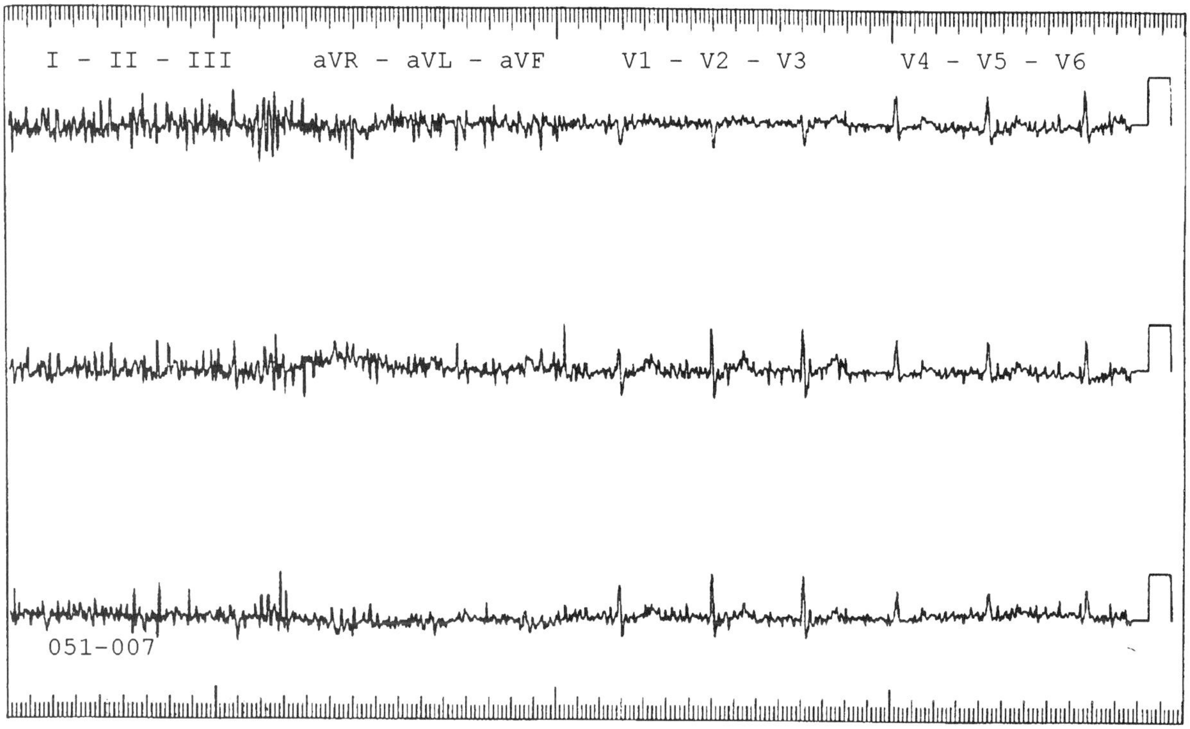

Muscle Tremor

```
--    75  --    08  40    see below
?±0    1:5    V1½    5:0     normal
              none
        probably normal
?+60   ±V1,    positive V2-6

(1) Supraventricular mechanism,
    rate 75, regular rhythm,
    probably sinus.  Atrial ac-
    tivity is not clear.
(2) Otherwise probably WNL, at
    worst only small ST-T ab-
    normalities

--Muscle tremor artifact  ob-
  scures detail.
```

Be as specific as possible in each element of the report. Atrial activity is not clear here, but a ventricular rate of 75 (the computer called it 128) with a regular rhythm ("rhythm" in the everyday sense of the word) and a QRS of supraventricular origin (its precise duration is arbitrary, but it is not wide) point strongly to the sinus node as the source. Alternatives to explain all of these features are few. They include sinus, rate 150 with 2:1 AV block, but that is an unlikely rate for 2:1 block, and assumes you don't see two P waves, more unlikely than uncomplicated sinus assuming you don't see one P. Atrial flutter with atrial rate 300 would work, too, but that would assume three unidentifiable Ps for each QRS. It may be junctional, but the rate is more like sinus. Judgment is always involved. It is usually not difficult to decide among these if you know the patient.

Muscle tremor is a very common artifact that often can be lessened by an attentive technician (102). It is characterized by chaotic spiking of the trace that varies in amplitude, "noise," different from the regular oscillations, "hum," of 60 cycle AC (EKG 69).

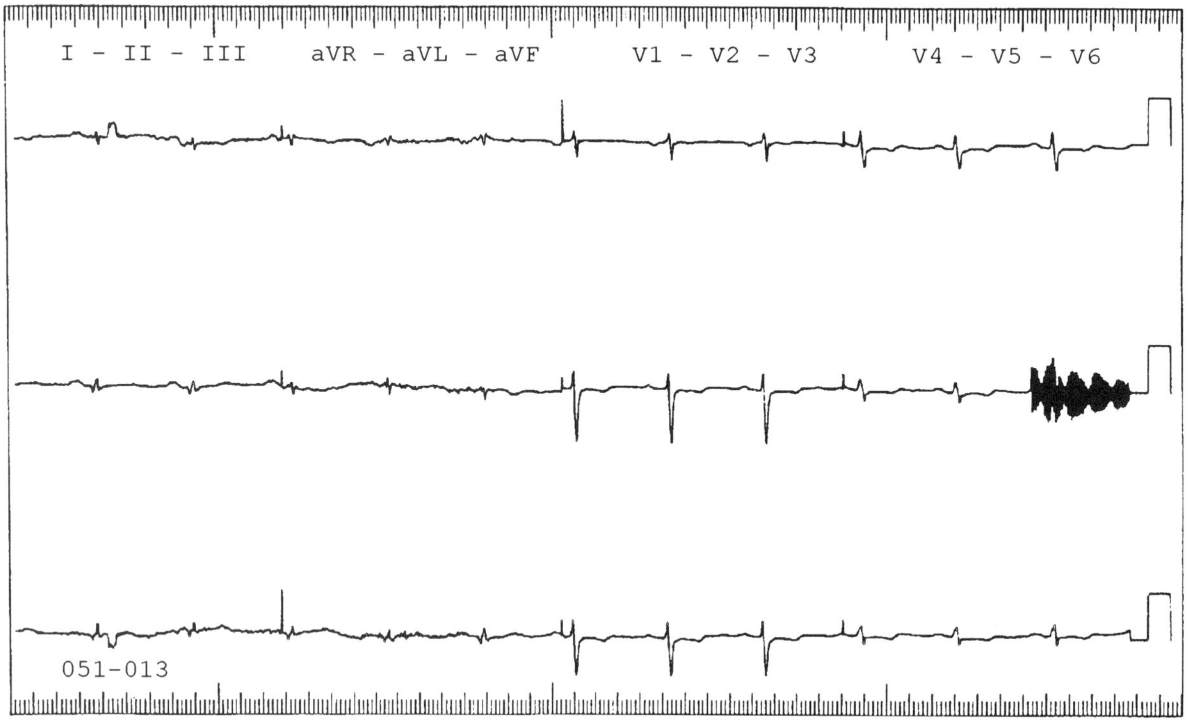

60-Cycle AC Interference, Low Voltage

Most electricity in the U.S. alternates polarity 60 times a second, broadcasting an absolutely regular signal that is intercepted by both the patient's body and the EKG machine. The right leg lead connects these, the "chassis" of the heart, the unknown (88, 99), and the chassis of the EKG machine, the recorder; the only variable in the system is the unknown. When this connection is not intact, the recorder shows the alternating current as "hum," distinguished from the "noise" of muscle tremor (insets), as well any other electrical events in the body. AC interference used to be a major problem, but has been contained so effectively by manufacturers of EKG machines (102) that it is rare now.

T voltage is low in this tracing (42, 228). Evidence for an old infarct is inconclusive. Nothing at all looks new.

70 70 20 08 ?40 sinus
?? (low) 2:4 V4 3:1 Q2,3,F
none
related to T
low isoelectric V1-6

(1) Sinus mechanism, rate 70
(2) ST-T abnormalities, non-specific
(3) Suggests old inferior mci

--60 cycle artifact obscures some detail.
--nothing at all looks new

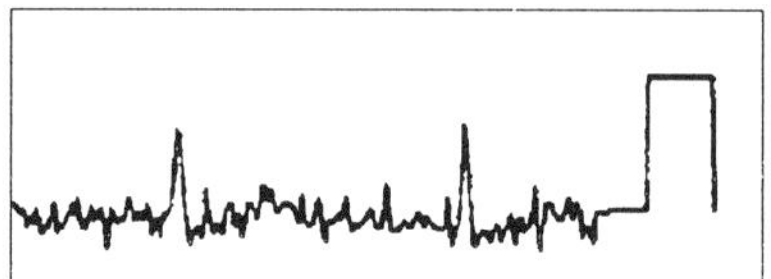
Muscle tremor (V5 EKG #68)

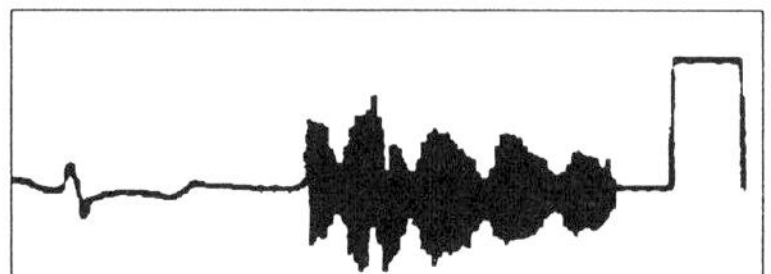
60 cycle AC (V5 from above)

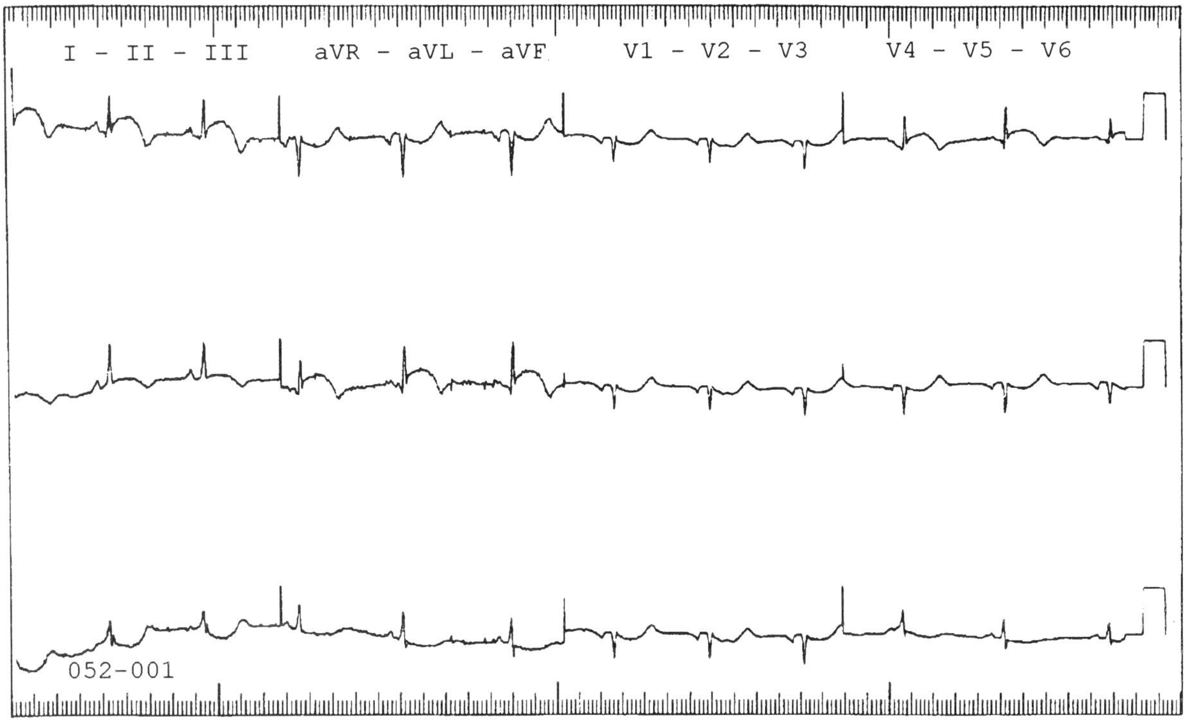

Infarction, Injury, Artifact

Description of the ST contour can be a challenge (45, 206). In this tracing it is arched in I, II, aVL, and V6. (Note that the leads labeled V4-5-6 are really V6-4-5) (109). Displacement is small, but J is clearly up in I, aVL, and V6, and there is no doubt that the pattern reflects myocardial injury. The opposite view of the same features, depression and sagging, is just suggested in Lead III.

Evidence for an infarct would be easy to miss, but, recognizing the misplacement of V leads indicated above, it is strong. P is not usually negative as far to the left as V4, but the progression of initial QRS contour (174) and the trend of T confirm that it is in this case. The criteria for a scar deep in the myocardium, abnormality of the initial part of QRS (175), are fulfilled in views from the front of the chest. This and the ST-T evidence of myocardial injury add up to a recent anterior myocardial infarct.

```
65    65    12    06    40     sinus
+45   0:5   V3½   4:1   QSV1-4, qV5
    slightly up 1, avL, V5
   sagging/flattened/arched
±180 low,   +V1-4,  neg V5,  ±V6

(1) Sinus mechanism, rate 65
(2) Ant myocardial infarct,
    probably of recent origin

--Description and interpreta-
  tion correct for  transposi-
  tion of V4 and V5.
```

Anybody can make a mistake, and few EKG technicians have been trained in the topographic anatomy of the chest. To recognize mislabeling of leads requires knowing what to expect. See the analogies of a pennant on a pole (Fig. 3-1) (44), and an elephant in a box (85).

EKG 71

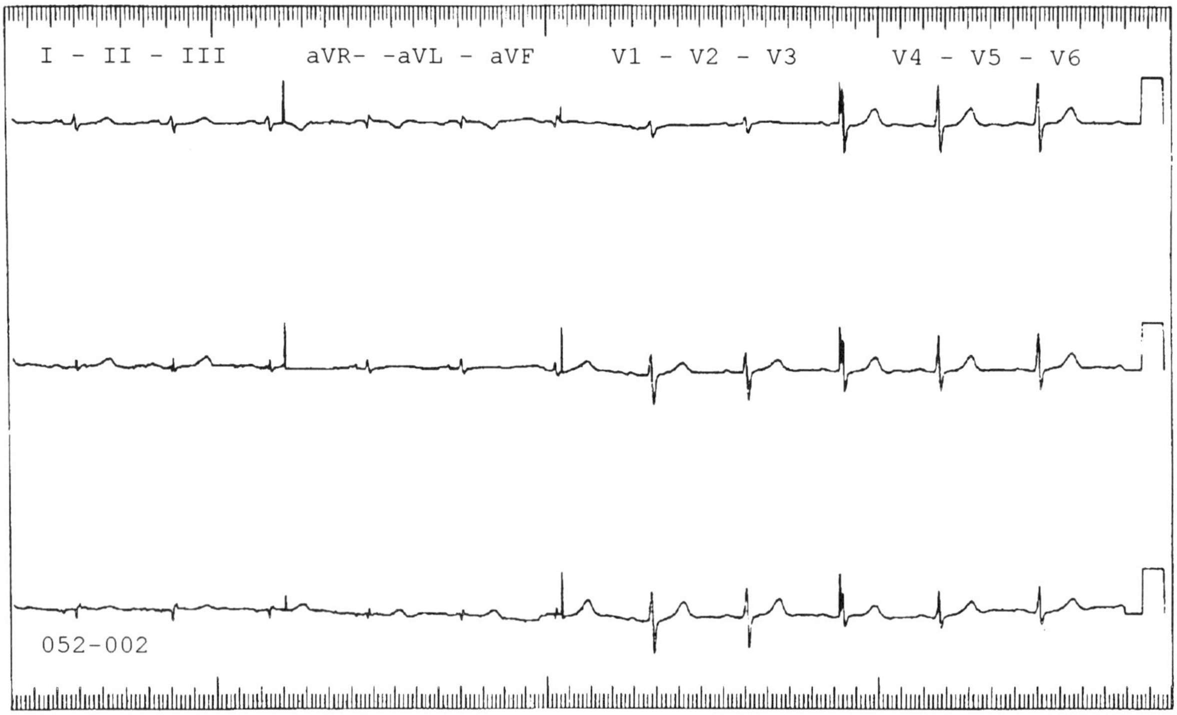

Low Voltage, within Normal Limits

```
70    70    20    06    40      sinus
??    1:2    V1-3    5:2     normal
              none
             normal
+45   ±V1       positive V2-6

(1) Sinus mechanism, rate 70
(2) Within normal limits
```

When voltage is described as low without specifying P, QRS, or T, it will be understood to mean that QRS amplitude is small. Amplitude can be expressed precisely, but what value defines low is rarely specified. A useful criterion is 0.5 mm or less (zenith to nadir) for the largest complex in Leads I, II, and III. [Why can't aVR, aVL, and aVF be judged by the same standard (38, 42, 88, 228)?] Amplitude in precordial leads is subject to such wide variation that no meaningful figure can be given.

However one chooses to define it, low voltage is a finding, not a diagnosis, comparable to short stature on physical examination. Orientation, duration, and contour must be considered, as well the stability of the finding, and the subject's habitus, pulmonary status, and other factors, before its importance can be evaluated (228). Somehow it has become traditional to see low voltage as suggesting pericardial effusion (228), but this is only one of many, many explanations, and rarely justified.

In this tracing, there is no abnormality of orientation duration, amplitude, or contour of P or ST-T, and QRS is normal except for amplitude.

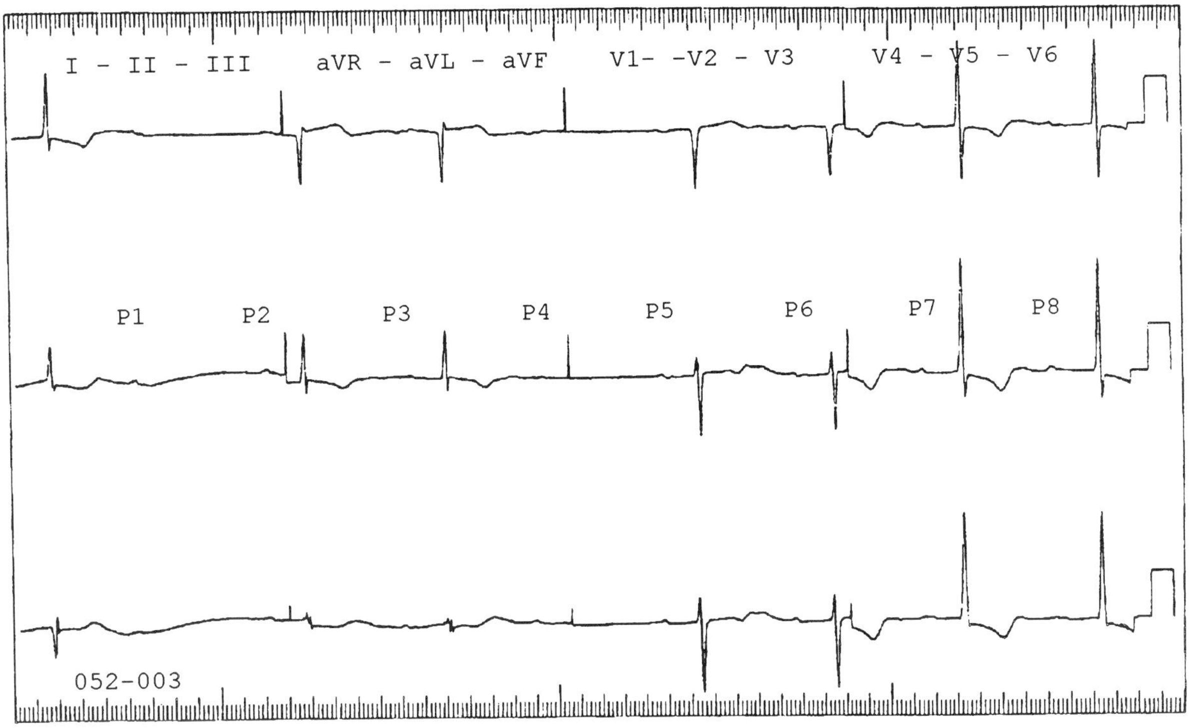

Second Degree AV Block (Type I?)

55 40 -- 08 44 see below
±0 0:12 V3½ 20:1 normal
slightly down V6
related to T
±180 +V1 low ±V2-3 neg V4-6

(1) Sinus mechanism, rate 55
(2) 2° AV block, prob Type I, ventricular rate about 40
(3) ST-T abnormalities, probably left ventricular overload

Second degree AV block is present when all QRSs are of supraventricular origin, but not all supraventricular impulses are conducted to the ventricles. The mechanism is sinus here, rate about 55, but Ps number one and four are not conducted. It is not altogether clear in this case whether PR grows longer with each successive beat until one is dropped, Wenckebach (Type I) block, or remains unchanged, Mobitz (Type II) (152). See EKGs 81 and 138.

U is prominent, especially in V2-3, but not abnormal.

The computer called inferior subendocardial injury, and there is indeed a little depression of ST in II and aVF. It is not clearly even abnormal by itself, but it does suggest coronary insufficiency, and that may explain the AV block. The patient's age and clinical status are important factors. The primary physician, who knows these, can put the EKG findings into clinical context.

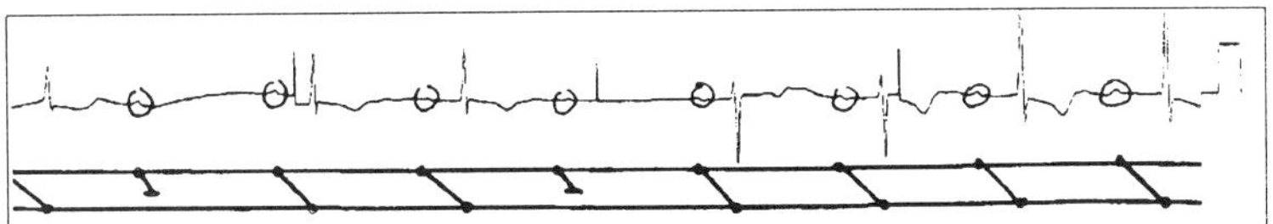

Englemann laddergram from above

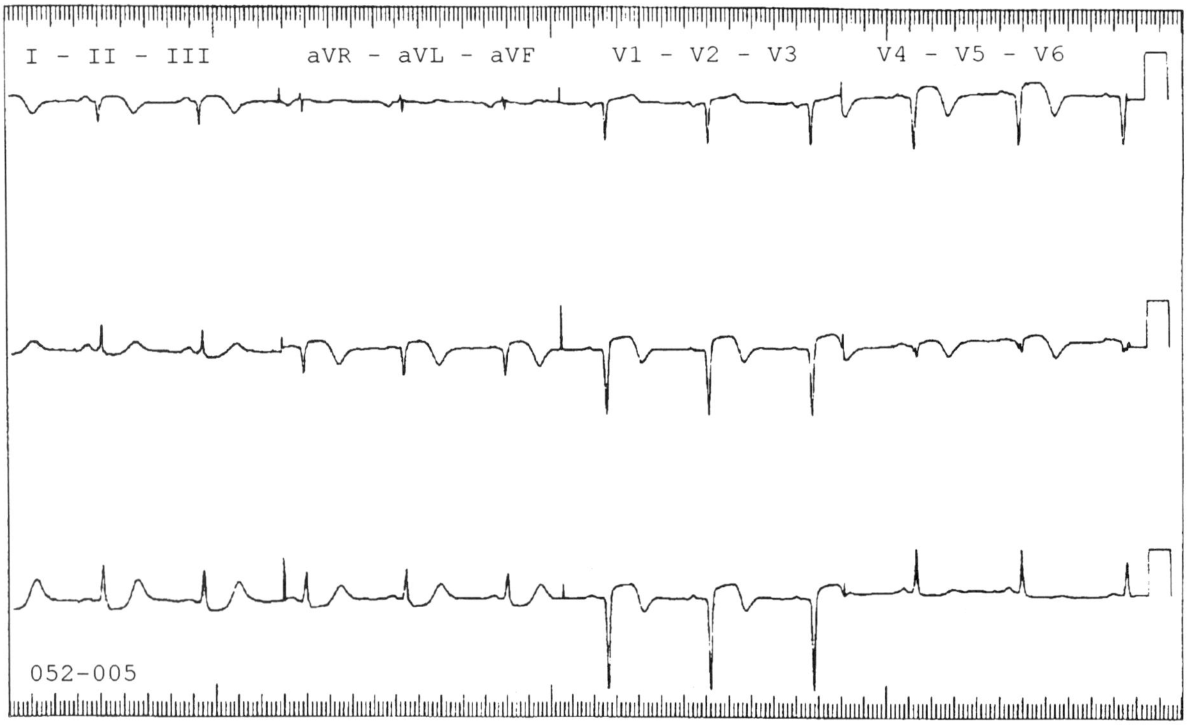

Acute Anterolateral Myocardial Infarct

```
65    65    16    08    40        sinus
+120   0:8   V5   10:0  QV2-4   QSV5
  up I,L,V2-5, down II,III,aVF
          sagging/arched
+120   +V1 low,   neg V2-5,    ±V6

(1) Sinus mechanism, rate 65
(2) Acute antero-lateral myo-
    cardial infarct
```

There are three components to the diagnosis of an infarct: evidence of the anatomic lesion itself, the view from which it is seen, and an estimate as to its age (173). In this tracing, the views from the front (V2-5) and left side (Lead I) of the patient, show as good QRS evidence of a deep scar as one is likely to see (174), and the ST-T pattern of injury implies a recent origin. The two characteristics of ST that indicate injury, displacement and contour, are especially well demonstrated. It is displaced (oriented) anteriorly and cephalad, as indicated by elevation in anterior leads, depression in inferior ones, and very little displacement at all in Lead I. Elevation and depression are not two features, but different projections of the same thing. Depending on the view, ST contour can be indicated as sagging, arched, or, in leads to which displacement is perpendicular, as V6 here, not remarkable. Lesions that show in V1-2-3 are commonly called septal, but the EKG does not show specific structures. There is only one point in play, and it describes the net of all forces without regard to their origin (78). The septum is a joint venture of both ventricles, not a separate structure.

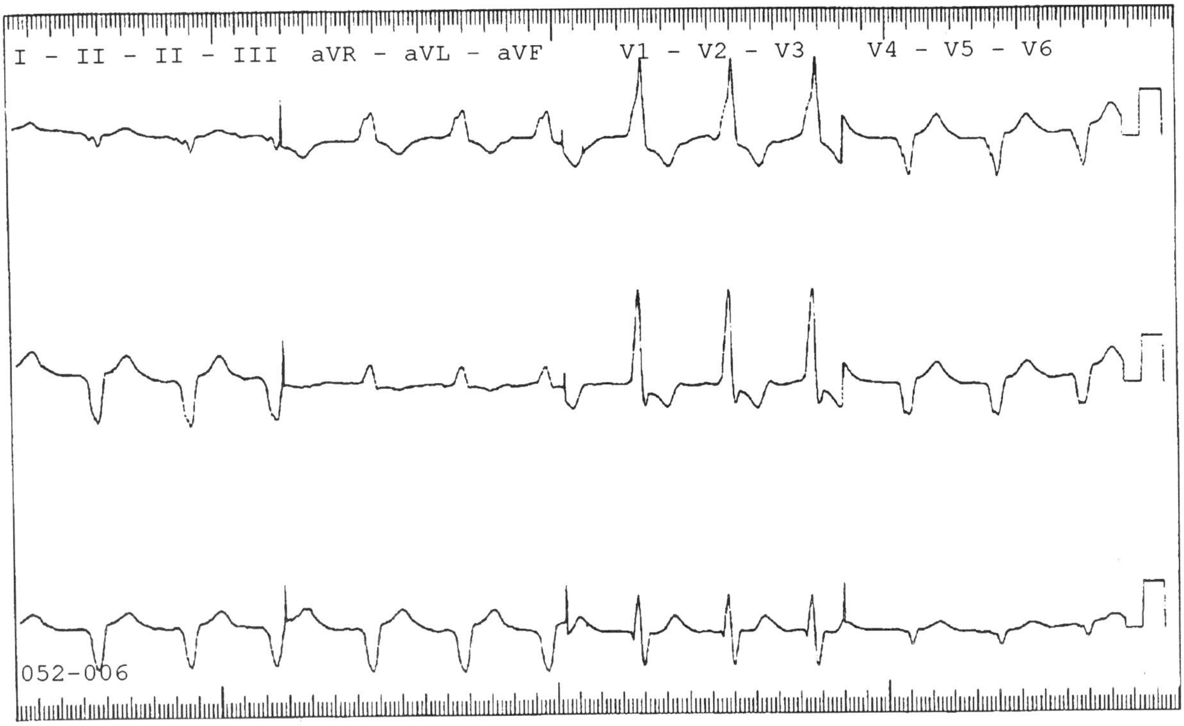

Complex EKG

The only thing unequivocal about this tracing is that the ventricles are beating, or at least electrically active, at a rate of about 75 beats per min with an almost regular rhythm. The rate, and statistics, suggest a sinus origin (123), and the slight variation in cycle length is not much against this; atrial fibrillation might work; atrial flutter, or a junctional origin, is less likely. Given that it is of supraventricular origin, there is an IV conduction defect, and the predominantly distal slur, expressed as an R wave in V1, suggests RBBB. The counterclockwise direction of the mean frontal QRS suggests LAFB. The early slur in QS II, III, and aVF suggests an inferior infarct; and the similar configuration in V4-6, an anterior one. The ST-T pattern may be secondary to the QRS deformity, no matter that its explanation. A ventricular origin of QRS could explain everything.

```
??    75  --  16  44   see below
-105  18:0  V3  0:3    diff slur
      slightly down V1-2
          related to T
+75   neg V1-2, pos V3-6, low V6

(1) Ventricular rate 75 with
    almost regular rhythm,
    probably sinus but atrial
    activity is not clear,
    almost as easily AF, less
    likely idioventricular
(2) Atypical IV cond defect,
    probably RBBB
(3) Old anterolateral mci, prob
(4) Old inf mci, prob, and/or
    left anterior hemiblock

--Nothing looks new
```

There is not much doubt that there is heart disease, but the pragmatic value of the findings depends on the clinical setting. They have to be put in context.

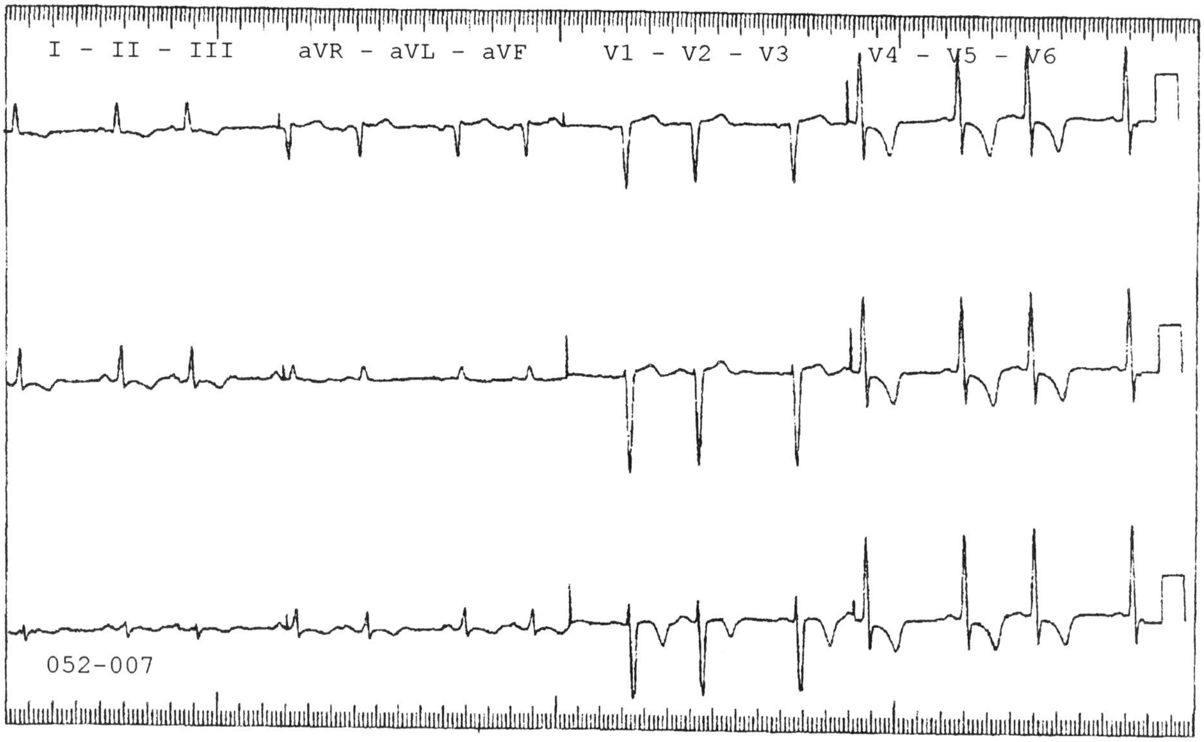

Bigeminy due to PACs

Mid-Precordial ST-T abnormality

The mechanism is sinus with normal AV conduction. The third beat is a PAC; its P is premature, different from sinus P, and its QRS-T is unchanged (inset) (127). PACs are so common in healthy people that they cannot be considered abnormal by themselves. In this case, one follows each sinus beat producing pairing of beats, bigeminy, twinning (129, 146). This may be manifest as palpitation, but is not very important as an incidental finding.

The impressive abnormality here is the negative precordial T that is deeper between V1 and V6 than in either V1 or V6, and symmetrical. This is one of those ST-T patterns that, though nonspecific, correlates well enough with symptoms to suggest myocardial ischemia (136) due to impairment of flow, coronary insufficiency, as distinct from that due to increase of demand as with left ventricular overload (211). Better examples are seen in EKGs 79 and 94. Seen from V6, the symmetry is less apparent, and left ventricular overload is in the differential. Either, both, or neither may be present.

```
80   80   16   10   40      see below
+30    0:12   V3½  18:5     normal
              none
          related to T
-120   +V1-2   neg V3-6 symmetric

(1) Sinus mechanism, rate 80
(2) Bigeminy due to PAC's
(3) ST-T abnormalities, probab-
    ly cor insuf and suggestive
    of left ventricular over-
    load also.
```

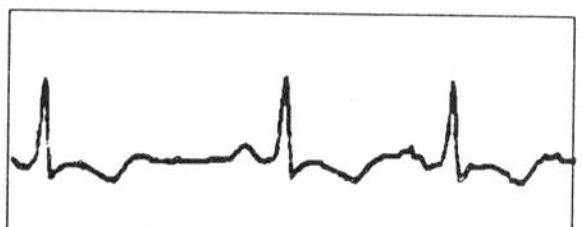

Lead III from above

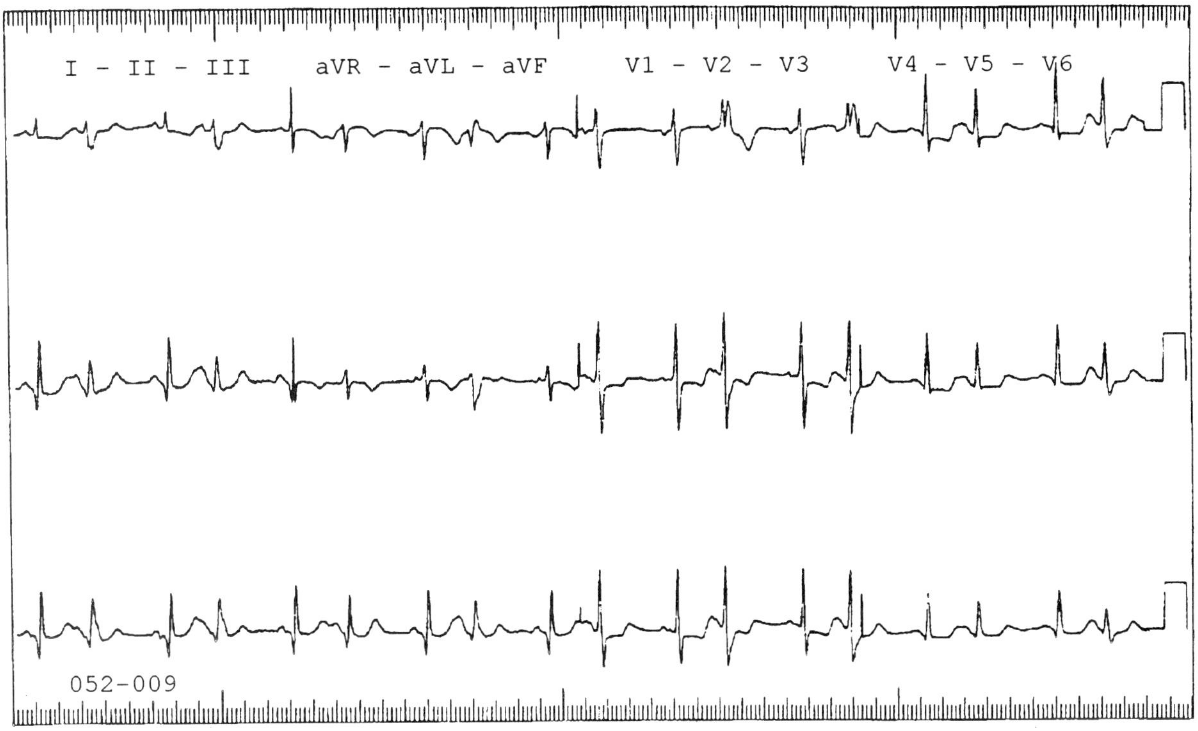

Bigeminy due to PACs (With Aberration), Inferior Myocardial Infarct, Flattened Depression of ST

```
110   110   12   08   36  sinus
                          with PAC's
+60   5:8   V2   8:0      Q2,3,F,V6
            down V3-6
        sagging/flattened
+90  low     isoelectric V1-6

(1) Sinus mechanism, rate 110
(2) Bigeminy due to PAC's
    (with aberration)
(3) ST-T abnormalities typical
    of subendocardial injury as
    with coronary insufficiency
(4) Old inferior myocardial in-
    farct, probable
```

The wide beats are PACs with aberration (169), not PVCs. Each is preceded by a P that is early and different from the sinus P. As here, aberration is usually in a RBBB pattern.

The inferior Q is prominent, but not very wide or irregular in contour. By itself, it is not clearly abnormal at all but does raise the question of an inferior infarct. Infarction is the ultimate result of coronary insufficiency, and the ST-T evidence suggestive of that (204) increases the likelihood that there is one. The absence of ST elevation in the leads that show the QRS abnormality suggests that the infarct, if there is one, is old. The injury pattern suggests a left anterior descending artery lesion. Angina in a patient with an old infarct would explain everything, but the clinical picture is all important in assessing the significance of the findings. Subendocardial injury need not mean angina pectoris (207). V6 is usually thought of as anterior, and Lead II as inferior, but the two are very close together in space and often show the same infarct. A line can be in more than one plane.

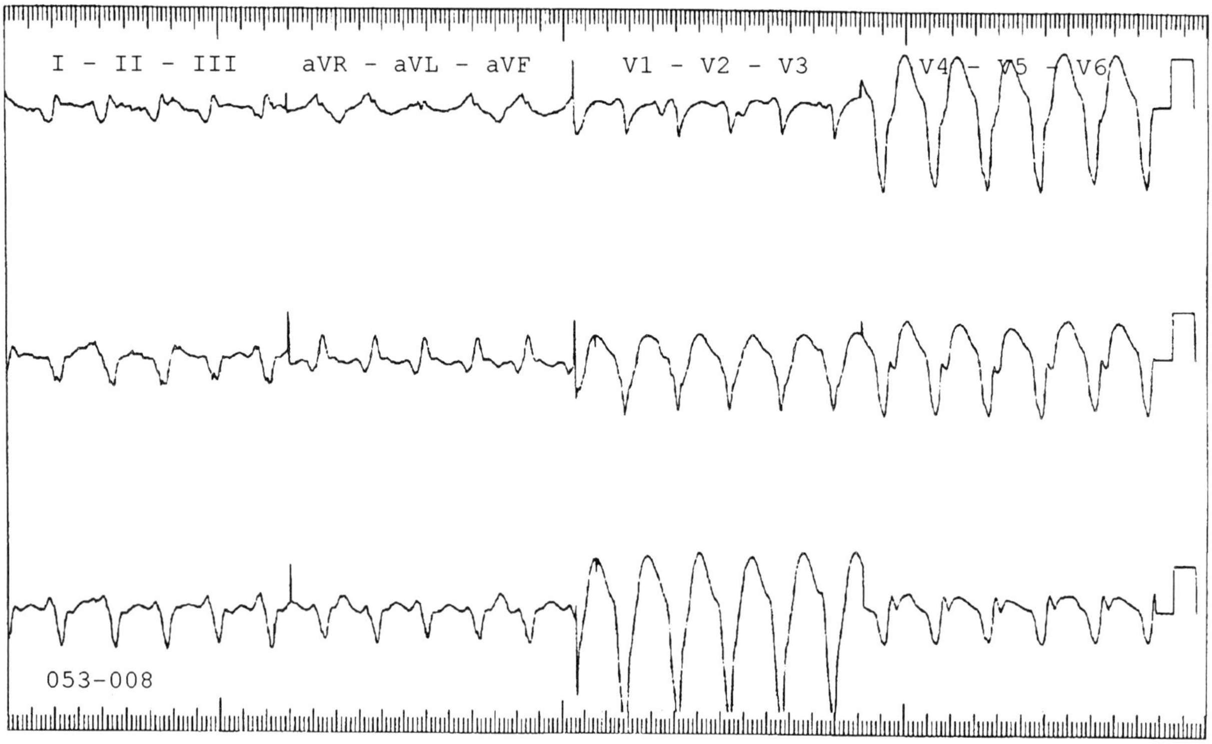

Ventricular Tachycardia

There are probably P waves, rate about 85, seen best in V1 (the negative waves beneath the 1 and the 2 of the labels V1 and V2), strong evidence that the atria are under the control of a sinus pacemaker, while the wide QRS, of bizarre configuration and at a rate greater than atrial, implies that the ventricles are paced from an intrinsic focus. "Ventricular tachycardia" covers both the locus and the rate. As the term is used, it suggests a rate much greater than 135, closer to 200, but locus and rate can be separated (144).

Another feature in favor of a ventricular origin of QRS in this case is the fact that it is monophasic and of the same sign all the way across the precordium.

```
-- 135   --   20   40    see below
-90   0:5   --   0:8  diffuse slur
              up V2-6
          arched/flattened
low     ±V1, positive V2-5   ±V6

(1) Ventricular tachycardia
```

Its rhythm is perfectly regular, and, though the traditional wisdom is that regular rhythm is more likely with supraventricular mechanisms than with ventricular, it may be found with either.

Distinction between ventricular tachycardia and supraventricular tachycardia with an intraventricular conduction defect is often arbitrary from the tracing alone, but the clinical setting usually leaves little doubt.

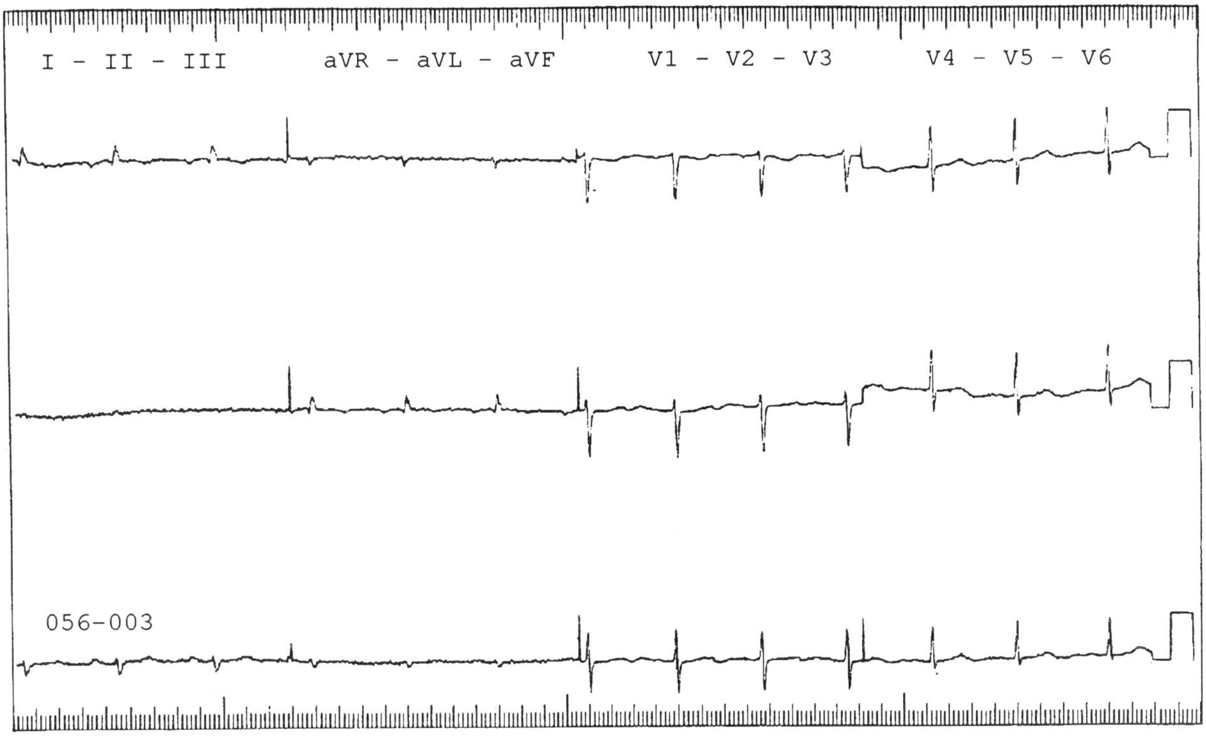

Crossed Right Arm and Leg Leads, Flat Line in Lead II

This is a very common artifact. Lead II is made with the left leg positive and the right arm negative. The right leg lead grounds the patient to the EKG machine (99) so that the only variable seen by the galvanometer is the unknown, the electrical activity of the heart. It will work wherever attached, and is not a component of any lead. The right arm lead, however, represents an apex of Einthoven's triangle (86). It is half of Leads I and II, and contributes to all the others except III. When on the right leg, it is attached to the same apex of the triangle as the left leg lead, the pubic symphysis, and Lead II, which measures the difference between left leg and right arm, finds none (104, 106, 108). Lead II is flat, Lead I is III upside down, and Lead III is unchanged. Leads aVR, aVL, and aVF are modified accordingly. The V leads are altered, too, but not to a clinically important extent. The tracing contains a lot of information, but is not complete.

75 75 20 06 40 sinus
-- 1:10 V3 8:1 normal
none
normal
-- ±V1-2 positive V3-6

(1) Sinus mechanism, rate 75
(1) Probably within normal limits, but incomplete

--recorded with right arm and leg leads transposed

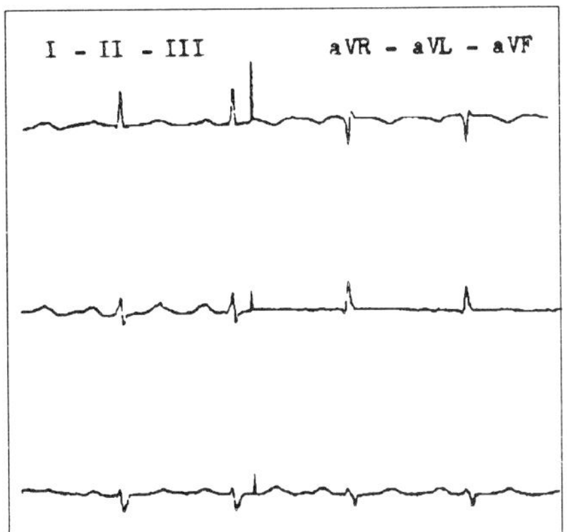

Frontal leads, control

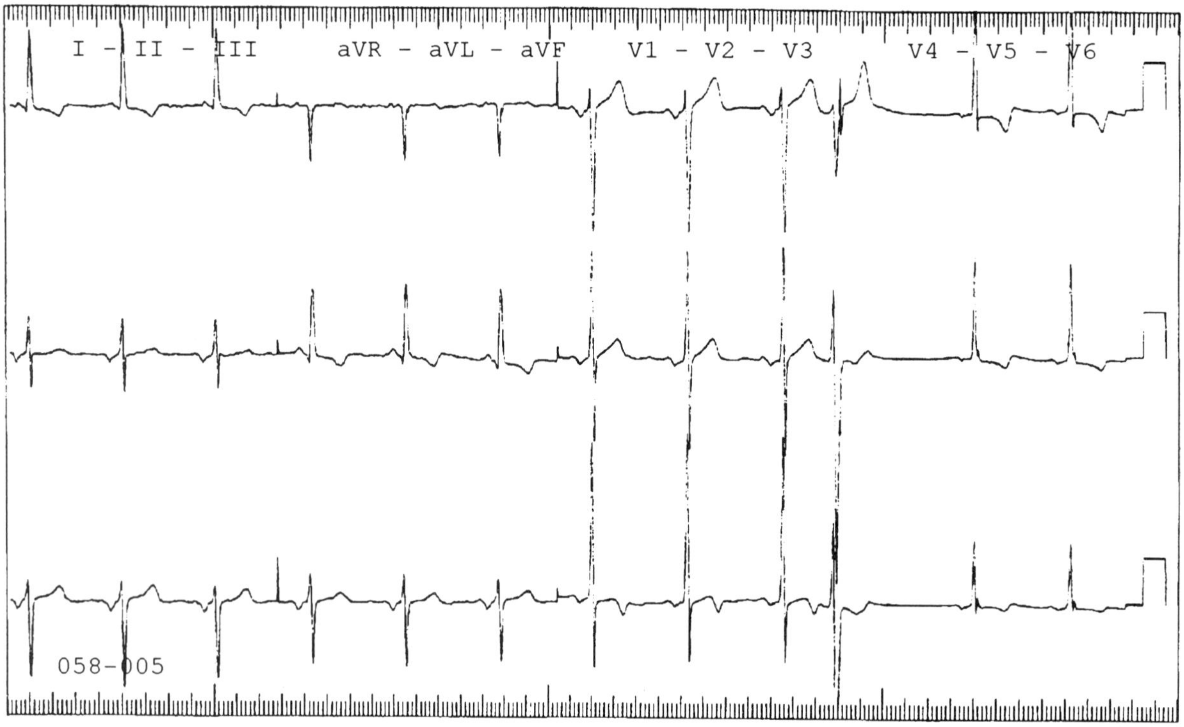

70	70	16	08	36	see below
-30	5:25	V1½	12:0		normal
		none			
		related to T			
low	+120	+V1-2	±V3	neg V2-6, deep V4	

(1) High junctional mechanism, rate 70
(2) ST-T abnormalities, probably coronary insufficiency, and suggestive of left ventricular overload also

High Junctional Mechanism
ST-T abnormalities

P is directed cephalad (negative in aVF)and precedes QRS. This indicates retrograde excitation of the atria from a low atrial, or high junctional, focus (125). Whether it is usurping, ("accelerated") or default is a judgment call; its rate is a fact. If P had followed QRS, the implication would have been of a low junctional origin.

The computer called left ventricular hypertrophy, but all computer programs overdo that, some using more than one criterion, a shotgun approach that is hard to justify. Whatever numbers are chosen, they must be validated by correlation with anatomic reality, and this is defined differently by different investigators. Few, if any, use enlargement of cells, the classic definition of hypertrophy. Applying the criteria of Sokolow and Lyon (192), a suggestion of left ventricular hypertrophy can be defended here, but there are many factors that govern QRS voltage (228), and there are better ways to recognize overwork of the left ventricle than the EKG (196). The ST-T pattern has elements to suggest both coronary insufficiency and left ventricular overload (211), the latter supporting the suspicion of left ventricular hypertrophy.

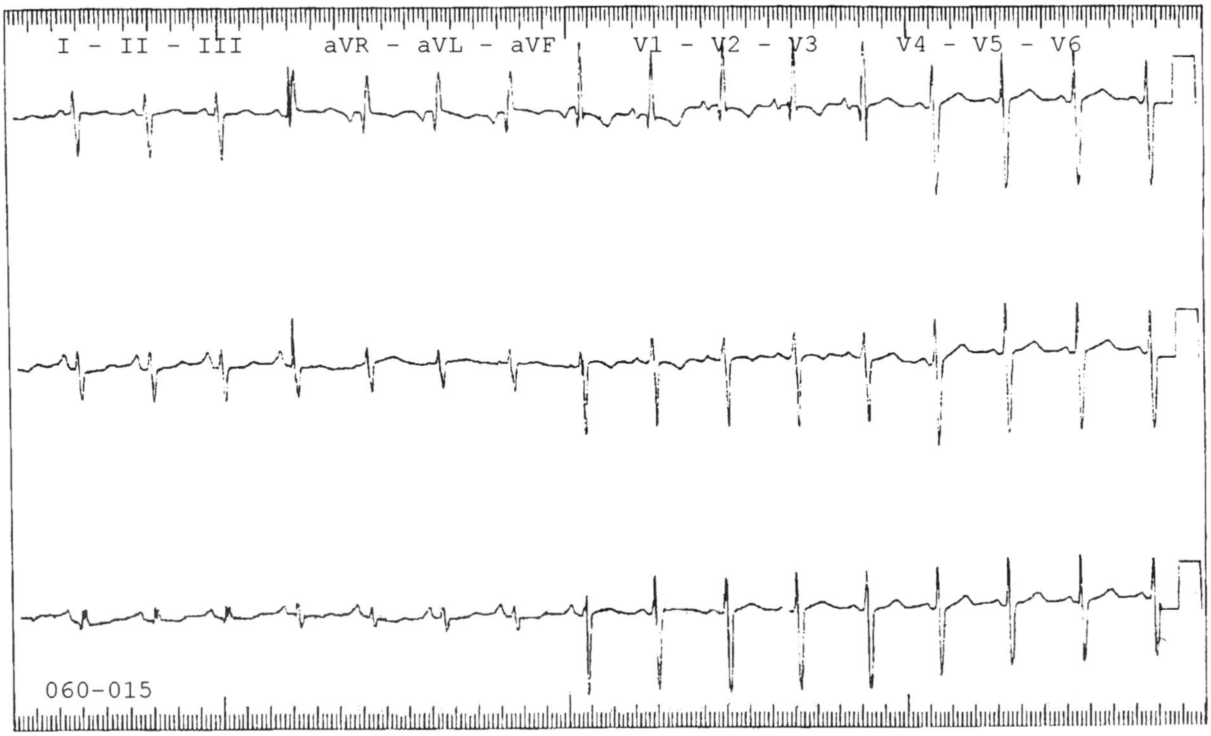

Right Ventricular Hypertrophy, Right Atrial Enlargement

```
95     95    12     08    36      ·sinus
±180   QR3:15   V1½   8:12     normal
                 none
              related to T
low     neg V1-2,   ±V3,     pos V4-6
P: prominent II, III, aVF

(1) Sinus mechanism, rate 95
(2) Right ventricular hypertrophy
(3) Right atrial enlargement
(4) Otherwise WNL
```

The mechanical function of the right and left ventricles can be separated to a large extent, but not their electrical characteristics. Simultaneous excitation of the ventricles, from endocardium outward, is well established (76). The concept of the IV septum between them is valid in a physical sense, but it is not a separate structure defined by cleavage planes. From an electrophysiologic point of view, the ventricles and septum are a unit, and the EKG is a record of the motion of a single point representing the net of all electrical activity in the body. In the normal heart, most of the myocardium is part of the left ventricle, and the force generated during depolarization of both, expressed as if it were an event rather than a process, the "electrical axis," reflects this. In most cases it is directed to the left and back. In this tracing, though, it is to the right and forward, implying that the right ventricle dominates; ergo, it must be hypertrophied (40, 193).

There are other explanations for exaggerated anterior forces (165), including, chiefly, right bundle branch block (159). The normal duration and contour of QRS rule that out in this case, but the two cannot always be separated so easily, and may coexist.

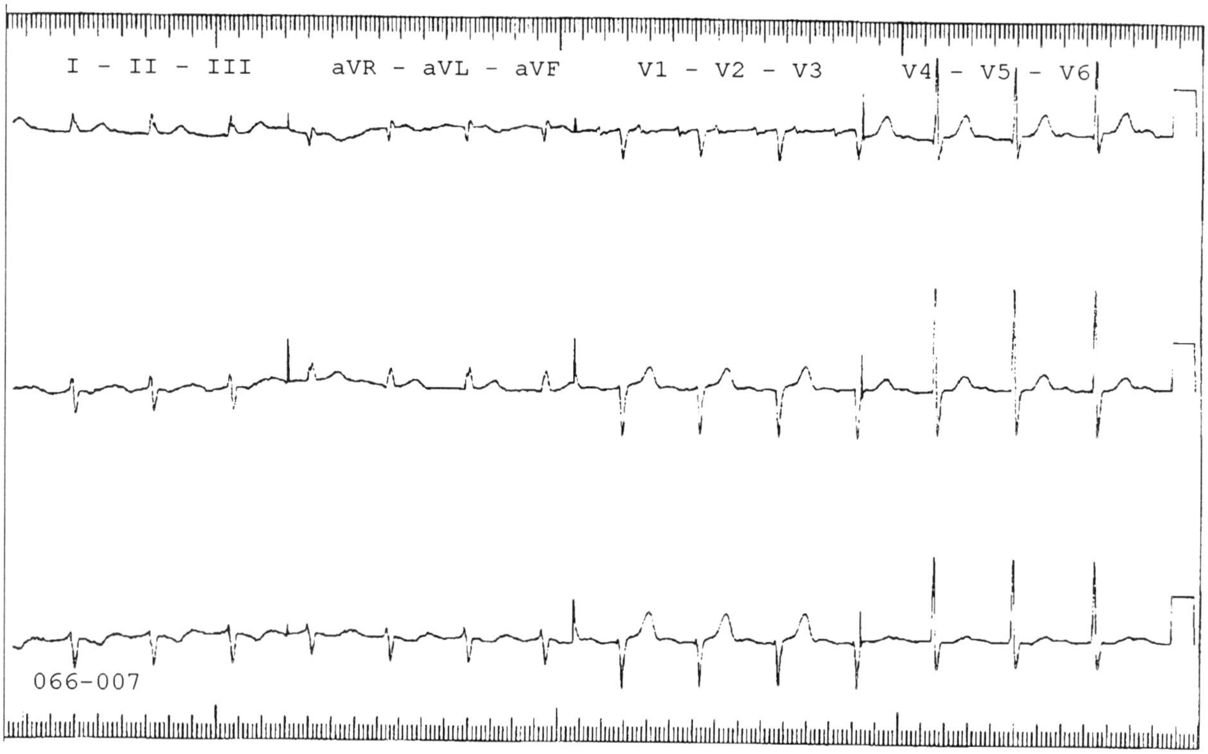

"PAT with Block"

A popular criterion for defining atrial flutter is continuous motion of the trace in a "sawtooth," or "picket fence" pattern in inferior leads, but what is continuous in one lead may not be in another. In this tracing, atrial activity cannot even be identified in Leads II, III, and aVF, but is clear in V1 (inset) where Ps that look very much like those of sinus origin are separated by a flat line. Their rate is against a sinus origin, but goes well with usurping ectopy. Nomenclature for usurping atrial ectopy is not consistent, often failing to differentiate between what is seen and what explains it. There is no single right name for the combination of findings in this tracing. The potential importance of the one chosen is that a continuous process (reentry, or circus conduction, the current explanation for classic flutter), and a discontinuous one (repetitive depolarization of an atrial focus, one explanation for atrial tachycardia), may dictate different therapy.

180 90 -- 08 36 see below
-45 0:5 V3½ 20:5 normal
none
normal
-45 ±V1 positive V2-6, low V6

(1) Atrial tachycardia with 2° AV block, 180/90
(3) Otherwise within normal limits

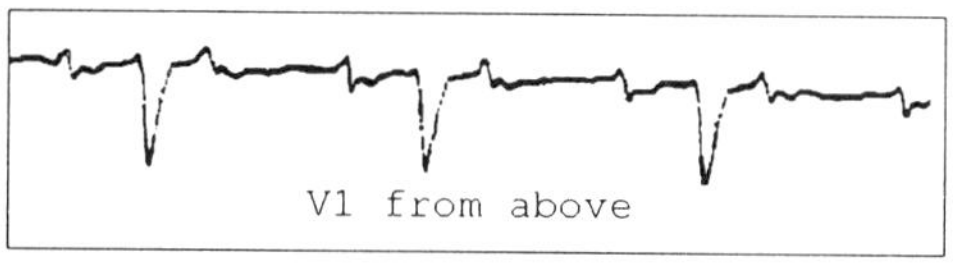

Second degree AV block with atrial rate less than 200 suggests impairment of AV conduction in addition to ectopy and contributes to the idea that digitalis excess may be a factor in "PAT with block" (129, 137). The computer suggested an anterior infarct, but the evidence for one is very small.

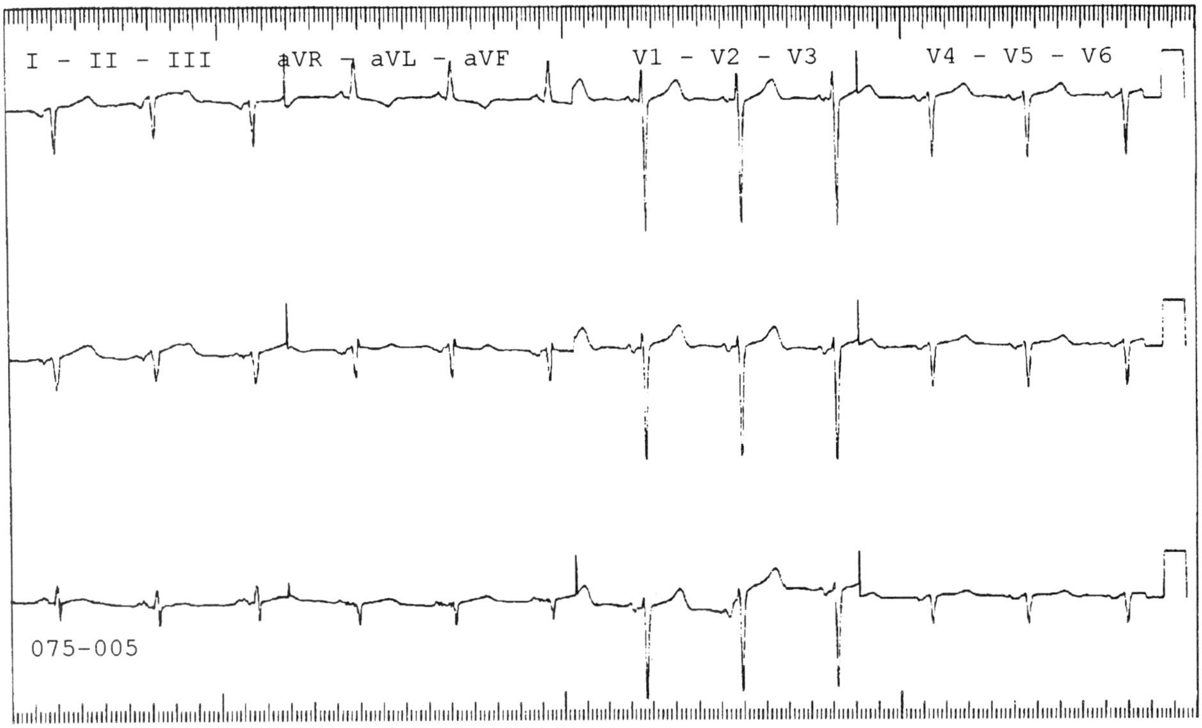

Dextrocardia

```
70     70     12     08     44      sinus
-150   5:20   --     1:5            normal
                  none
              related to T
+45      positive V1-6, low V5-6

(1) Sinus mechanism, rate 70
(2) Dextrocardia
(3) ST-T abnormalities suggest-
    ive of "left" (systemic)
    ventricular overload
```

Dextrocardia comes in several versions. Unmodified, the term refers to the mirror image form as part of situs inversus, as in this case. Findings in the frontal leads are the same as those with crossed arm leads. Left chest leads simulate those from the right chest in normal hearts, with diminishing amplitude and increasing negativity of QRS from V1 through V6. V1 and V2 are reversed, but this may be hard to detect. *Positions for precordial leads do not change because of dextrocardia* (97). Dextrocardia has no effect of the galvanometric connections for the V leads; it makes no difference in what order the extremity leads are connected to form the central terminal of zero potential (88).

Other explanations for parts of this picture include right ventricular enlargement, left posterior fascicular block, and crossed arm leads with precordial leads in reverse order or on the right side of the chest. Distinction among these is not usually difficult. When there is heart disease in addition to dextrocardia, the problem can be complicated.

The evidence for "left" (systemic) ventricular overload here is the wide QRS-T angle with T of normal amplitude, duration, and contour.

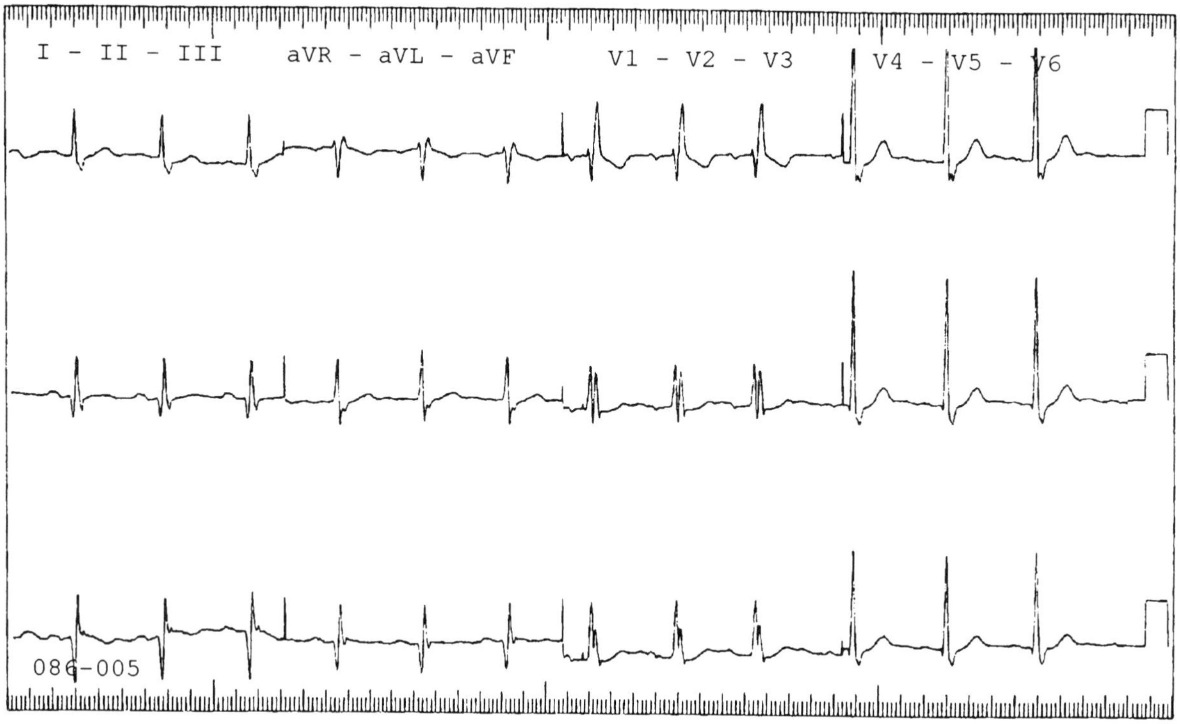

Right Bundle Branch Block, Old Inferior Myocardial Infarct

```
75    75    20    12    40      sinus
--, rSR 1:5:10, --, 20:3,BSTDRA
                           Q2,3,F
         slightly down V3
              normal
low ±0     neg V1    ±V2    +V3-6

(1) Sinus mechanism, rate 75
(2) Right bundle branch block
(3) Old inferior MCI
```

There is only one point on the paper at a time, and its position at any instant is a result of all the electrical forces that exist at that moment. It may reflect the effects of multiple lesions, but cannot, by itself, be interpreted as evidence of more than one. For instance, either left anterior fascicular block or an inferior infarct can explain "left axis deviation," but the axis treats the complex as an event rather than the process that it is, and to attribute its abnormal orientation to two things at the same time does not make sense (164). The difference between LAHB and an inferior infarct is in QRS contour, and, to a less extent, duration. Distinction is often arbitrary.

The situation with right bundle branch block is different. A lesion that affects only the early events in myocardial excitation does not interfere with recognition of one that changes only the terminal ones. The EKG diagnosis of myocardial infarction depends on abnormality of initial QRS forces (170); right bundle branch block; on abnormality of terminal forces.

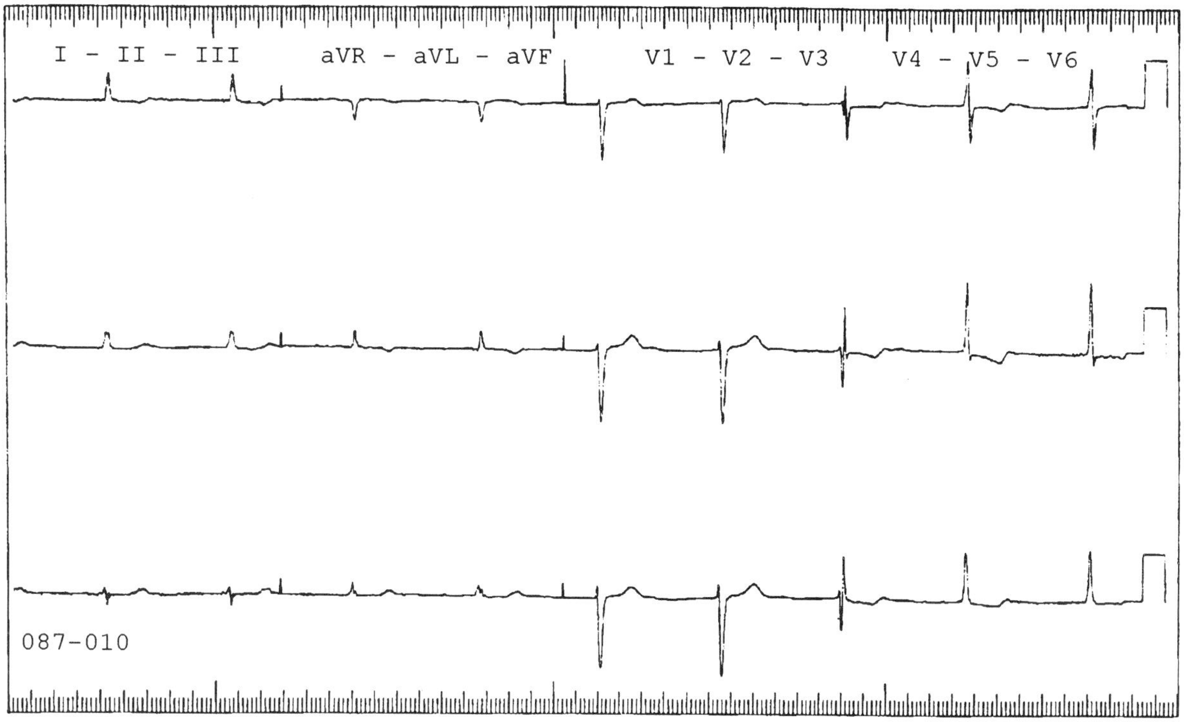

Mid-Junctional Mechanism

QRS is of supraventricular origin (not wide) and its rhythm is regular. Atrial activity is not identifiable, and this may be because P, or *f*, waves are too small to be seen, because there is no atrial activity, or because P coincides with QRS and is not separable from it. To call it mid-junctional assumes the last of these, an opinion. If a tracing from the same patient showing P waves of sinus origin is available, as the one in the box at the left, made later the same day, the interpretation is a near certainty. It may be that to distinguish among high, middle, and low junctional origins adds little, but it can be done. High junctional mechanisms, also called low atrial (EKG 79), are common, and, by themselves, can be considered a variant of normal. Those from a low focus (His bundle?, EKGs 60 and 66) are less common, and are more likely to be abnormal. Mid-junctional mechanisms are rare. Whether any of these is usurping (abnormal) or default (compensatory) is a judgment; the rate is a fact (125).

-- 55 -- 08 44 see below
+30 1:10 V4 10:0 normal
none
related to T
+105 low +V1-3 ±V4 neg V5-6

(1) Supraventricular mech, rate 55, with regular rhythm, prob mid-junctional. Atrial activity is not identifiable.
(2) ST-T abnormalities, suggestive of left ventricular overload, but small.

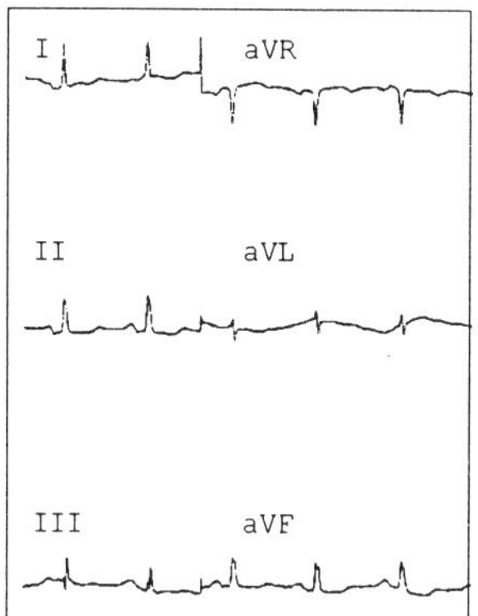

Control for above

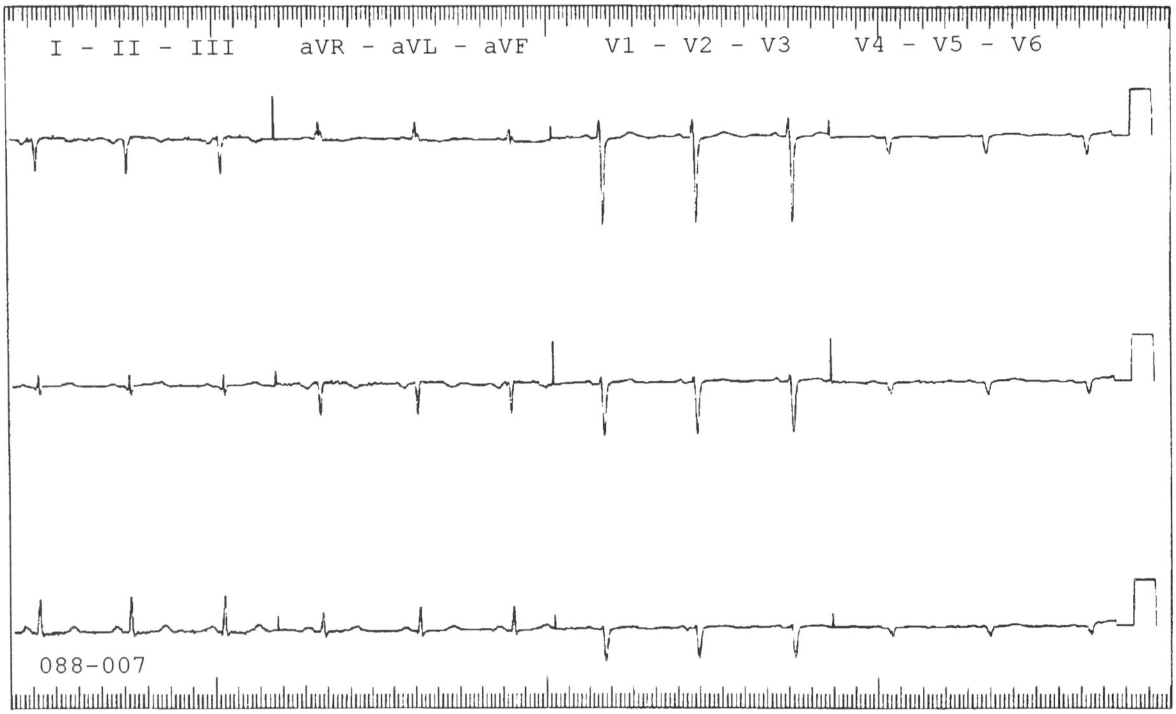

Dextrocardia

70	70	12	06	40	sinus
+150	5:20	--	0:2		normal

none
normal
+105 low, pos V1-2 low, ±V3-6

(1) Sinus mechanism, rate 70
(2) Dextrocardia
(3) Otherwise within normal limits

The term "dextrocardia" can be applied to a wide variety of congenital lesions, but, unqualified, is understood to refer to the mirror-image anomaly (Type I, "true" dextrocardia) that is part of the larger picture known as situs inversus, in which all the viscera are transposed; the left, or arterial, atrium and ventricle are on the right, and vice versa. The heart is otherwise normal.

Frontal plane leads of the electrocardiogram are indistinguishable from those seen with crossed arm leads (P, QRS, and T are directed to the right), but the picture in leads V1 and V2 (equidistant from the midline on opposite sides) is reversed, and V3-6 are the same as V3R-V6R with a normal heart; i.e., P, QRS, and T grow smaller and more nearly completely negative from V3 to V6. As in this case, P may be so small that it cannot be described in detail.

Chest lead positions are not changed for dextrocardia (97, 107).

The differential includes right ventricular enlargement, and crossed arm leads with precordial leads in reverse order or on the right side.

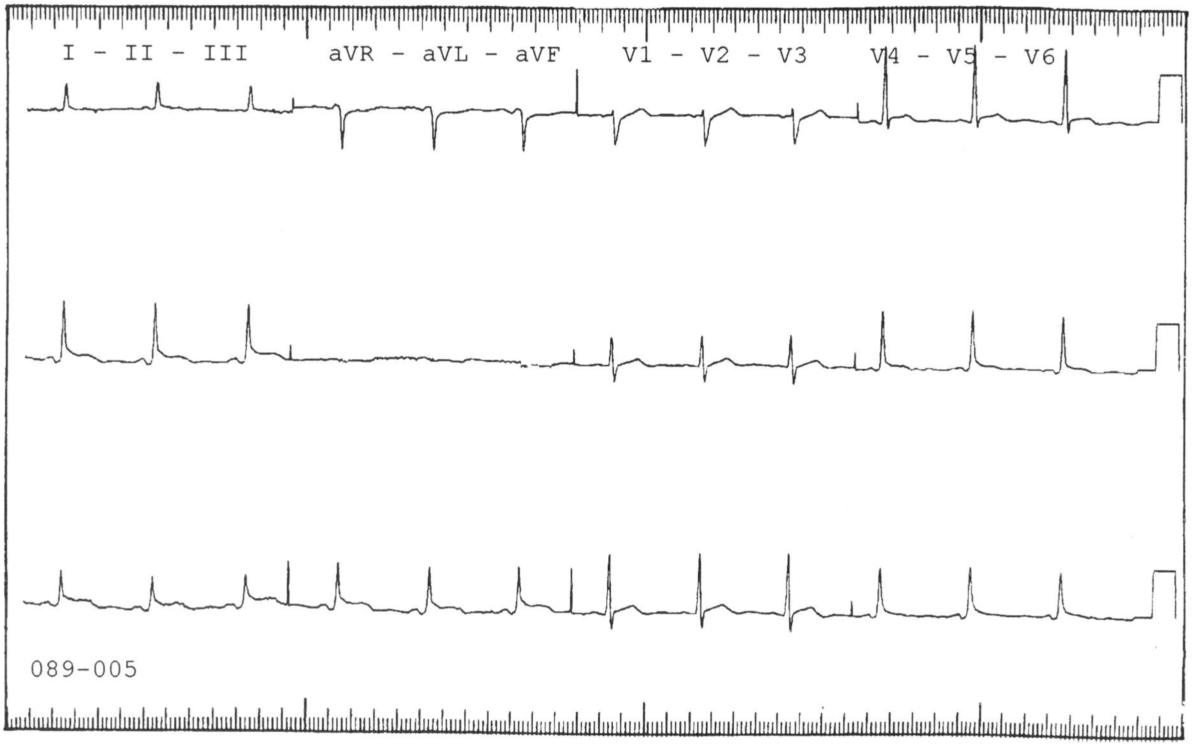

Pericarditis

```
75   75    12    08    36       sinus
+60    2:6    V1½    10:0    normal
   up 2,3,F,V5-6  down aVR
           flattened
low      pos V1-4 low,       ±V5-6

(1) Sinus mechanism, rate 75
(2) ST-T abnormalities typical
    of subepicardial injury as
    with pericarditis
```

Abnormal ST displacement means that the myocardium is injured, its electrophysiologic function is impaired (202). When the injured tissue is subjacent to the epicardium, as with pericarditis, displacement is toward the outer surface of the ventricles, its orientation close to that of QRS. This is almost always some combination of leftward, caudad, and anterior, producing elevation in leads I, aVL, II, V6, aVF, III, and/or V4-6, depending on where the inflammation is. Depression in aVR may not show, but there is only one point in play, and if it is toward some part of the body it is away form another. The amplitude of displacement is small (as a fraction of QRS amplitude, and as compared to that seen with acute myocardial infarction), and, combined with low T voltage, this makes for flattening of the ST segment. The quantitative difference between the ST-T pattern of pericarditis and that of an acute myocardial infarct; e.g., EKGs 59 and 73, is presumably related to the mass of tissue involved. In pericarditis, injury is imposed from the outside and involves only the tissue immediately subjacent to the epicardium; with an infarct, injury begins deep and involvement of superficial layers implies extension outward to include a greater mass of tissue (44, 204, 208).

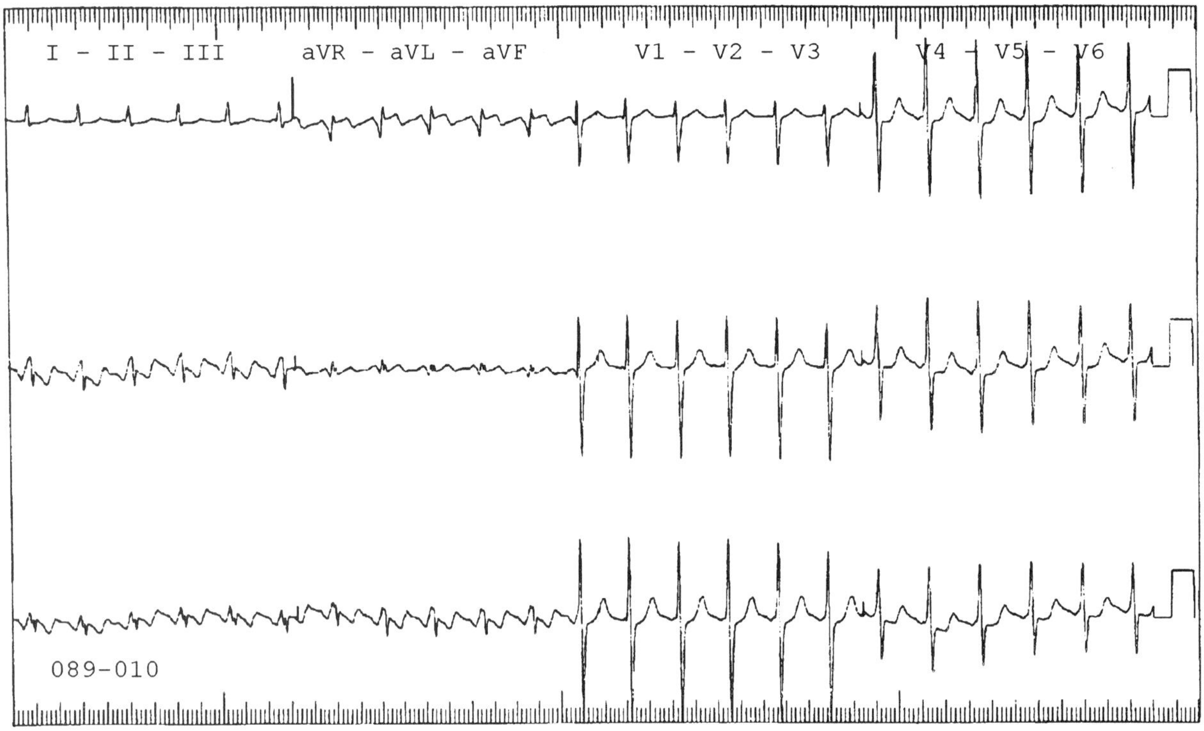

Atrial Flutter, Subendocardial Injury

```
270  135  --  08  32  see below
+60?  4:10  V4  12:8      normal
        up aVR, down V5-6
            flattened
Insep from ST       Positive V1-6

(1) Atrial flutter, 270/135
(2) ST-T abnormalities, typical
    of subendocardial injury as
    with coronary insufficiency
```

Atrial flutter is defined as that condition in which the rate of repetitive atrial ectopy exceeds the ability of the AV conduction system to transmit 1:1. Translated to the EKG, this says that there are P waves at a rate of more than about 200/min with regular rhythm, and second degree AV block (129). If there is also impairment of AV conduction, AV block may occur at a slower atrial rate. Stated differently, there is usurping ectopy with regular rhythm and second degree AV block. The means by which the ectopy is sustained is not specified. The AV block is a normal result of greater input into the AV junction than it can handle. There are two explanations for perpetuation of the atrial activity; a continuous process, reentry, and a discontinuous one, repetitive firing of a single focus. This definition includes "atrial tachycardia with block" (129), and leaves little room for "1:1 flutter." Whether these should be treated as separate entities is far from clear, the difference apparently depends on intrinsic features of the P waves, and these cannot always be seen well enough to be sure about them (119, 136).

The back side of the ST displacement of subendocardial injury, elevation in aVR, is clearer here than in most cases.

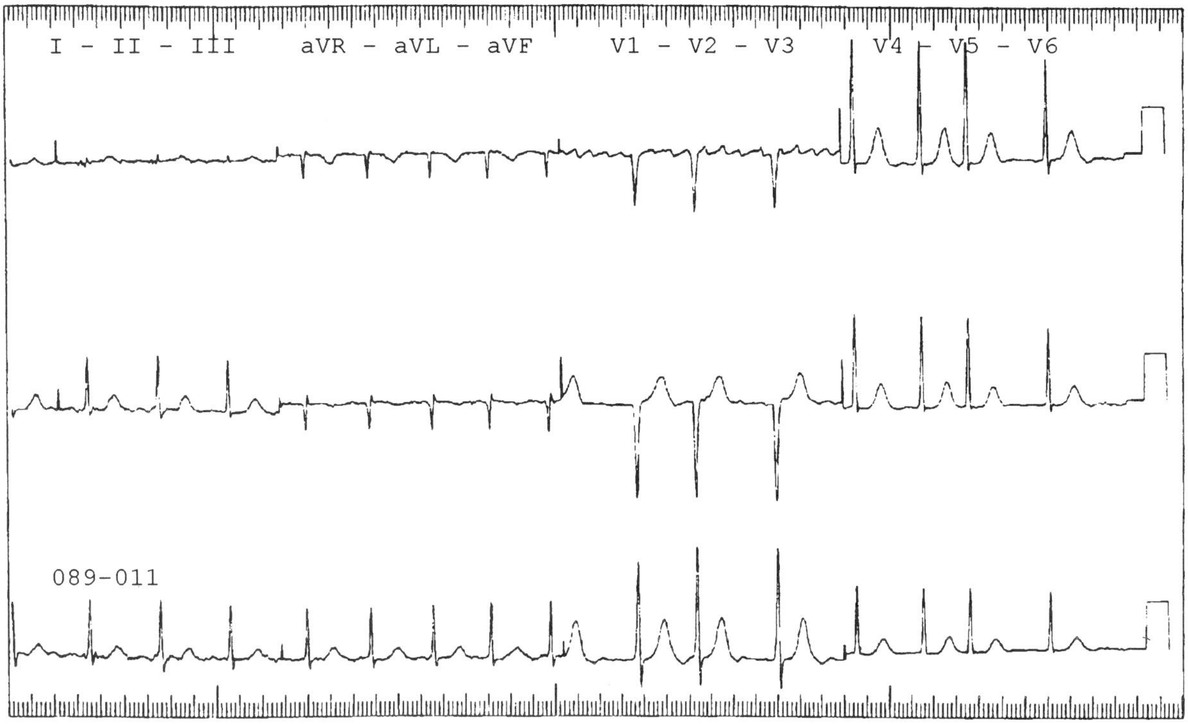

Atrial Fibrillation

```
--  100  --   08  36    see below
+90   0:10    V2½   15:0  QSV1-2
              none
              normal
+60    ± V1         positive V2-6

(1) AF, vent rate about 100
(2) Otherwise probably WNL

--The QS in V2 may be evidence
  of an old scar, but nothing
  at all looks new.
```

Atrial fibrillation is present when the trace is not the same between any two consecutive ventricular complexes in a given lead (19, 27, 131). The word "fibrillation," especially if pronounced to rhyme with fiber, tells what to look for. The unorganized action of fibers, or fascicles, presents a pattern of *f* waves that are fibrillary, unpredictable in size, shape, and timing, but smooth as contrasted with the sharp, spiked record of striated muscle tremor (EKG 68), with which it may be confused. *f* waves may be fine or coarse, or, as here, in between. When they are coarse and relatively large, distinction between flutter and fibrillation is not always clear, and probably not important. Both represent very rapid atrial ectopy with second degree AV block (132).

This tracing is otherwise probably with normal limits. The computer called an old anterior infarct, presumably on the basis of the QSV1-2, and that may be correct, but those complexes are too clean and narrow to be abnormal by themselves. The clinical history is critical...as always. To accept a computer readout as a substitute for judgment puts the patient at inappropriate risk.

EKG 89

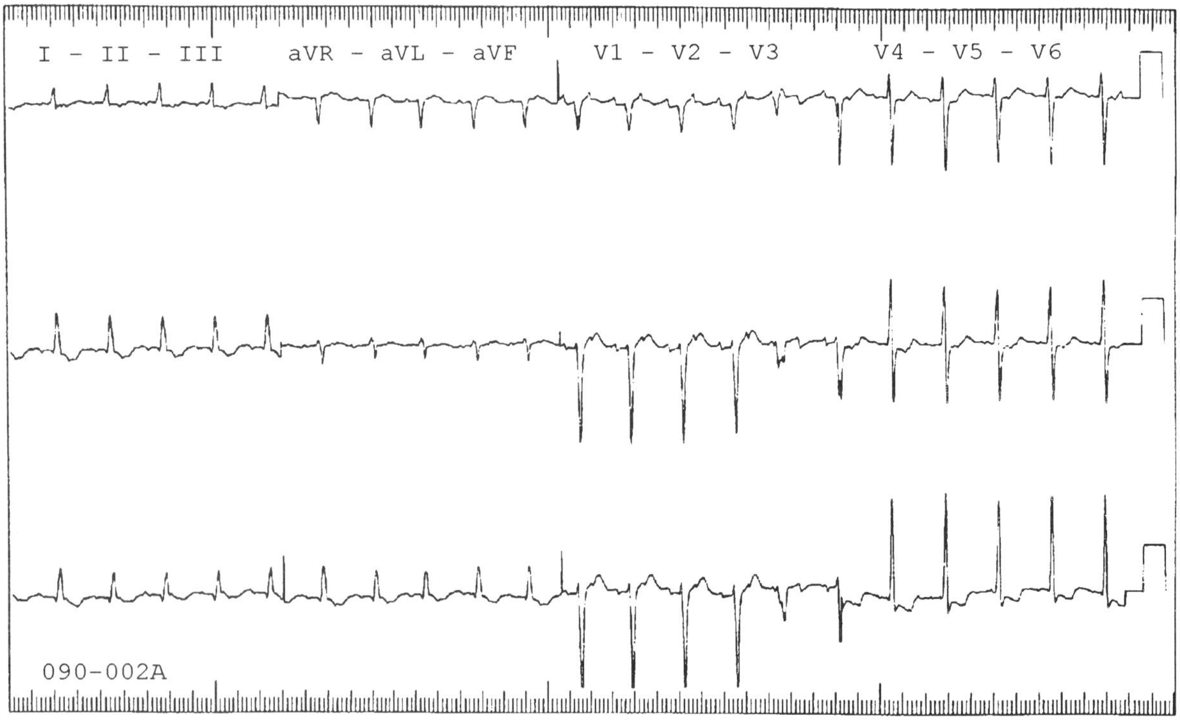


```
260  130  --  08  28  see below
+60  0:5   V5   20:2      normal
       slightly down V4-6
            flattened
-105  ±V1, pos V2-5 low, neg V6

(1) Atrial flutter, 260/130
(2) ST-T abnormalities with
    elements to suggest both
    LVO and cor insufficiency
```

Atrial Flutter

This is a good example of atrial flutter (129), defined as usurping atrial ectopy with regular rhythm and second degree AV block, a definition that includes common and uncommon forms, fixed and varying AV conduction, and what some would call atrial tachycardia with block. Atrial activity may show as a continuously undulating trace with a "picket fence" appearance in II, III, and aVF, or the trace may be flat between Ps. The definition above implies nothing about how the ectopy was initiated or sustained, or whether it may be short lived or chronic. It just names what is seen in the tracing. The answers to the other considerations may influence decisions as to the course of action to be taken, but must be supplied by the patient's doctor, aware of the available options and applying judgment as to which is in the patient's best interests. In this tracing, the computer noted "unusual P axis, possible ectopic atrial tachycardia", useful observations but not an interpretation. Anything is possible, any mechanism not of sinus origin is ectopic, and, having noted that the ventricular rate is 130, to say that it is fast (tachy) adds nothing.

See also EKGs 90–93 from the same patient.

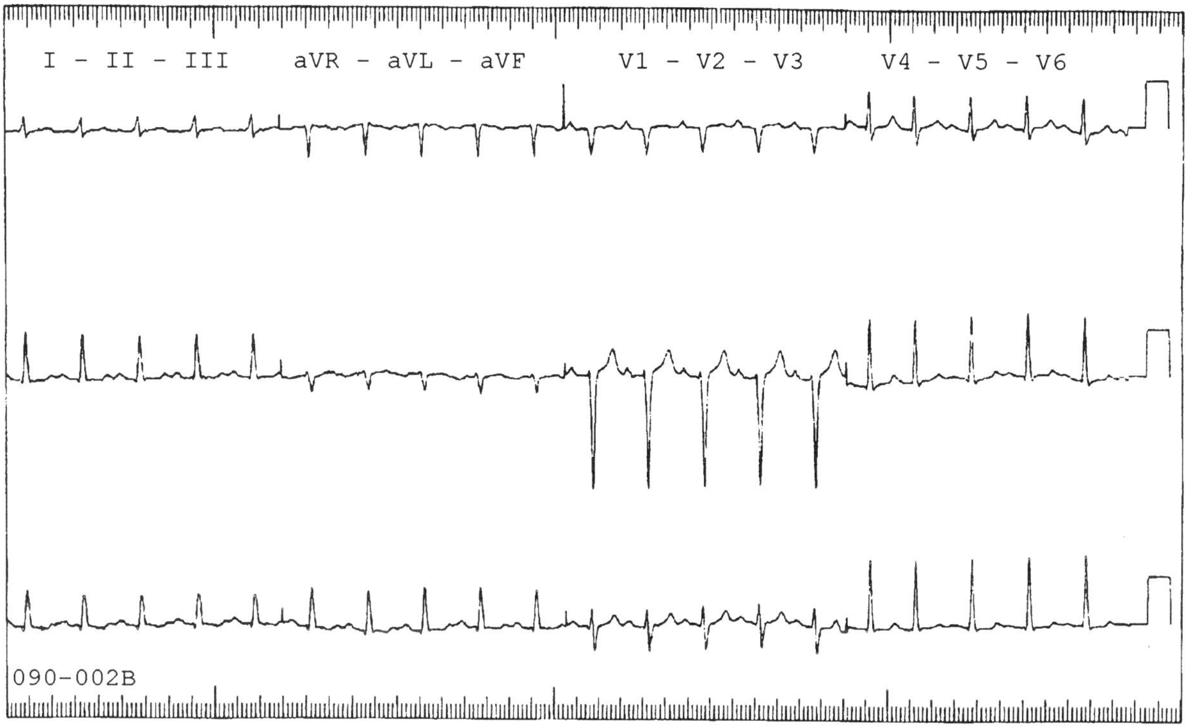

Sinus Mechanism, ST-T Abnormalities, Nonspecific

```
120    120   16    08    32     sinus
+75    0:5     V3    15:0     normal
                none
          related to T
low    ±V1      pos V2-4      ±V5-6

(1) Sinus mechanism, rate 120,
    with one PAC
(2) ST-T abnormalities, non-
    specific

--just low T voltage, not far
  from normal
```

It is worth calling attention to some things that are so routine that they are not always thought of as potentially important. First, though small, P waves are large enough to tell that they are clearly oriented caudad and ventrad (positive in aVF and V1), indicating a sinus origin (27, 70, 123). Their rhythm is regular within the limits of normal change with respiration, and their rate is 120/min. Also, to cite a PR interval at all is to say that each QRS is a result of the same impulse that produced the preceding P. There is one PAC, the fourth beat from the end of the tracing.

T voltage is low (50), a minimal and completely nonspecific abnormality (201). This was not noted by the computer, but the criterion the program uses to define low is not known.

See also EKGs 89 and 91–93 from the same patient.

EKG 91

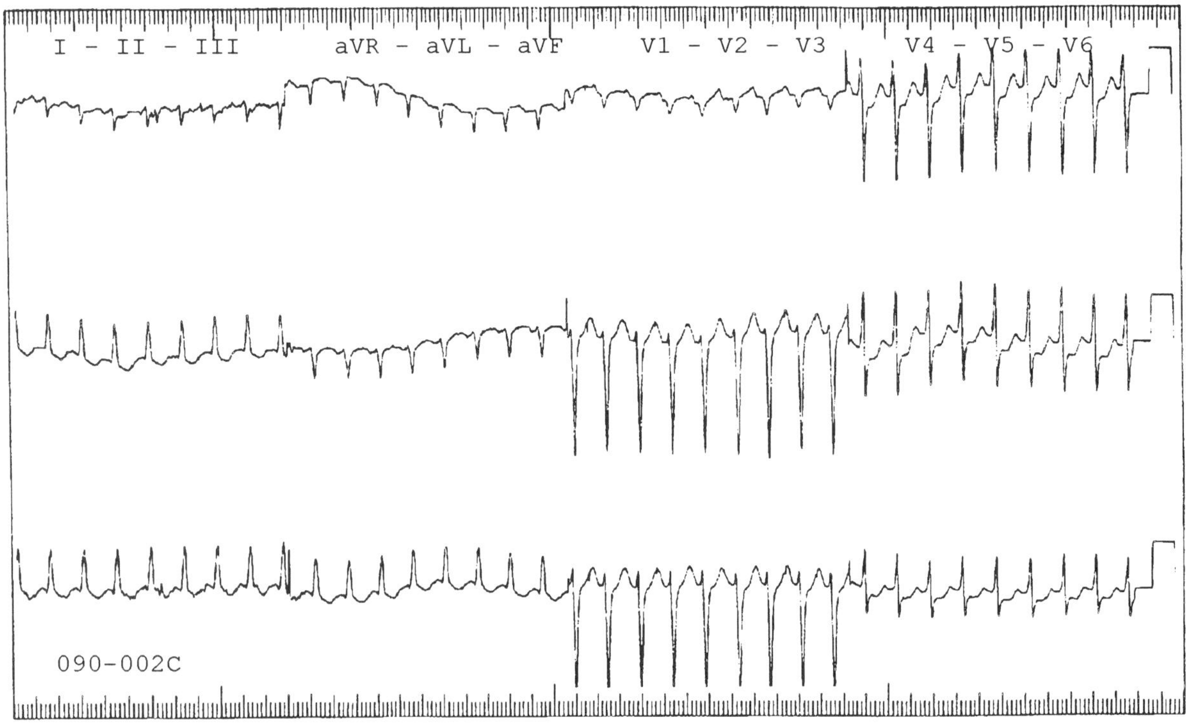

"1:1 Flutter," "SVT," "AVNR," etc.

```
200   200   08   ?24         see below
+105    0:3   V4½    8:3    normal
            down V4-6
            flattened
low -90   ?+V1    +V2-6    low V6

(1) Ectopic supraventricular
    mechanism, rate 205, with
    regular rhythm, probably
    atrial in origin.  Atrial
    activity is not altogether
    clear
(2) ST-T abnormalities typical
    of subendocardial injury as
    with coronary insufficiency
```

The mechanism in this tracing is of supraventricular origin (25), rate about 200, with regular ventricular rhythm. To be more specific from EKG findings alone would require description of atrial activity, and that is not an option here. A more directly applicable name depends on judgment and the clinical setting. The rate nearly precludes a sinus origin (123), and any origin other than sinus is ectopic. The regularity of ventricular rhythm is against atrial fibrillation (132). It may be junctional, with retrograde P too small to see, or lost in QRS (234). Remember, there is only one point on the paper (121). The term "accelerated junctional mechanism" is sometimes heard, but usually for much slower rates than this, and "accelerated," like "tachy," adds nothing when the rate is specified. "AVNR" (AV nodal reentry), offers a putative explanation for unspecified findings (134, 138). "1:1 flutter" (129) implies what used to be called atrial tachycardia, assumes P waves, and begs the question of defining flutter. The ST-T pattern is typical of subendocardial injury (202, 206). To call this just "SVT" is not to be as precise as possible. See also EKGs 90 and 92–93 from the same patient.

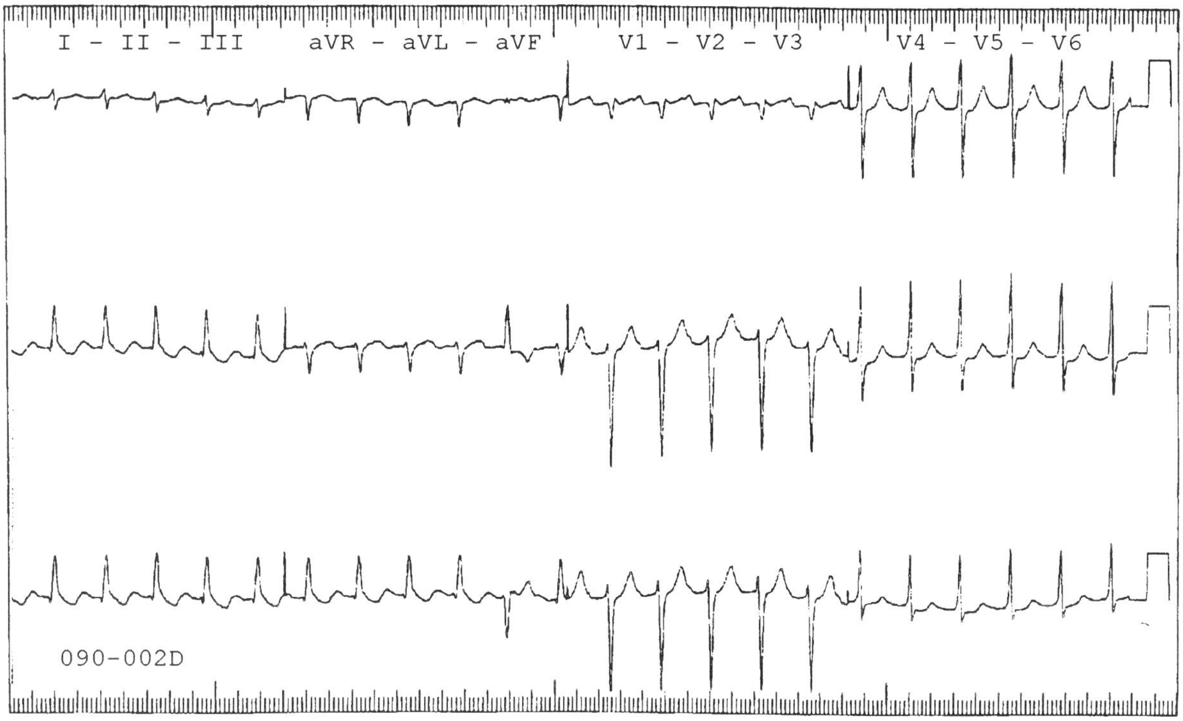

Atrial Flutter

```
270  135   --   08   32  see below
+90    0:3    V4½    12:2    normal
      slightly down V5-6
     straightened/sagging
-75   ±V1     pos V2-6     low V6

(1) Atrial flutter, 270/135
(2) ST-T abnormalities, sug-
    gestive of cor insuf, but
    small.
```

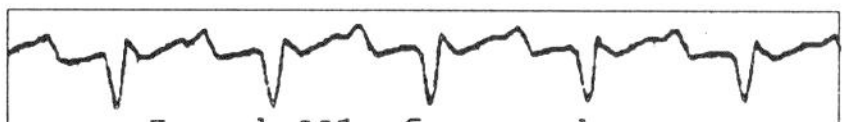

Recognition of the mechanism here calls for a clear understanding of just what a P is (27, 70), and of what is meant by "atrial flutter" (129). Atria and ventricles may function independently, even simultaneously, and there is only one point on the paper recording both. The computer called this sinus, but it is not; there are two Ps for each QRS, one overlapping the last part of every other QRS (inset). The only lead in which this "extra" one can be seen with confidence is V1, where its distal half is continuous with QRS and could be mistaken for small terminal R The feature that identifies it as a P is its downstroke which is exactly the same as that of the more readily identifiable biphasic ±P overlapping the end of T. Other points that this tracing illustrates are the critical importance of defining the baseline by some criterion other than extrapolation from either TU segment or PQ, and the problem of defining the onset of P, and, thus, the length of PR.

See also EKGs 90–91 and 93 from the same patient.

The Problem of Naming Usurping Atrial Ectopy

V1 from EKGs 89, 90, 91, and 92, original size

P waves are seen best in V1 in all four tracings, illustrating different forms of supraventricular tachycardia. They have been arranged on this page for easy comparison of the differences in morphology of P that can occur, even in the same lead, reflecting the locus of the focus driving the atria.

One shows a sinus mechanism. There are two examples of flutter, and the meaning of "SVT" is ill defined.

The evidence of subendocardial injury in EKG 91 may be related to shortening of diastole with the very rapid rate.

Review the 12-lead tracings and note that the mechanism is not the only thing that changes. Orientation, amplitude, and contour of QRS and ST-T vary also. All these tracings are from the same patient. Tracing A was made March 1; B, November 4 of the preceding year; C and D, 13 minutes apart on November 9, five days after B.

EKG findings are not always constant. Awareness of this increases with experience at describing all aspects of every tracing in a series.

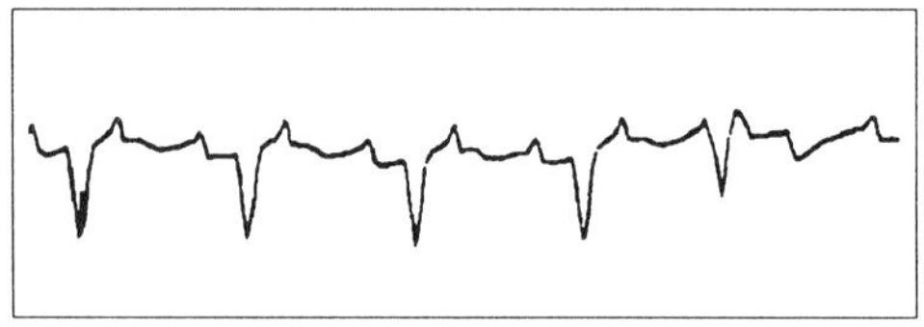

A V1 from EKG #89
Atrial flutter, 260/130

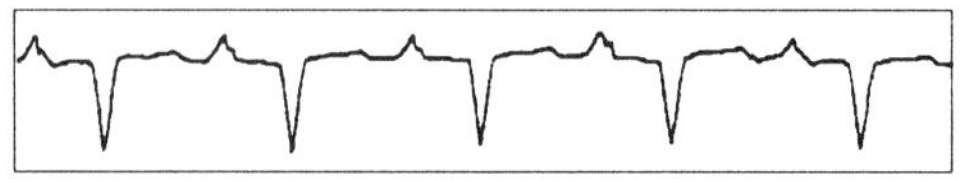

B V1 from EKG #90
Sinus mechanism, rate 120

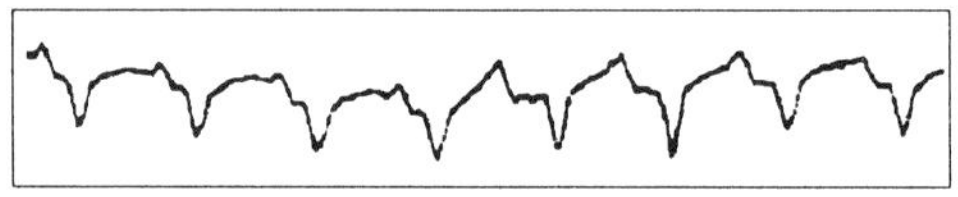

C V1 from EKG #91
"1:1 flutter","SVT",rate 205

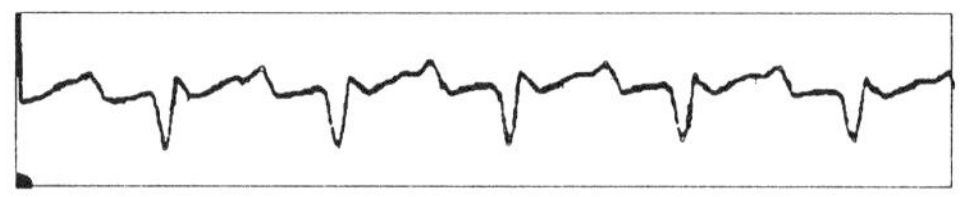

D V1 from EKG #92
Atrial flutter, 270/135

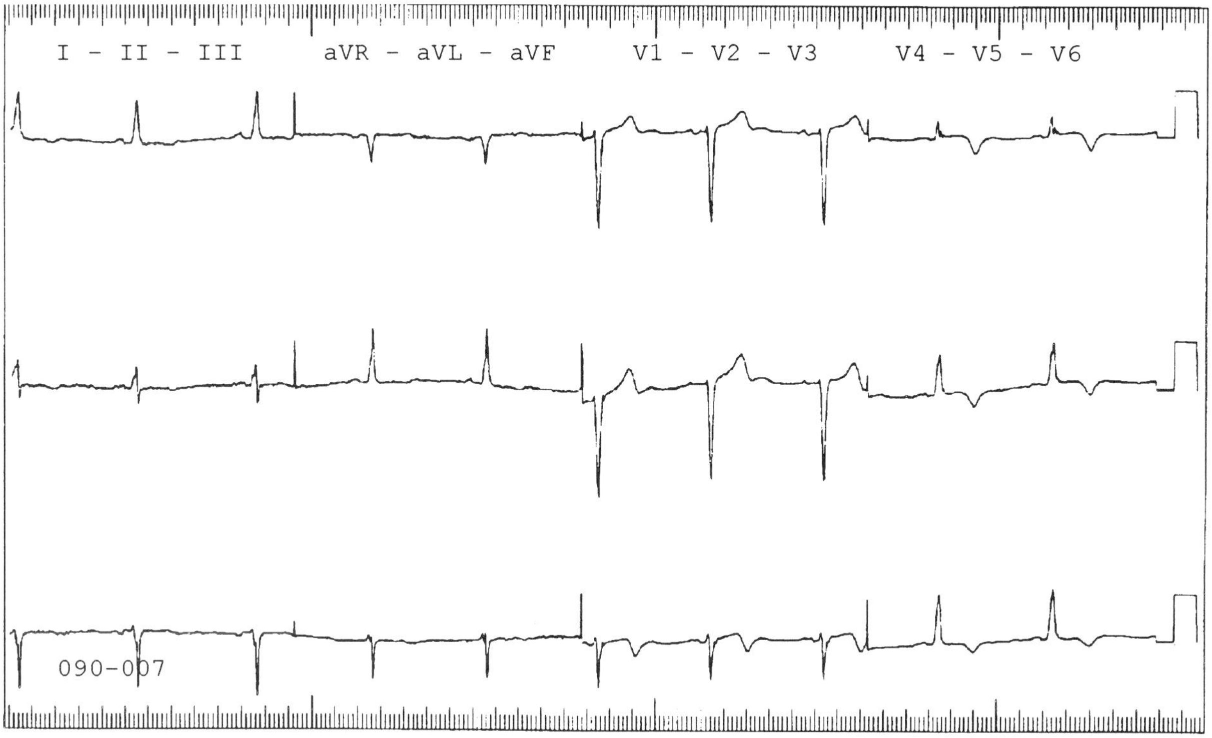

Mid-Precordial T Negativity

60	60	16	10	40	sinus
-15	1:10	V3½	10:0		normal
		none			
	related to T (see below)				
low	pos V1-2, neg V3-6, symmetrical				

(1) Sinus mechanism, rate 60
(2) ST-T abnormalities, probably evidence of coronary insufficiency

All ST-T abnormalities are nonspecific, but some fall into patterns that are useful, and this is one of them, suggesting coronary insufficiency. The repolarization complex is a continuous curve whose proximal part, ST, can be analyzed separately from its distal part, T (43). In this tracing, its duration, the QT interval, is normal, there is no ST displacement, and ST contour is described best as a function of T. T is abnormal in that it is oriented dorsad, deeper in leads between V1 and V6 than in either of those, and symmetrical (211). Clinical experience justifies interpreting this picture as suggestive of coronary insufficiency in most instances. Negative T waves are often called "inverted" and seen as evidence of ischemia. Ischemia, discrepancy between supply and demand for blood (really for oxygen), is the final common pathway by which most EKG abnormalities in adults are mediated, but the tracing shows its results; e.g., atrial fibrillation, myocardial infarction, bundle branch block, or ST-T patterns, not ischemia per se. The etymologic implication of the word is impairment of flow, and this is what most of us are likely to hear, but demand is equally important, and increase in that, usually left ventricular overload, produces a different pattern (see EKGs 7 and 112).

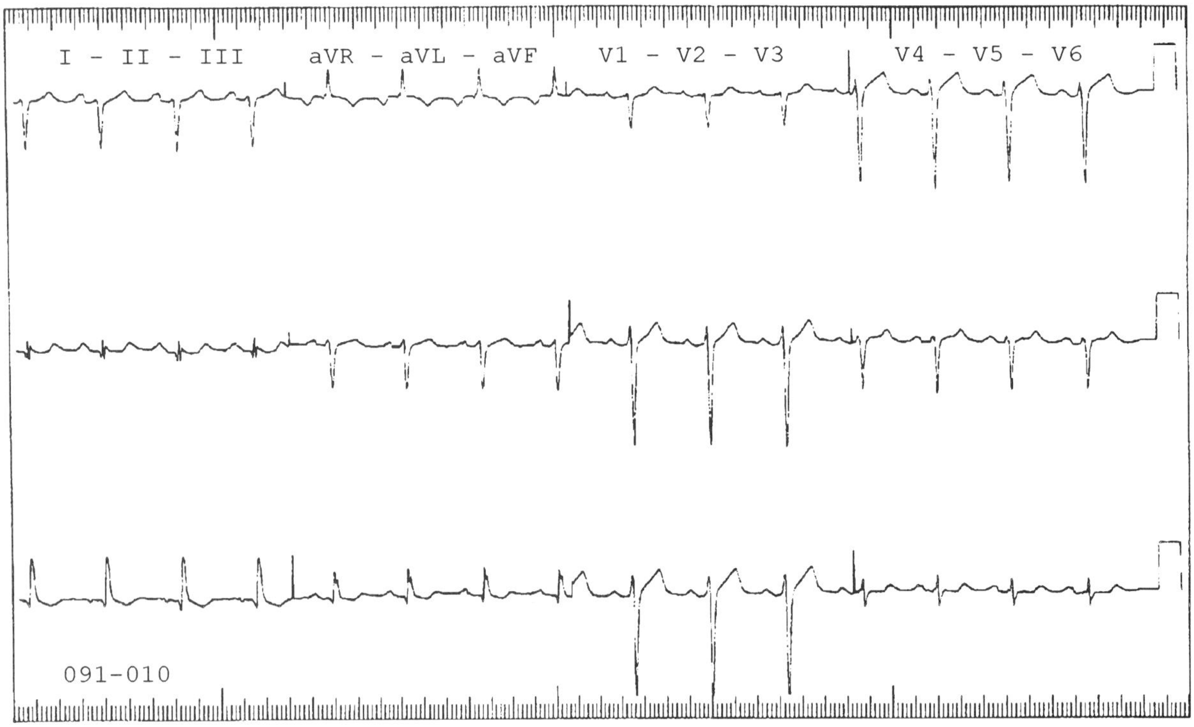

Left Posterior Fascicular Block

90	90	20	08	36	sinus
+150	1:7	V6	4:3		normal
		none			
		normal			
±0		positive V1-6			

(1) Sinus mechanism, rate 90
(2) Left posterior fascicular block
(3) Otherwise WNL

Left anterior fascicular block (EKGs 36 and 39) is widely accepted as an explanation for marked "left axis deviation" when initial forces are normal and there is no other explanation for it, but left posterior fascicular block (165) is invoked only rarely for the comparable picture with "right axis deviation" (MFQRS more clockwise than about +120°), and the idea of left anterior septal fascicular block (165) has not caught on at all. All three seem to make sense, but proof of any of them is tenuous at best. There is no reasonable doubt about the anatomic and physiologic reality of right and left bundles (though not many of us have ever seen either), but demonstration of anatomically discrete components of them, much less blocking of one, necessary for validation of the EKG diagnosis, is hard to come by.

The proposed criteria for LPFB (marked clockwise direction of MFQRS with normal initial QRS forces) overlap those for both normal and right ventricular enlargement so much, and the blood supply in the hypothesized area is so much more redundant than that in the anterior myocardium, that a diagnosis of LPFP is rarely justified (165).

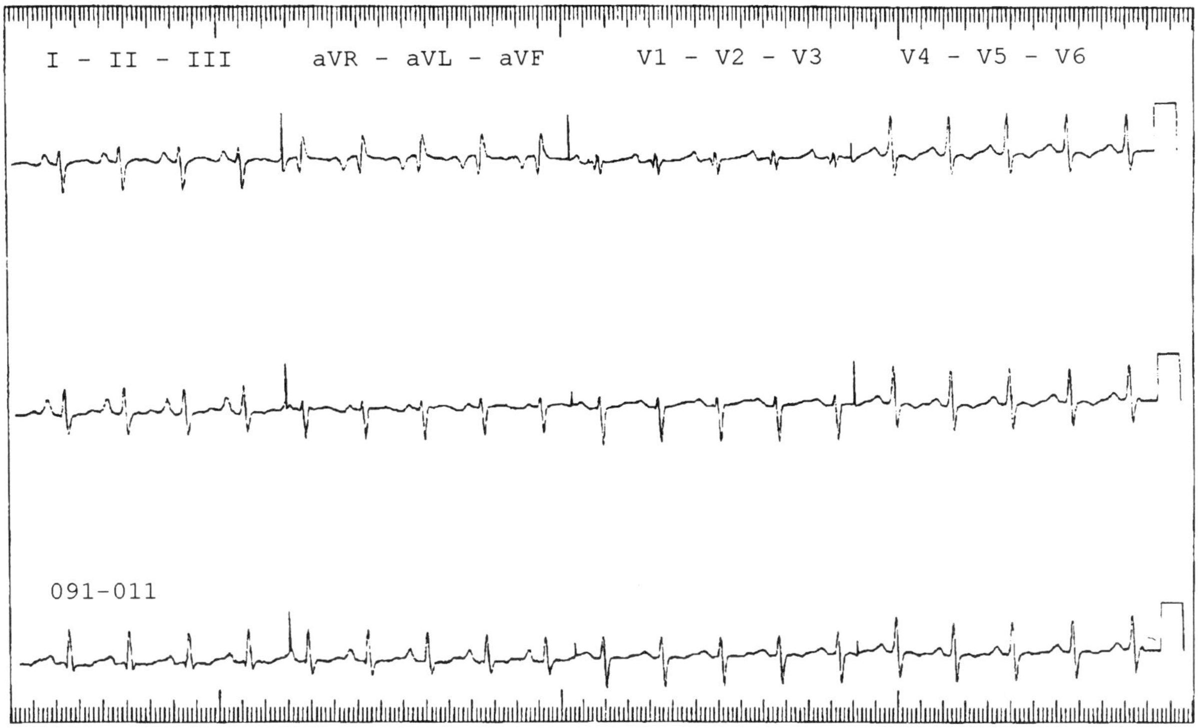

Right Atrial Enlargement, Right Ventricular Enlargement

```
115   115   16   08    --      sinus
+135   QRS 1:1:2   --   8:5 normal
                none
          related to T
low            ± V1-6
P: prominent, peaked II, III, F

(1) Sinus mechanism, rate 115
(2) Right atrial enlargement
(3) Right ventricular enlarge-
    ment
(4) ST-T abnormalities, non-
    specific
```

The atria are depolarized sequentially, right first, followed by left, an important difference from the simultaneous depolarization of the ventricles. The process is directed leftward and downward, initially ventrad, and terminally dorsad, explaining the small notch in P2 just past its peak, and the plus/minus configuration in V1, a pattern found, in some degree, in most of the P waves in this collection. When an atrium is required to pump more volume per time (flow), or work against increased resistance, it responds by becoming larger, either hypertrophy and/or dilatation. In the case of the right atrium, this shows in the initial component. The notch becomes smaller, and the result is a prominent, peaked, nearly symmetrical P in II, III, and aVF, with or without a comparable increase in initial positivity in V1 (29, 287, 232).

Evidence of enlargement of the right ventricle (40, 193) (EKGs 80 and 96), as here, strengthens the diagnosis of right atrial enlargement.

T voltage is low in this tracing, a minimal abnormality not related specifically to either of the other lesions.

EKG 97

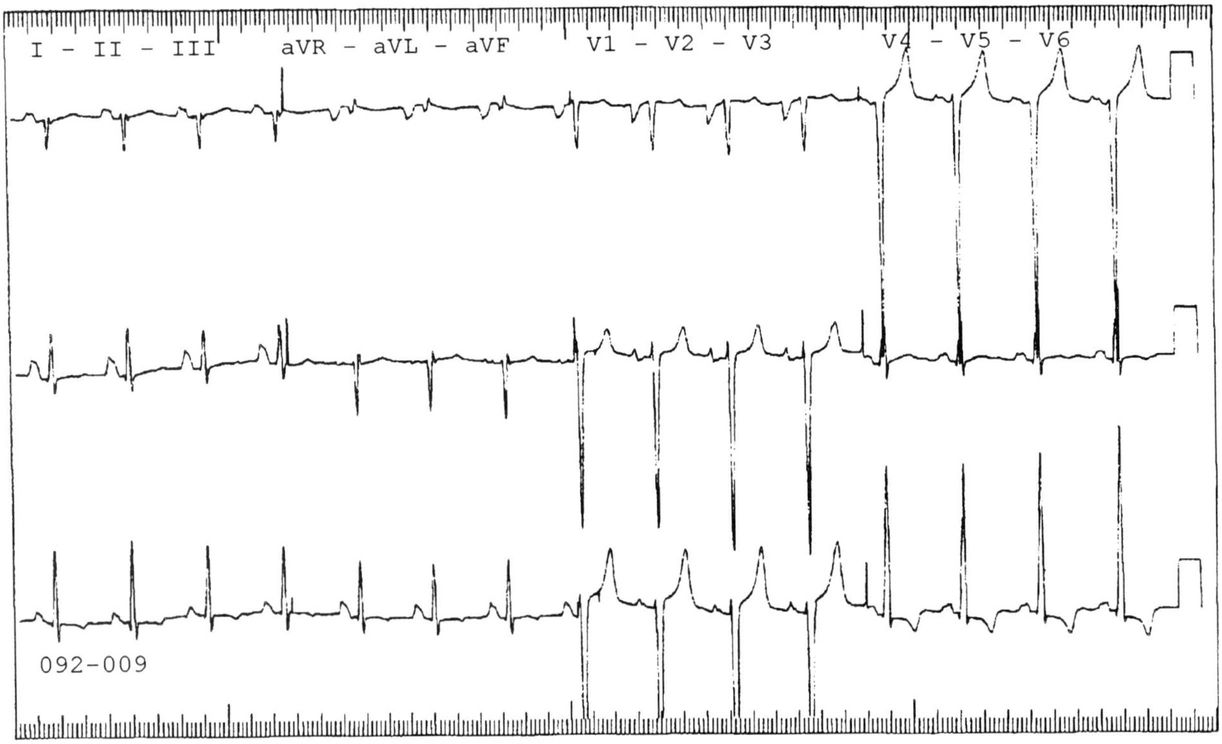

Right Atrial Enlargement, Left Atrial Enlargement

90	90	16	08	36	sinus
+120	0:10	V5	35:2		normal
		slightly down V6 related to T			
low	±V1	+V2-4	±V5		neg V6

(1) Sinus mechanism, rate 90
(2) Right atrial enlargement
(3) Left atrial enlargement
(4) ST-T abns, suggestive of left ventricular overload

"Enlargement" does not distinguish between dilatation and hypertrophy. EKG evidence of atrial enlargement probably reflects mostly dilatation, change in volume rather in mass. Not only is it likely to be transient, often changing within hours in response to change in the lungs, which hypertrophy would not be expected to do, but also atrial hypertrophy is hard to define quantitatively, even at autopsy. Both the prominent, peaked P2,3,F, pointing to the right atrium, and the large, terminal, negative component of PV1, pointing to the left (29, 187, 232), are beyond cavil in this tracing. The plain visibility of both is a beautiful example of the relevance of Einthoven's hypotheses (86), and of the importance of thinking in three dimensions (87). The first part of P originates in the right atrium and is parallel to the frontal plane; the last part, in the left, and perpendicular to the frontal plane. There is no cancellation of potential (181), a fundamental that, applied to QRS, precludes recognition of hypertrophy of both ventricles. Nonetheless, the "right axis deviation" (37, 226), and an ST-T pattern suggestive left ventricular overload (211), in this tracing may imply overload of both (148). Note the inconstancy of QRS voltage in V5 and V6.

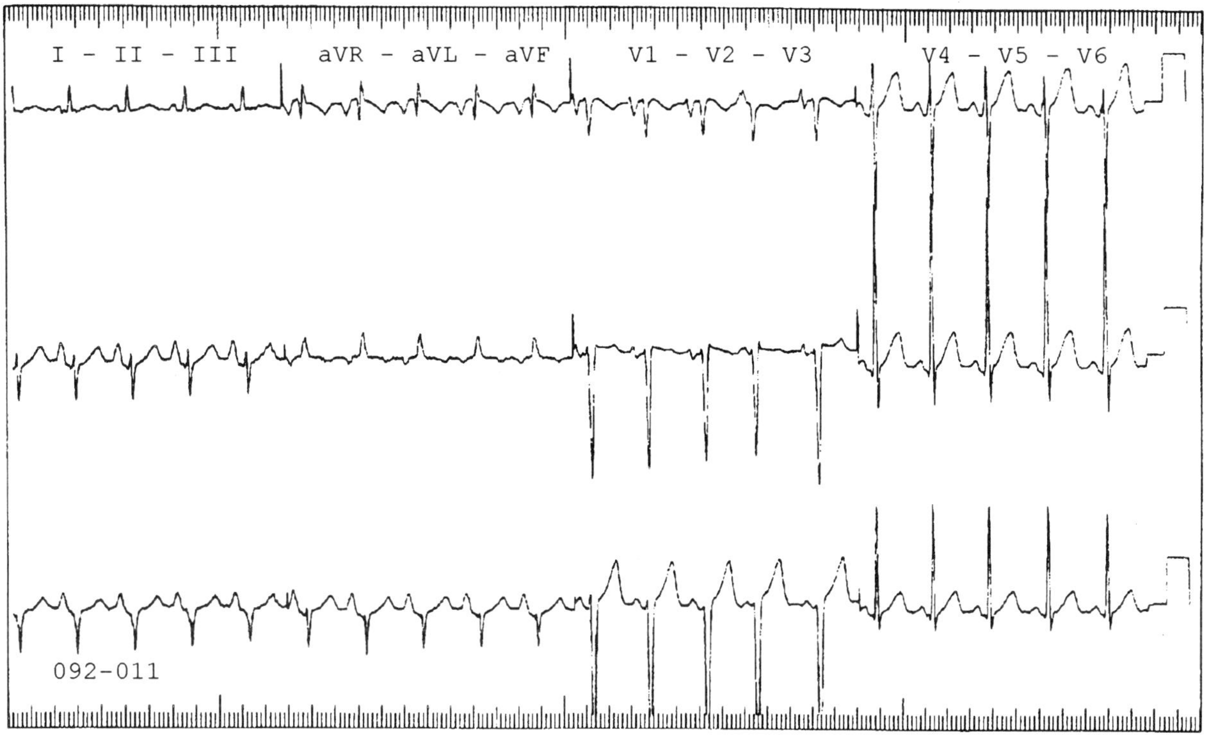

Right Atrial Enlargement, Left Anterior Fascicular Block

An impulse arising in the sinus node spreads centrifugally over the atria, progressing leftward and downward, initially anteriorly, dominated by the right atrium, and finally posteriorly, ending in the left. The atria act electrically as a curved plane, i.e., no thickness. Abnormalities of both atria can be recognized in the same tracing. The ventricles, in contrast, depolarize simultaneously, radially, through a considerable thickness. The position of the trace at any instant during the QRS represents the net of both, but cannot be interpreted as evidence of two things; recognition of biventricular hypertrophy is beyond the limits of the method.

Prominent, peaking of P2 and P3 (inset) was correlated with lung disease very early in the history of electrocardiography, and became known as "P pulmonale." aVF is included now. The pattern is explained by loss of compliance of the right ventricle, which increases the resistance against which the atrium works, but does not change QRS. Evidence in this tracing for an old inferior infarct, and/or left anterior fascicular block, is equivocal (164).

```
120    120    12    08    32   sinus
-60    0:7    V3½    20:3     QS3,F
              none
             normal
+75   neg V1     ±V2      pos V3-6
P: tall, peaked II, III, aVF,
   prominent terminal negativ-
   ity V1

(1) Sinus mechanism, rate 120
(2) Right atrial enlargement
(3) Left ant fascicular block,
    and/or old inf mci, prob
(4) Left atrial enl, probable
(5) Otherwise WNL
```

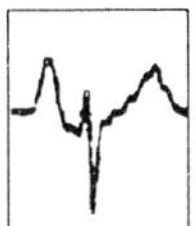

Lead II

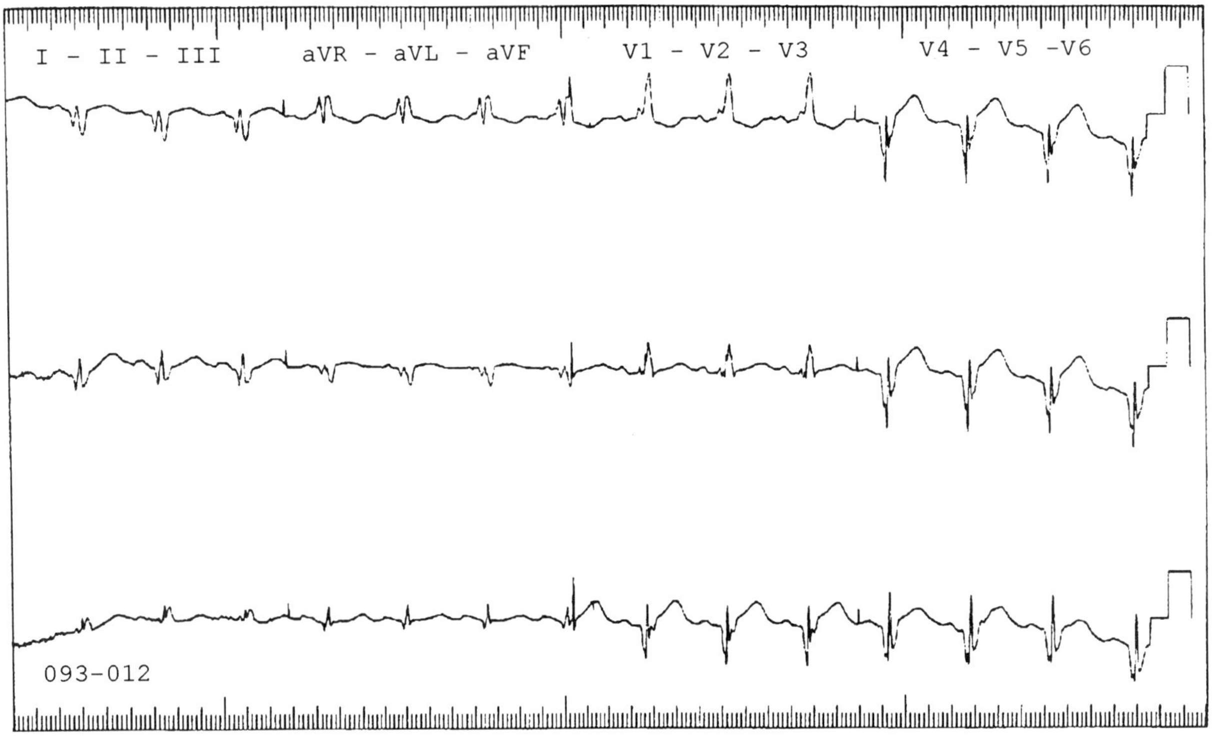

Right Bundle Branch Block, Anterolateral Myocardial Infarct

```
85   85   16   10   40      sinus
+135,10:0,V3,QRS6:6:5  Q1,L,V3-6
          up V4-6
       related to T
low+60   flat V1-2,   pos V3-6

(1) Sinus mechanism, rate 85
(2) Right bundle branch block
(3) Anterolateral myo infarct,
    age indeterminate
```

There are several possible explanations for widening of QRS, i.e., slowing of ventricular depolarization (168). In this case, the abnormality is limited to the last part of the process. Excitation there is slow, directed to the right and forward, and produces a contour that is a little irregular. Stated differently, there is a broad, slurred S in Lead I, and a similar terminal R in V1, findings easily understood as evidence of block of the right bundle branch (159).

Myocardial infarction produces changes in the initial part of QRS (174), seen here as an abnormal Q in V3-6, the front of the chest, anterior, and I and aVL, the left side of the chest, lateral (177). (The view from V6 can be considered either anterior and/or lateral; a line can be in more than one plane.) The age of the infarct is indeterminate because, though ST is displaced, suggesting a recent origin, its contour is not clearly abnormal.

There is (or there may be) such a thing, though ill defined, as peri-infarction block (168, 184), and that may be a factor here in addition to RBBB.

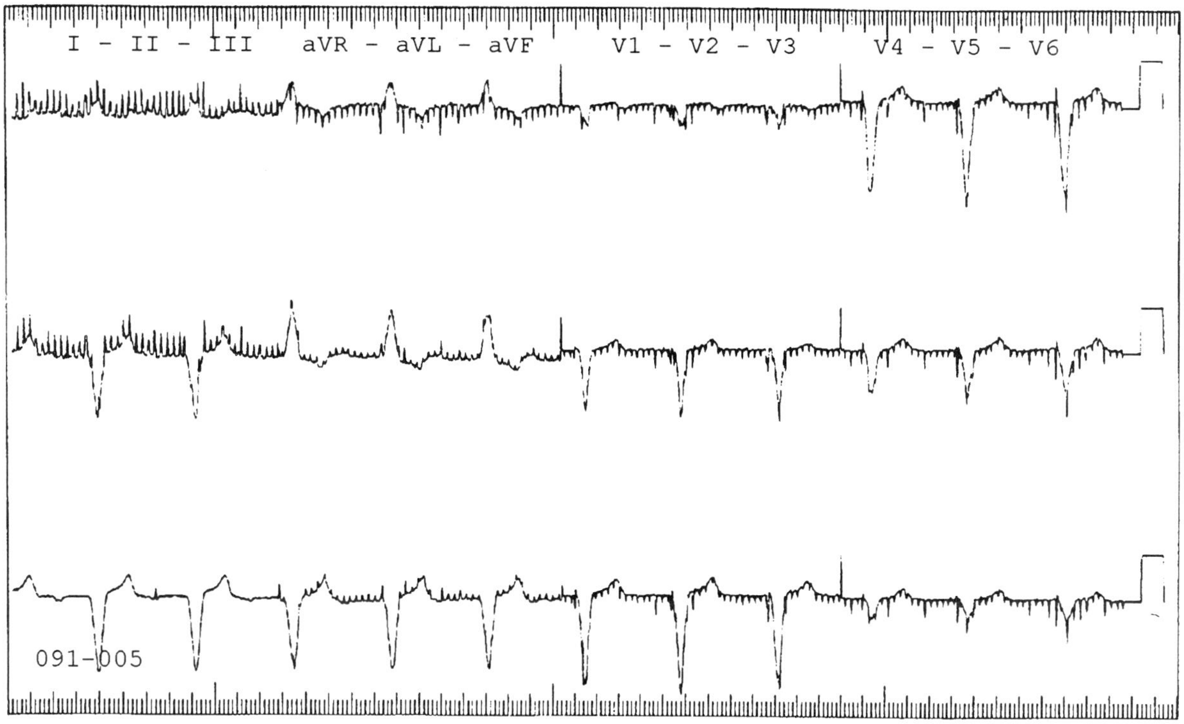

Minute Ventilation Pacemaker

--	70	--	44+	see below
-75	0:3	--	0:5	diff slur

none
not remarkable
+90 neg V1 pos V2-6

(1) Atrial activity is not clear
(2) Artificial ventricular PM capturing regularly, rate 70

--The spike at 25/sec is a function of this pacemaker.

A minute ventilation pacemaker generates a signal at a rate of 25/s, the artifact in this tracing that is received at another point in the system and correlated with respiratory rate. Increase in respiratory rate is taken as evidence of the need for more oxygen, and results in a greater rate of the stimulus delivered to the ventricles. Limitations of the method include other explanations for tachypnea, e.g., reaction to exercise and response to movements not related to respiration. The pacemaker is capturing regularly in this tracing, but its spike is not always distinct from the 25-cps one. Atrial activity is not clear; the small negative wave 0.32 s. before the first QRS in Lead III may be a P.

Presence of the artifact in Leads I and II, and not III (the two spikes in Lead III are of uncertain origin), implies imperfect connection of the patient cable to the right arm. In a tracing made the day after this one, the only spike was that of the pacemaker introducing each QRS. QRSs were the same as here. Atrial activity was still not clear.

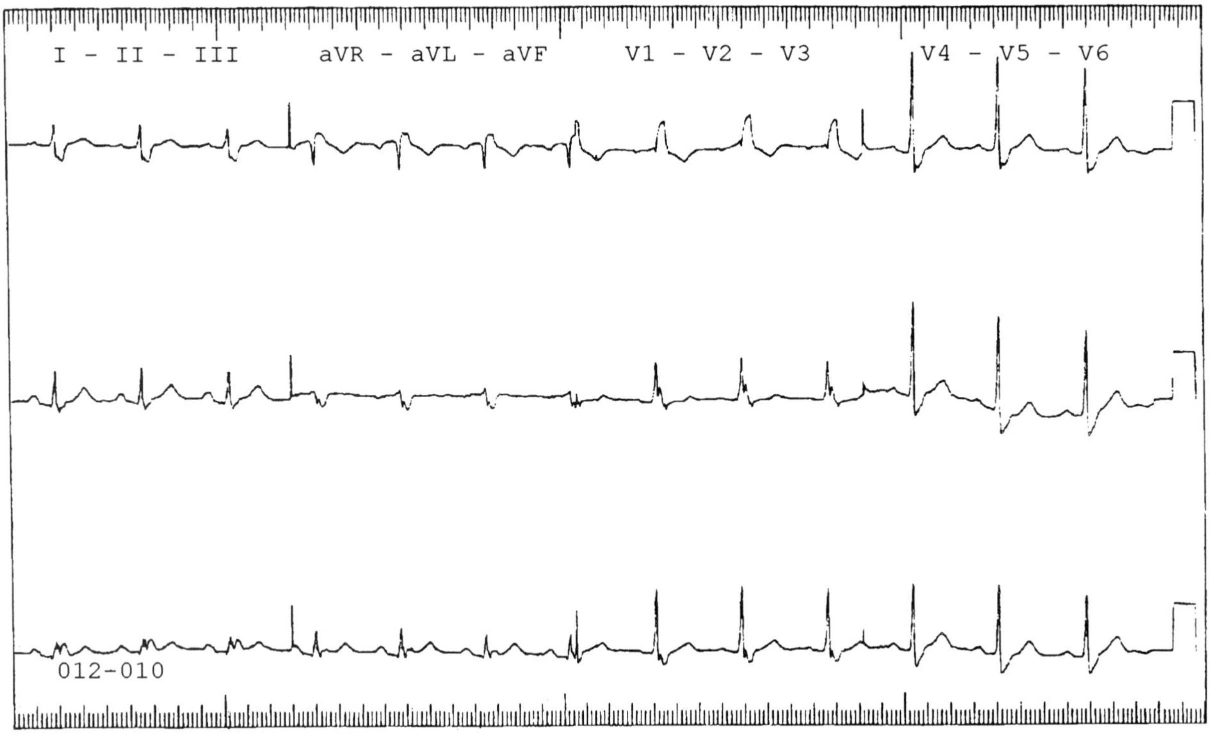

Right Bundle Branch Block

This is typical right bundle branch block, and within normal limits in all other respects (159). QRS is wide as a result of change limited to its distal part. It begins with sharp angles and straight lines, indicating normal pathways and rate, but ends with wide, blunted, curves that are of abnormal contour, ragged/slurred/notched, indicating a slower rate and an abnormal course whose direction, rightward and ventrad, implies delayed activation of the right ventricle, something that would be the logical result of block of the right branch of the bundle of His.

ST-T is of normal duration, amplitude, and contour, and oriented opposite the blocked part of QRS, suggesting that myocardial function is unimpaired.

```
80    80    20    16    40     sinus
--   rsR/1:1:6   --   15:5   BSTDRA
              none
             normal
+60   neg V1   ±V2   positive V3-6

(1) Sinus mechanism, rate 80
(2) Right bundle branch block
(3) Otherwise WNL
```

To give a figure for the frontal QRS axis in this tracing would be specious, Procrustean, beyond the limits of the method. QRSV1 could be described as either rsR, 1:1:6, or just an R wave, 6:0.

The diagnosis of bundle branch block identifies a local lesion in a specific structure, but says nothing about its etiology or permanence.

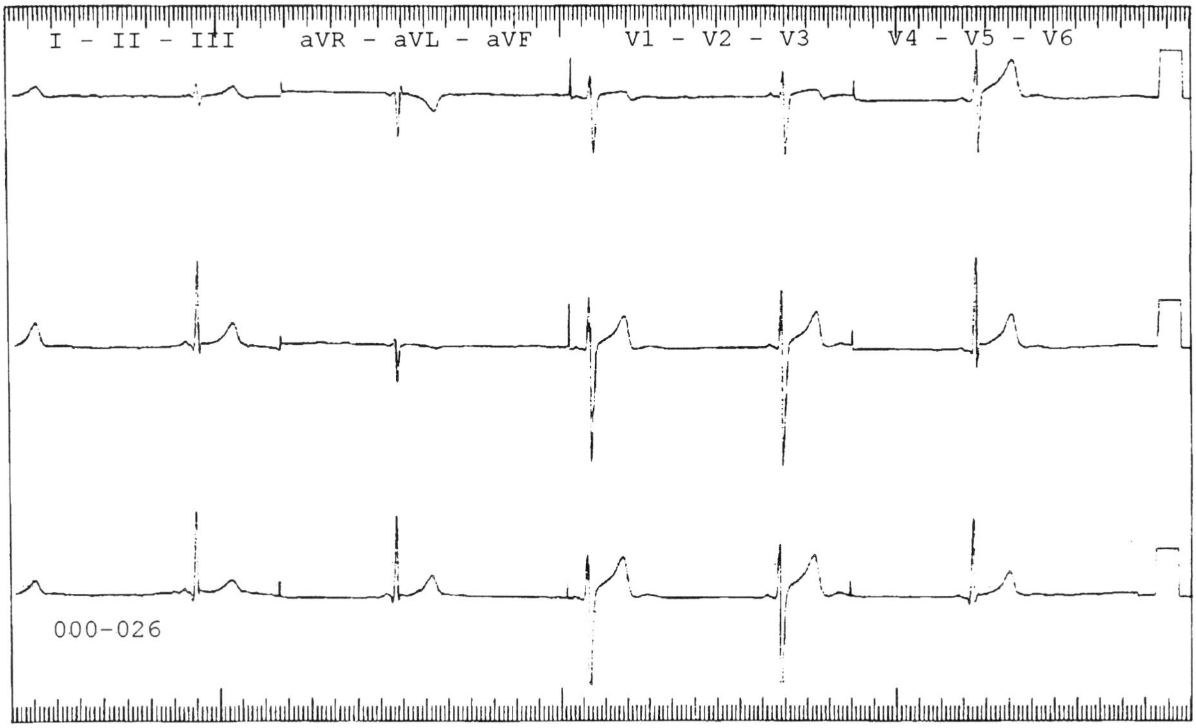

Sinus Bradycardia, Within Normal Limits

35 35 12 08 44 sinus
+75 5:12 V4 15:1 normal
slightly up V2-6
normal
+60 ±V1 positive V2-6

(1) Sinus mechanism, rate 35, with normal AV conduction
(2) Within normal limits

The doctor who ordered the tracing already knew the rate and rhythm, and did not need to be told that it was slow. What the EKG shows that cannot be known otherwise is the mechanism. If the patient is a 21-year-old athlete with no complaints, someone whose EKG was made for insurance purposes, or who is on medication known to slow heart rate, little significance would be attached to a rate this slow. If, however, the patient is 70-years-old and has a history of seizures, the rate raises the question of AV block, and the information in the tracing is critical. When the one reporting it does not know the clinical setting, it is useful to add that AV conduction is normal. The computer program in this case failed to recognize the P waves and called the mechanism "junctional bradycardia." In the absence of detectable atrial activity, with a ventricular rate this slow, and a narrow QRS, that would be a reasonable interpretation of the mechanism (19, 125, 243), but to add that 35 is slow is superfluous. P waves are small, but their orientation, duration, amplitude, and contour are normal, there is one for each QRS, and PR is not prolonged. QRS and ST-T are normal, and so is the tracing.

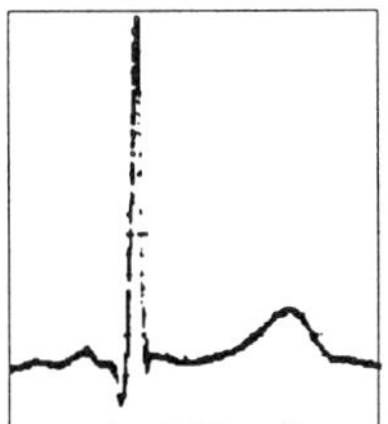
Lead III from above

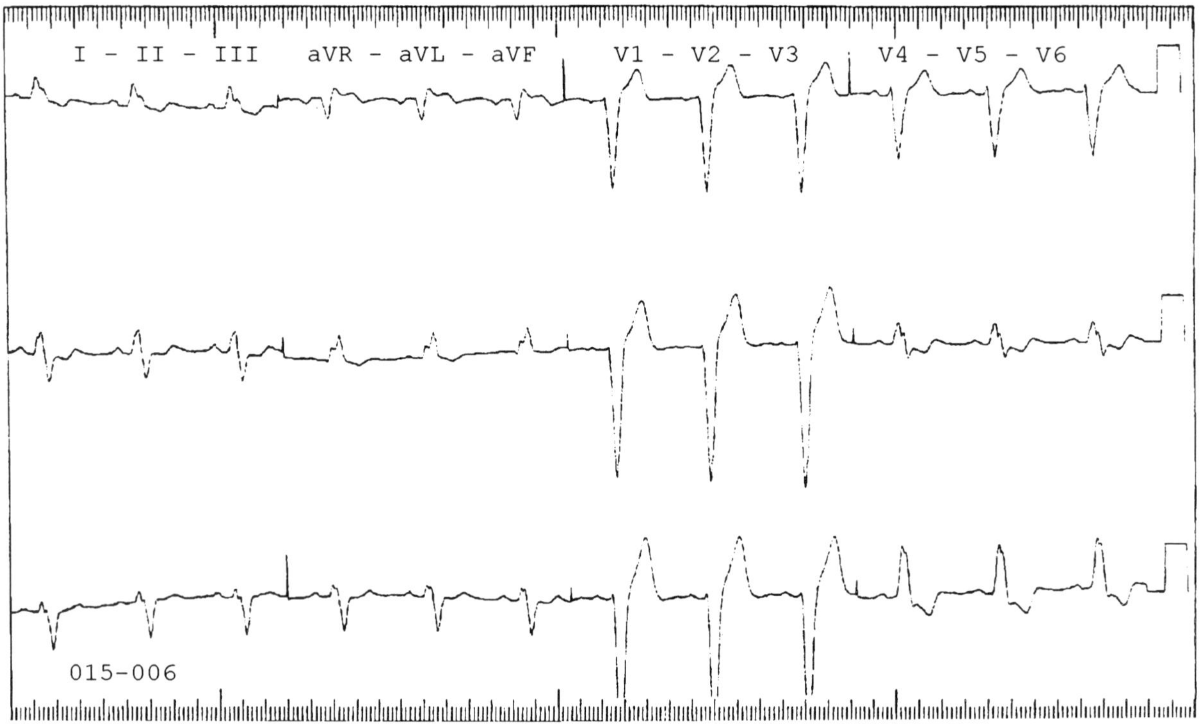

Left Bundle Branch Block

```
70    70    16    16    40     sinus
-30    0:20    V4½    10:0     DSLP
      down V5-6, sl up aVR
           related to T
low ?+120   +V1-4,   ±V5,   neg V6

(1) Sinus mechanism, rate 70
(2) Left bundle branch block
(3) Otherwise prob WNL

--The ST-T pattern is equivocal.
  It may represent coronary
  insufficiency.
```

This tracing is typical of left bundle branch block (complete, proximal, predivisional), a very common finding. There are two abnormalities, duration and contour of QRS. It is wide (168), and its contour can be described, in leads to which QRS is nearly parallel, as an initial stroke almost perpendicular to the baseline, a ragged top that is more or less horizontal, and a straight return stroke nearly parallel to the initial one. Its orientation is not an important consideration, but most of the ventricular myocardium is in the left ventricle, and, as in the normal heart, the QRS is usually directed to the left and back. The characteristic pattern is seen best in leads whose positive poles on the left, I, aVL, II, and V6, or, for the opposite view, anterior, V1

ST-T is hard to describe in tracings with bundle branch block, but, given normal myocardial electrophysiology, it is usually directed opposite to the blocked part of QRS. In this case, the depression in left leads is enough to raise a question of coronary insufficiency.

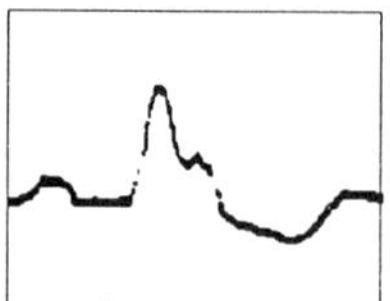
I from above

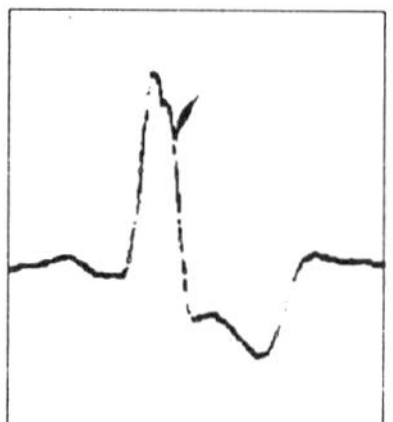
V6 from above

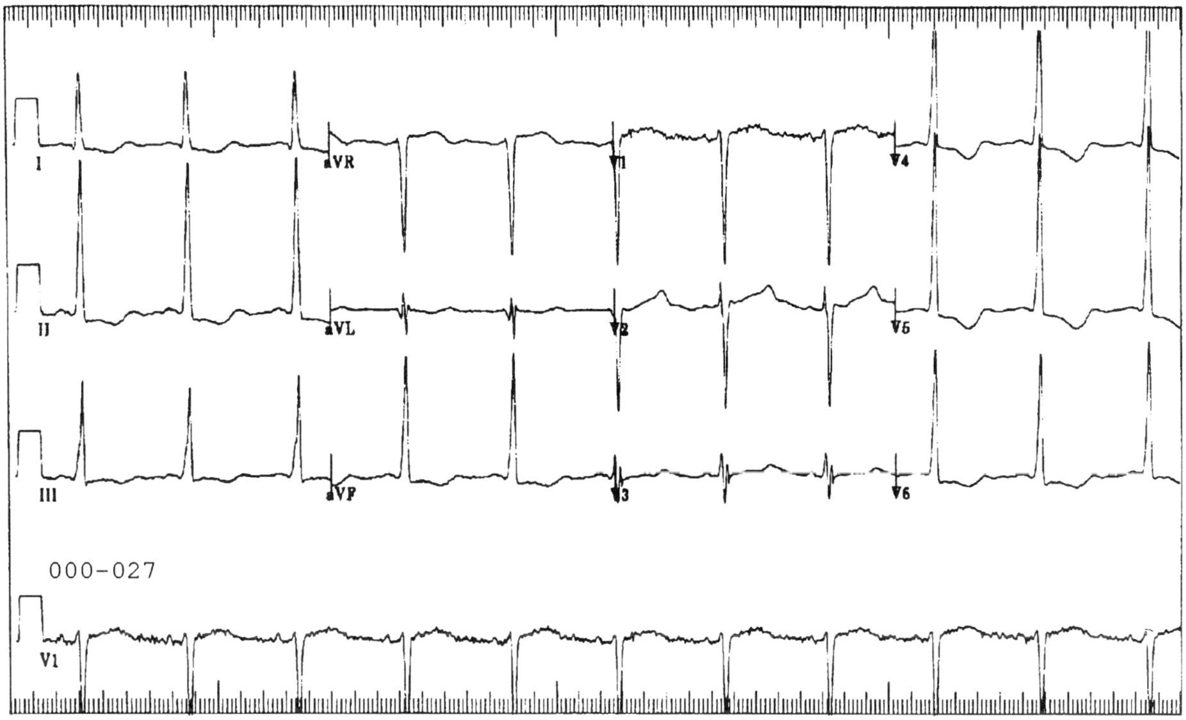

Left Ventricular Hypertrophy and Strain

```
65    65    16    10    ?44     sinus
+60    1:25    V3    25:1     normal
     slightly down II, V5-6
             normal
low   ±V1, +V2, ±V3, neg V4-6
U: inseparable from T

(1) Sinus mechanism, rate 65
(2) Left ventricular hypertrophy
(3) ST-T abnormalities, prob LVO
```

Hypertrophy of a muscle, increase in cell size, is a response to an increase in demand for work, overload. It is an anatomic change, and may or may not be identifiable in the EKG. When it is, it shows in the QRS; specifically, its ampli-tude. Overload, or strain, a functional change, precedes hyper-trophy and produces change in the more sensitive and less specific repolarization complex (189). Demand for work by a ventricle may be increased by lesions that increase the resistance to its output, those that require it to pump a greater than normal flow, or both. In either case, hypertrophy is secondary, a compensatory response, necessary for maintenance of normal cardiac output. These lesions are all identifiable by physical examination (196), and, assuming this was done before the tracing was ordered, the electrocardiographic diagnosis of left ventricular hypertrophy adds little. Perception of it as evidence of primary disease puts the patient at risk of at least unnecessary procedures. Many criteria for EKG evidence of left ventricular hypertrophy are available in the literature, but some do not distinguish between the physiologic lesion, strain, and its anatomic consequence, hypertrophy. Criteria for the anatomic reality of hypertrophy, by which EKG findings must validated, vary widely.

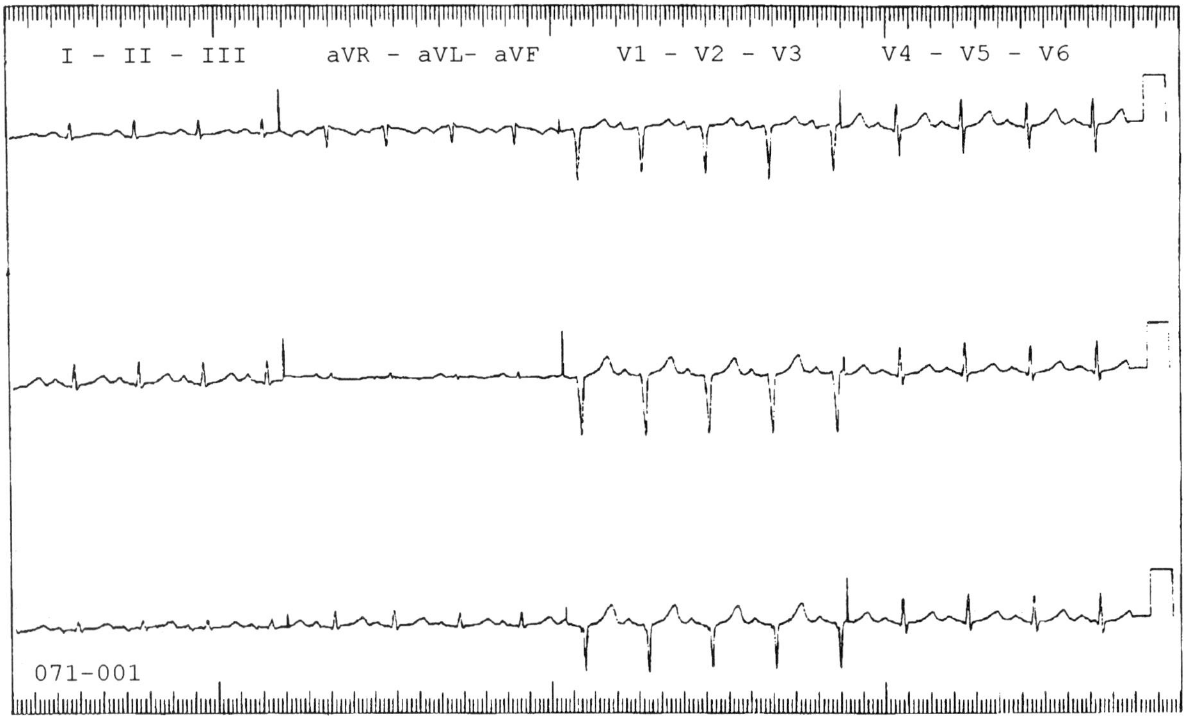

Old Anterior Myocardial Infarct

```
105   105   20   08   40  sinus
+60, 0:10, V4, 6:2, early notch
                           QSV3
             none
            normal
+60        positive V1-6

(1) Sinus mechanism, rate 105
(2) Old ant myo infarct prob
(3) Otherwise WNL

--Nothing looks new.
```

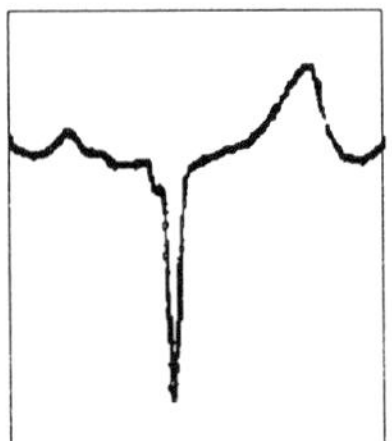

Notch in QSV3 from above

This is a good example of the importance of a tiny component of a tracing con-sidered in context; in this case, abnormality of the initial part of the QRS, a notch in V3. Notches can be found in the QRS in many (most?) tracings in one lead or another, and usually have no clinical application (42). When they are in the very earliest part of the complex, though, representing activation of the innermost part of the ventricular myocardium, where the distal end of the wedge-shaped lesion of an infarct would be expected (177), their importance is increased. The pattern in this tracing would probably be included in the term "poor progression of the R wave" (175) by those who accept that as meaningful, and some computer programs describe the complex in V3 as a Q wave, but it is a QS.

Despite the inconsistency of terminology, most computer programs are very good at recognizing anterior infarcts. They are too sensitive to inferior ones, but this is because it is much more difficult to specify criteria for them (175).

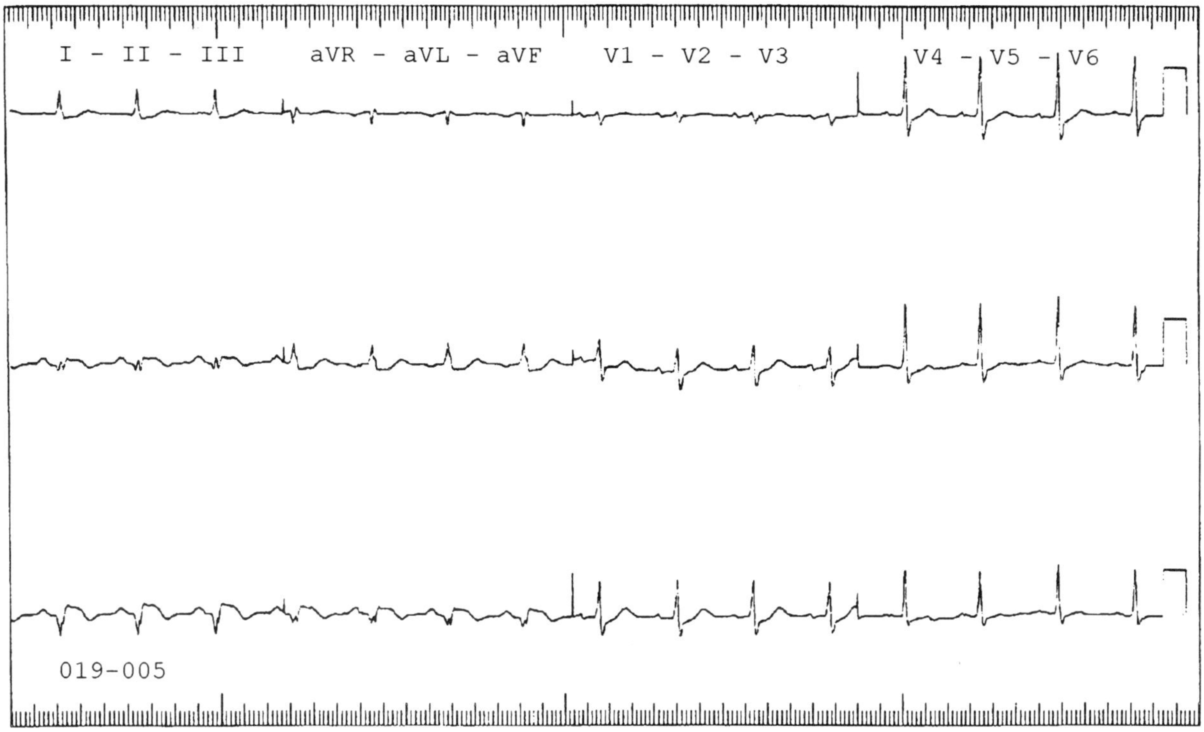

Acute Inferior Myocardial Infarct

```
90    90    16    08    36     sinus
-30   1:1   V1-2    10:1     Q2,3,F
      up 2,3,F, down V3
  arched, inseparable from T
low  ±V1,    pos V2-5 low,    ±V6

(1) Sinus mechanism, rate 90
(2) Acute inferior myocardial
    infarct
```

All three criteria for EKG diagnosis of a myocardial infarct are satisfied here; evidence of a scar deep in the myocardium (initial QRS abnormality), the view from which it is seen (inferior), and a basis for suspecting its age (ST displacement) (173, 181). These features, strictly speaking, cannot be said to show an infarct; that implies etiology. Other explanations are possible for the QRS abnormality and for the ST-T abnormality separately, but very few for the combination. When both are present, the interpretation that they represent an infarct is actionable unless there is compelling evidence for a better explanation. When it fits the clinical picture, its validity approaches 100%. The third feature, the view from which the evidence is seen, is much less important.

Note that the evidence of injury, ST displacement, shows as depression in V3 and elevation in Lead III, two views of the same thing, not both inferior superficial injury and anterior deep injury (204). The tracing represents the course through time and space of only one point (70).

EKG 107

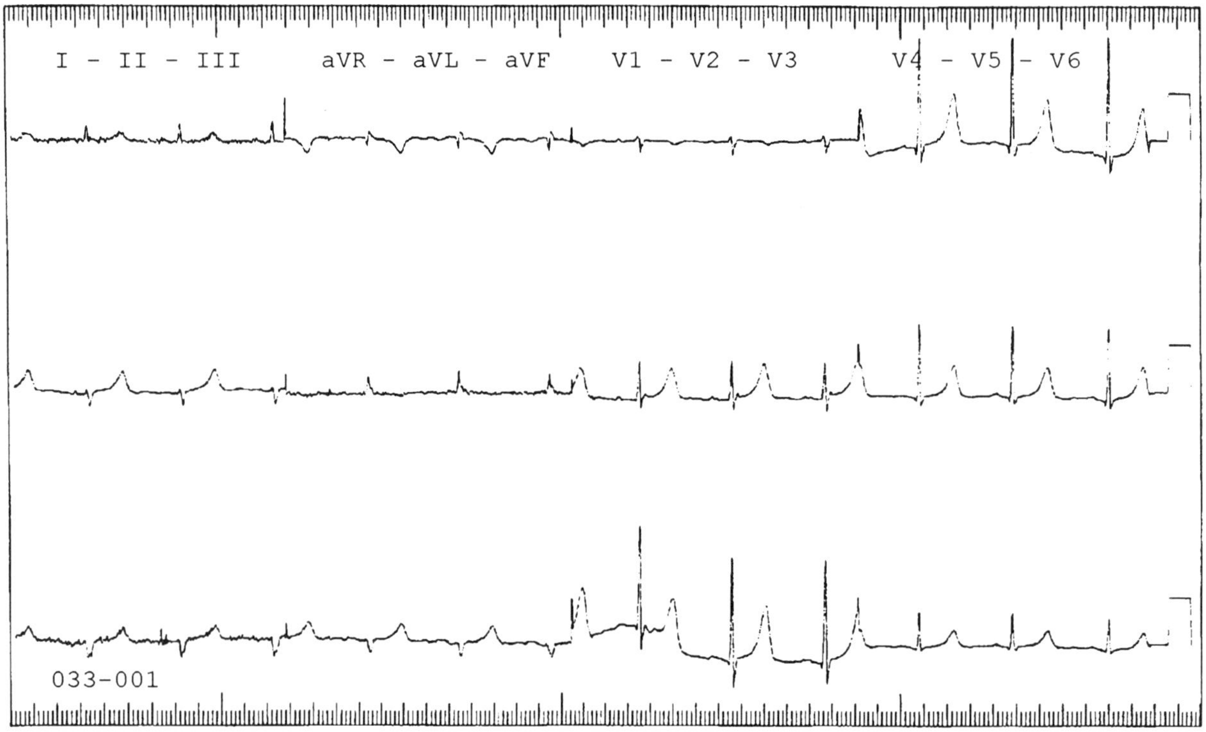

Probably Within Normal Limits

```
75    75    16    08    40      sinus
low   -60   1:2   V1    7:0    normal
                  none
                 normal
+60      ±V1    positive V2-6 tall

(1) Sinus mechanism, rate 75
(2) Prob within normal limits

--Evidence for left anterior
  fascicular block, and/or an
  old inf myo infarct, is  equi-
  vocal.  Nothing looks new.
--Precordial T is tall but not
  abnormal by itself.
--The clinical setting and
  stability of the findings are
  important unknowns.
```

The report of a tracing must always identify mechanism, structure, and function, individually and collectively, as precisely as possible, but should not be Procrustean. "Bracketing" can be used to indicate the range within which each falls (58), and, as in this tracing, supplementary comment can be used to clarify any ambiguity.

The frontal QRS at about –60° may be abnormal, but it is not reasonable to list all possible explanations for this (226), or to reprise the limits of the methods for its determination. Clinical judgment recognizes the two most likely possibilities as inferior infarction and left anterior fascicular block. Choice depends on normality or abnormality of initial QRS forces (184), and that simply is not clear in this case. If ST were elevated in II, III, and aVF, infarction would be much more likely, and, if there were evidence for right atrial enlargement, right ventricular enlargement would have to be included in the differential, but neither of these is present. T is tall in leads in which it is nearly parallel to QRS, and a bit more symmetrical than usual. Again, this may be abnormal (210), but is not clearly so.

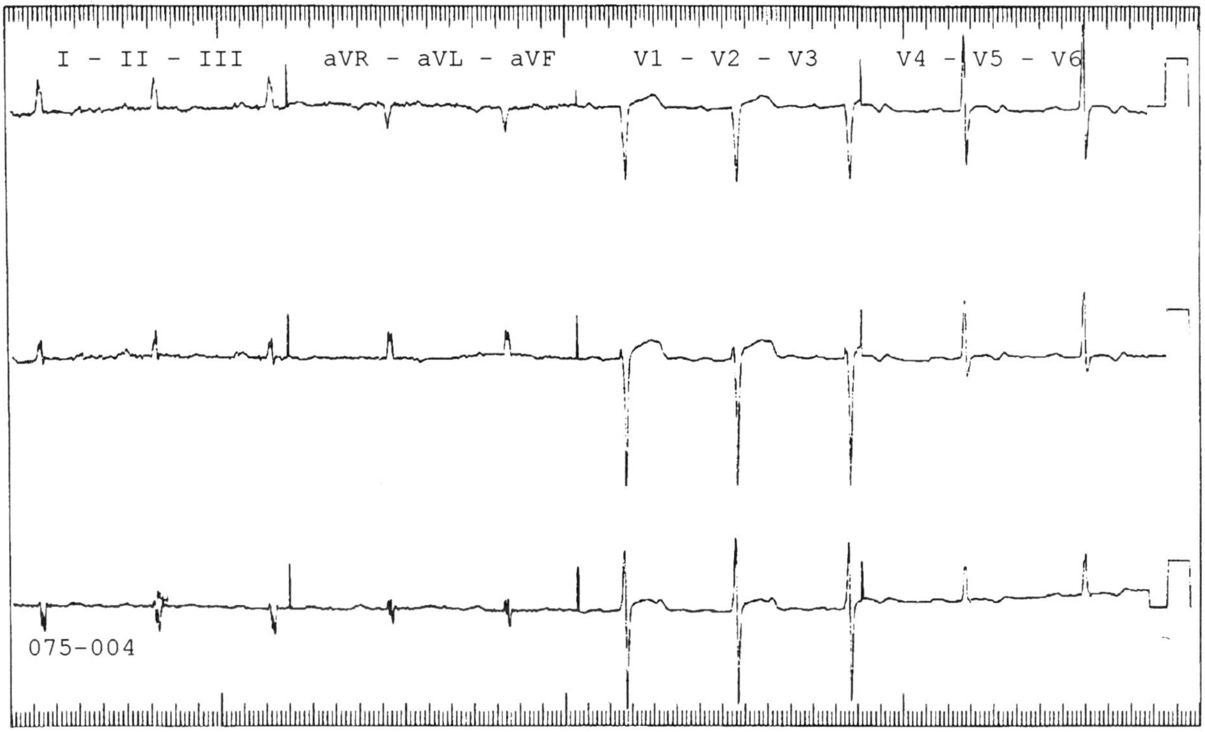

ST-T Abnormalities; Notches

Abnormalities limited to the ST-T complex are never specific, but the more proximal they are (ST), the more likely they are to be meaningful; the more distal (T), inconsequential. There are two features in this tracing that call for comment, low T voltage in leads with tall QRSs, and a notch in T (50, 213).

A notch (transient change in direction) in P, especially in Lead II, is normal, probably representing the change from dominance of the right atrium to that of left, the same thing seen as reversal of polarity in V1 (27). Notches are common in QRS (42). This is easy to understand when one sees the EKG recorded in two dimensions at the same time, a vectorcardiogram (90) (EKG 149). This form emphasizes the irregularities in the course of the point in time and space that the tracing represents.

60 60 20 08 40 sinus
±0 0:15 V3 8:0 normal
none
related to T
Low positive V1-2 ±V3-6

(1) Sinus mechanism, rate 60
(2) ST-T abnormalities, non-specific

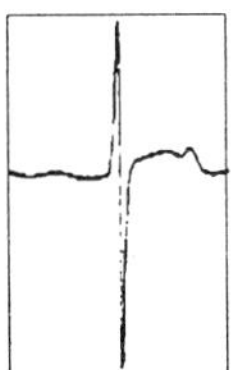

V2 from above

Notches in T are less common. They may be evidence of a superimposed P or U, or may simply represent the limits of the method.

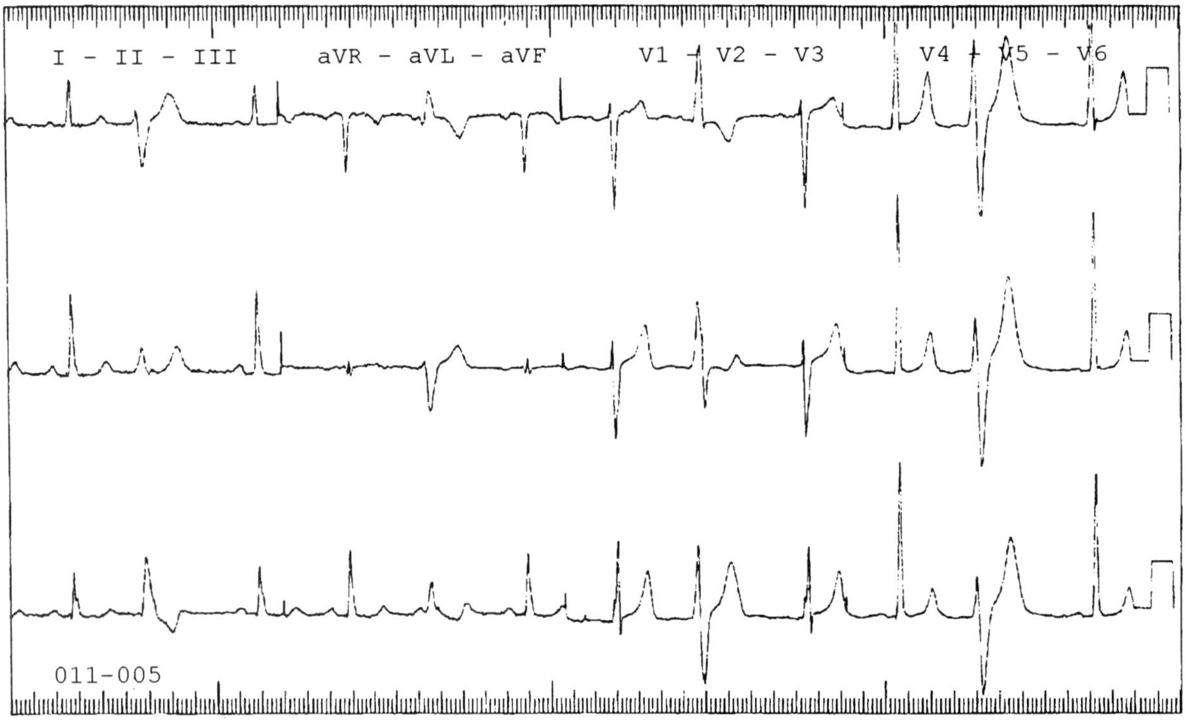

Bigeminy due to PVCs

75 75 16 10 40 sinus/PVC's
+60 0:12 V2½ 30:0 normal
none
normal
+30 positive V1-6

(1) Sinus mechanism, rate 75,
with normal AV conduction
(2) Bigeminy due to PVC's
(3) Otherwise WNL

"Bigeminy" implies an abnormality of rhythm, using the word in its usual sense, i.e., beats are not evenly spaced, but occur in pairs. The usual explanations for this are: a premature beat, either atrial or ventricular in origin, following each beat conducted beat; second degree AV block with 3:2 conduction; or escape-capture mechanisms in which a lower pacemaker, typically junctional, escapes at a rate just slower than the sinus rate, and is followed closely by a sinus beat (129, 142, 146). Strictly speaking, this tracing can be said to show only frequent PVCs since one sinus beat is not paired with a PVC. Note the "end-diastolic" PVC (inset)(143).

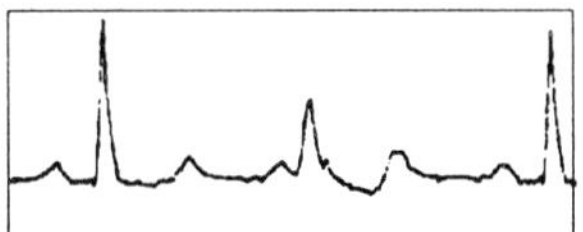
End-diastolic PVC
Lead II from above

Precordial Ts are tall but of normal contour, a common pattern of no clinical importance. The computer called left ventricular hypertrophy, an interpretation badly overdone by most programs. The clinician who must deal with this statement in an EKG readout/report should know not only what numbers in the tracing produced it, but also what criteria for clinical reality were used to validate them. Left ventricular hypertrophy, and lesions that explain it, are detected better by physical examination than EKG.

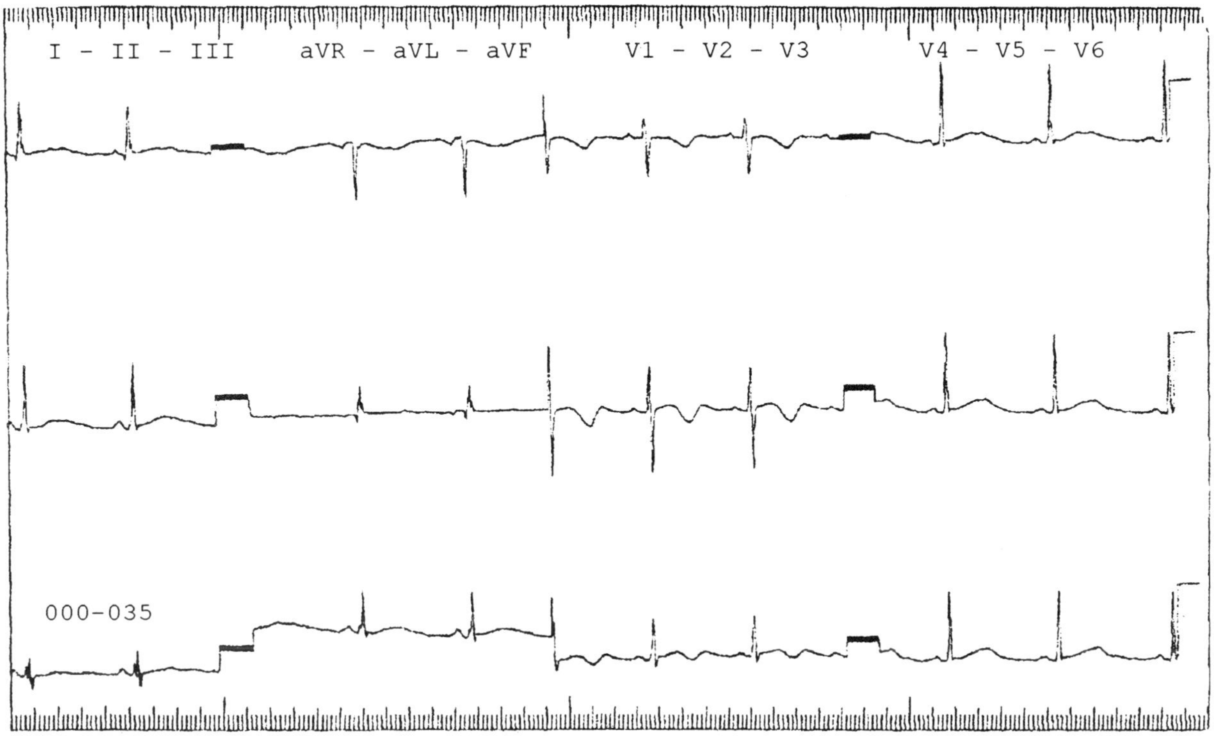

Long QT, Prominent U

```
65    65    16    06    40      sinus
+30   4:8   V2    10:0          normal
                 none
                normal
low    neg V1-2       pos V3-6 low
U: prominent, pos V2-6

(1) Sinus mechanism, rate 65
(2) ST-T-U abnormalities, non-
    specific

--Prominence of U, continuous
  with T, suggests a "long QT
  syndrome".
```

Duration of the QT interval is a measure of the time required for ventricular repolarization and is considered in analysis of every tracing (11, 23, 202). Like the orientation, amplitude, and contour of its components, ST and T, it is influenced by many, many factors. To describe it as long is to imply an abnormality, a finding to be interpreted in context; a long QT is a finding, a nonspecific ST-T abnormality, not a diagnosis. It does not take much experience to realize the limits of the method of its estimation, and to "correct" such an inherently ill-defined value by mathematic manipulation, the QTc, adds very little (24).

When QT is seen as very long, more than about 0.44 sec, there is a good chance that there is a U wave merged with T and what is being measured is really a QU. In a patient with a history of syncope, as in this one, this suggests a useful, if incompletely understood, clinical diagnosis, paroxysmal ventricular fibrillation, one of the "Long QT Syndromes" (134).

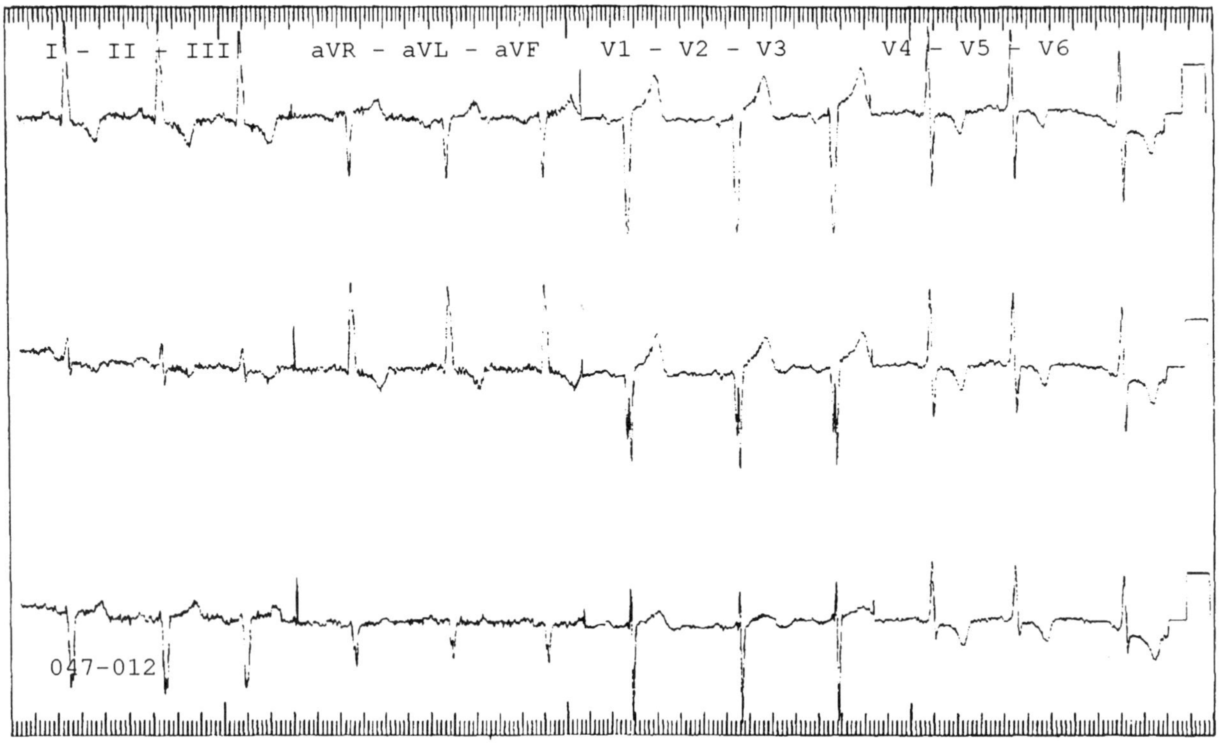

ST-T Abnormalities, Probably LVO, Old Anterior Infarct, Probable

70	70	16	10	40	sinus
-30	1:25	V4	10:3		QSV2
		none			
		related to T			
±180	pos V1-2	±V3		neg V5-6	

(1) Sinus mechanism, rate 70
(2) ST-T abnormalities, probably left ventricular overload
(3) Suggests old anterior myocardial infarct

The evidence here for a disproportionate load faced by the left ventricle, strain, or overload, is in the T wave. ST-T is of normal duration (QT), and substantially normal amplitude and contour, but T is oriented widely apart from QRS. Most computer programs will call this "ischemia." Ischemia is the ultimate means by which most EKG abnormalities in adults are produced, and it may result from exaggeration of the need for blood (oxygen), diminution in its supply, or both (136). The tracing shows the abnormality, not what brought it about. The combination of findings in this tracing is not specific for anything, but correlates well with increased load (189). The computer called left ventricular hypertrophy. Hypertrophy is a consequence of overload, and may be present, but left ventricular hypertrophy is one of the things all computer programs call too easily. The evidence here is minimal (192). Suffice it to say that the EKG diagnosis of left ventricular hypertrophy is not to be taken at face value. Some of the notches in the QRS represent muscle tremor, but the large one on the downstroke of QSV2 following an rS in V1 suggests myocardial scarring, presumably an infarct.

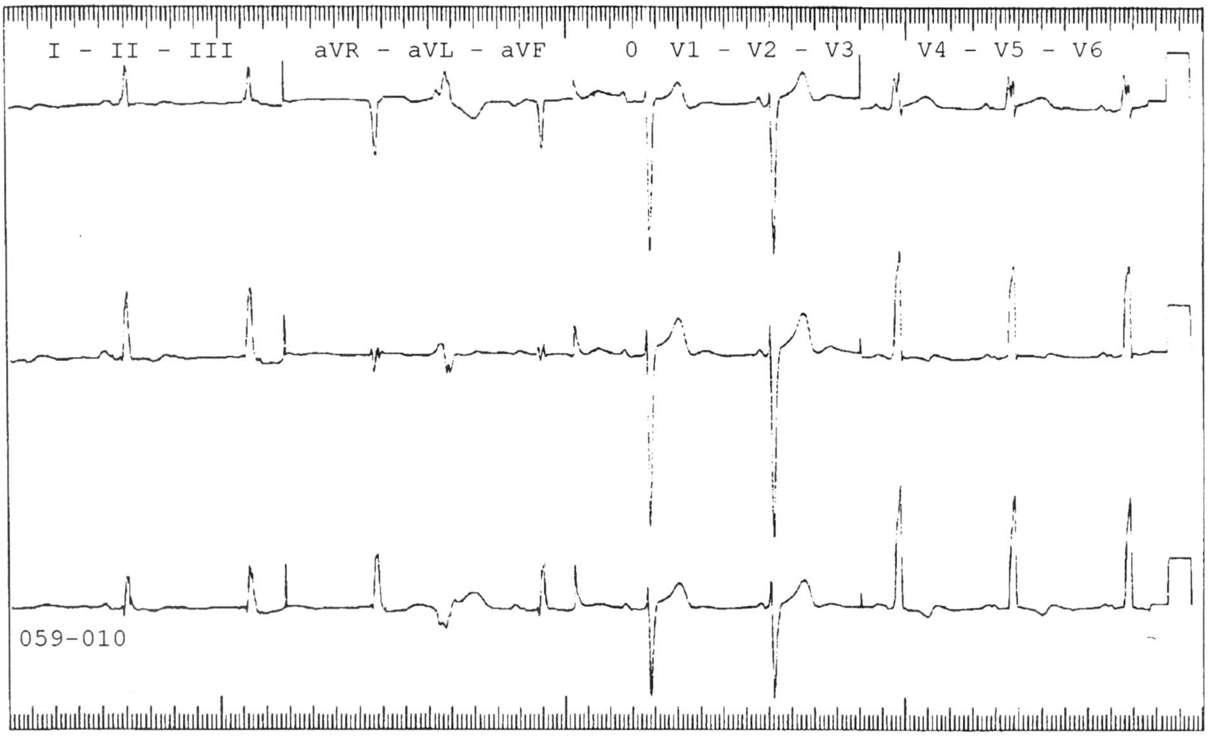

Isorhythmic Dissociation, ST-T Abnormalities

```
60   60     16    10   40      sinus
+60  2:30    V3-1/2   25:0  normal
                 none
              related to T
low    +V1-4,   ±V5,   neg V6  low

(1) Sinus mechanism, rate 60,
    with PVC's
(2) ST-T abnormalities suggest-
    ive of left ventricular
    overload
(3) Left ventricular hyper-
    trophy, probable
```

This tracing illustrates several limits of the method. First, the mechanism. It is basically sinus, the (normal) notch in the first P in Lead II, and the (small) terminal negativity of the first one in V1, are typical of a sinus origin (27). No P is identifiable before the third QRS, unless the tiny notch at the beginning of that complex in Lead I represents a P merged with a QRS of junctional origin. This explanation is supported by the very short PR in the second beat in V1-2-3 that would go well with a premature junctional beat, isorhythmic dissociation (134). There is only one PVC (142), and that is not enough to call abnormal.

The relatively great QRS voltage suggests left ventricular hypertrophy (192), a weak measure of hypertrophy but the only one of any value in the EKG. In this case it is supported by the wide QRS-T angle without other ST-T abnormality, a pattern suggestive of left ventricular strain, or overload. Hypertrophy follows strain, strain leads to hypertrophy; the two findings complement each other and point to the left ventricle as the seat of disproportionate hemodynamic burden. QRS notching suggests patchy fibrosis.

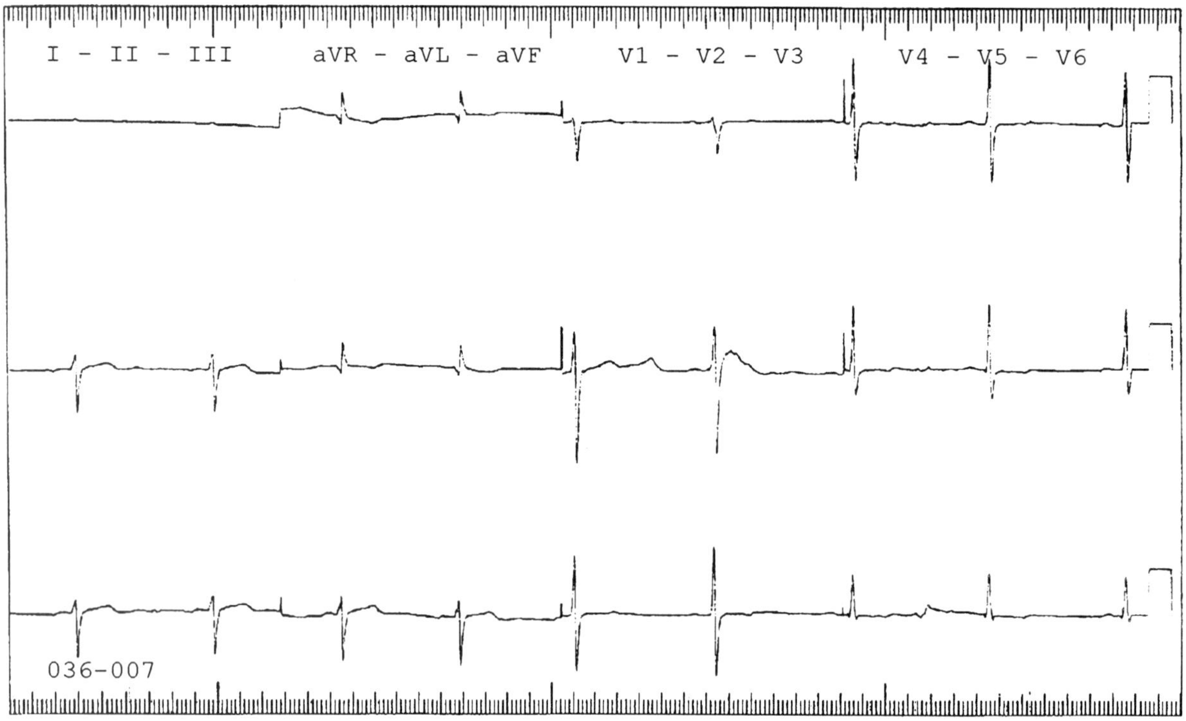

Artifact

Flat line, Lead I

50	50	20	08	40	sinus
?-90	1:8	V3-4	8:1		normal
		none			
		related to T			
?+90	±V1		+V2	±V3-6	

(1) Sinus mechanism, rate 50
(2) ST-T abnormalities, non-specific
(3) Incomplete; recorded with arm leads on legs and vice versa

First, distinguish between "lead," the graphic representation of a dipole, and "lead," a wire (243). Second, recognize that sometimes it is difficult to be sure whether a line is absolutely flat, meaning no information in that lead, or nearly flat, as when complexes are very small, and/or when all forces are perpendicular to it. A lead, dipole, expresses the difference in potential between the two points defined by its positive and negative poles. In leads I, II, and III, each of these points is an unknown, the difference between it and neutral, the B point. All the others have a V in their names, implying that their negative poles are, in effect, at the B point itself (8, 30, 115) This is an application of basic electrophysiology learned by all medical students in their first year (88), and it works. No difference in potential between the two electrodes of a lead means that both must be on the same point (95, 107). In this case, the components of Lead I (a dipole), the arm leads (wires) were attached to the legs, and vice versa. The legs (linear conductors) are connected to Einthoven's triangle at the same point. The right leg lead, a wire, grounds the chassis of the unknown, the body, to the chassis of the recorder, the EKG machine (88, 99, 242) and works no matter where it is attached.

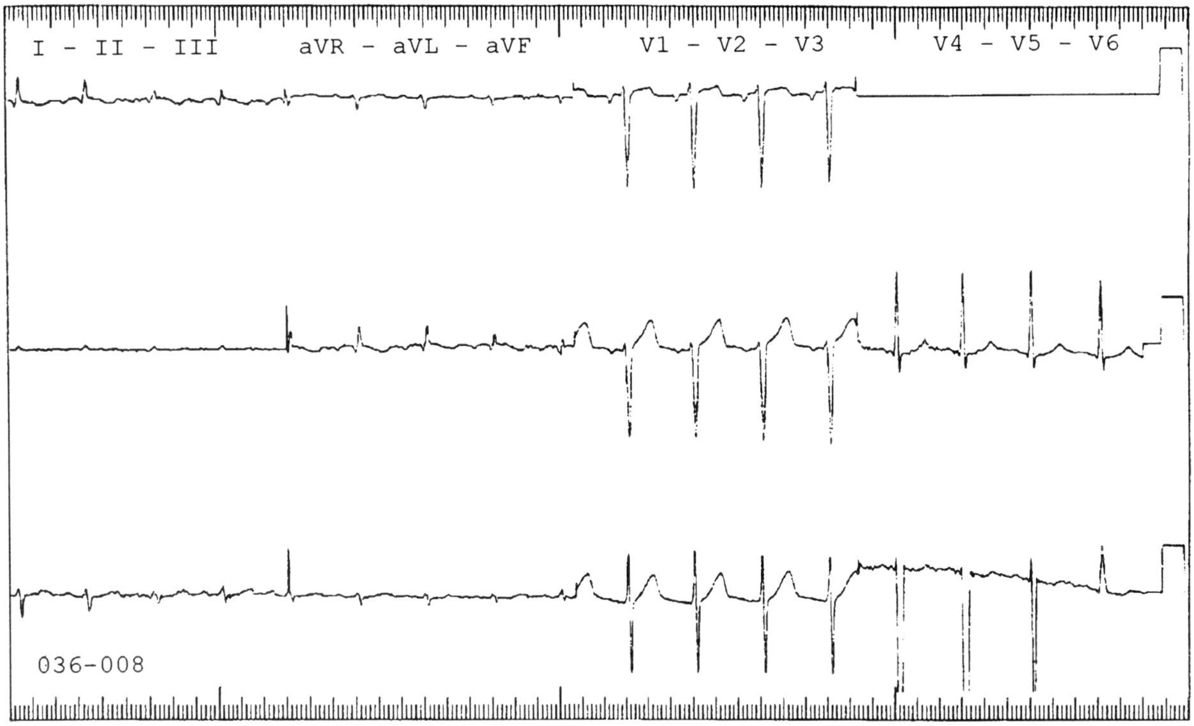

Artifact

Flat line

```
100   100   16    08    40    sinus
?-30  2:20  ??      ?:?     normal
              none
          related to T
?+150     ±V1      +V2-5       ±V6
P: Prominent terminal neg V1

(1) Sinus mechanism, rate 100
(2) Suggests LAE
(3) Otherwise probably WNL or
     at worst only small ST-T
     abnormalities.

--Incomplete; recorded with
  right arm and leg leads
  crossed.  V4 is missing
```

Absence of information in a V lead means that its electrode is not attached to the body; in a "bipolar" lead (86), that both ends are attached to the same the same apex of Einthoven's triangle (67, 86, 95, 107). In this case, the right arm and leg leads are crossed, and V4 is not connected.

The right leg lead "grounds" the body to the EKG machine, and works wherever it is placed, but with both components of Lead II connected to the same point, the symphysis pubis, there is no potential difference between them. Sometimes the limits of the method come into play, and "flat" may mean only very low voltage, and/or orientation of all forces perpendicular to that lead. Similarly there may be tiny deflections that represent "cross-channel chatter" (do you remember eight-track tape players?); the system is not perfect. The V4 electrode was simply not applied, perhaps its site was bandaged. The explanation for difference in QRSs in V6 is not apparent, but it is important to recognize that it must represent a technical problem, not evidence of an infarct as it was labeled by the computer program.

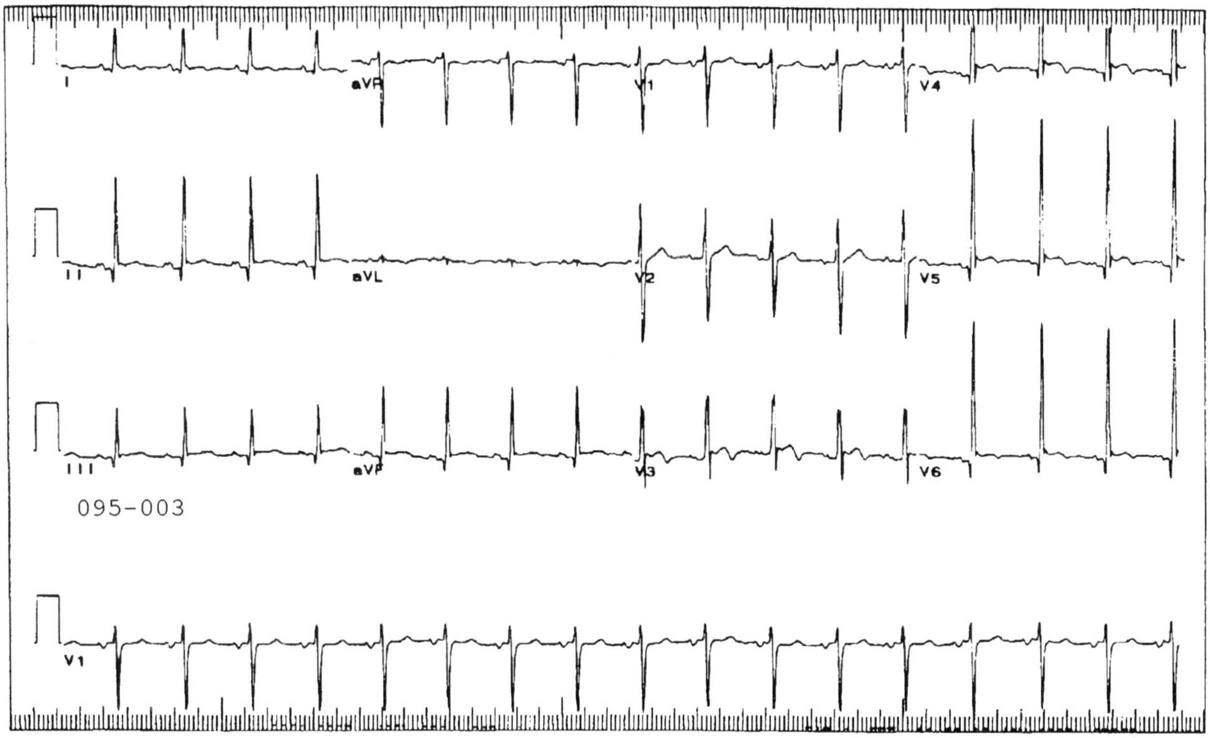

Pericarditis

```
105    105    12    08  32     sinus
+60    3:15   V2    25:0     normal
   slightly up 2,3,F, V3-6
         flattened
low  pos V1-2  neg V3-4,  ±V5-6

(1) Sinus mechanism, rate 105
(2) ST-T abns typical of sub-
    epicardial injury as with
    pericarditis
```

The important finding in this tracing is abnormal ST displacement; ST is not at the baseline and its contour is not normal (44, 205). Displacement is so small that its precise orientation is not clear, but is generally left, down, and anterior as indicated by elevation in II and V3-6. This pattern is sometimes described as "global" elevation, a term that does not make sense objectively. There is only one point in play, and if that is toward one place on the body it is away from another. The lead system does not include views from the right back, and the distribution of the inflammation responsible for the findings is likely to be diffuse. Sometimes, in similar tracings, ST is slightly depressed in aVR. The implication is myocardial injury limited to the tissue immediately subjacent to the epicardium. The similar, but much more marked, ST abnormality of acute myocardial infarction presumably represents involvement of more muscle by extension of the effects of coronary insufficiency from their beginning deep in the myocardium outward toward the arterial lesion (208). The computer came close on this one. It called pericarditis *or* injury, confusing the finding, injury, with an explanation for it. (It did not call ischemia.)

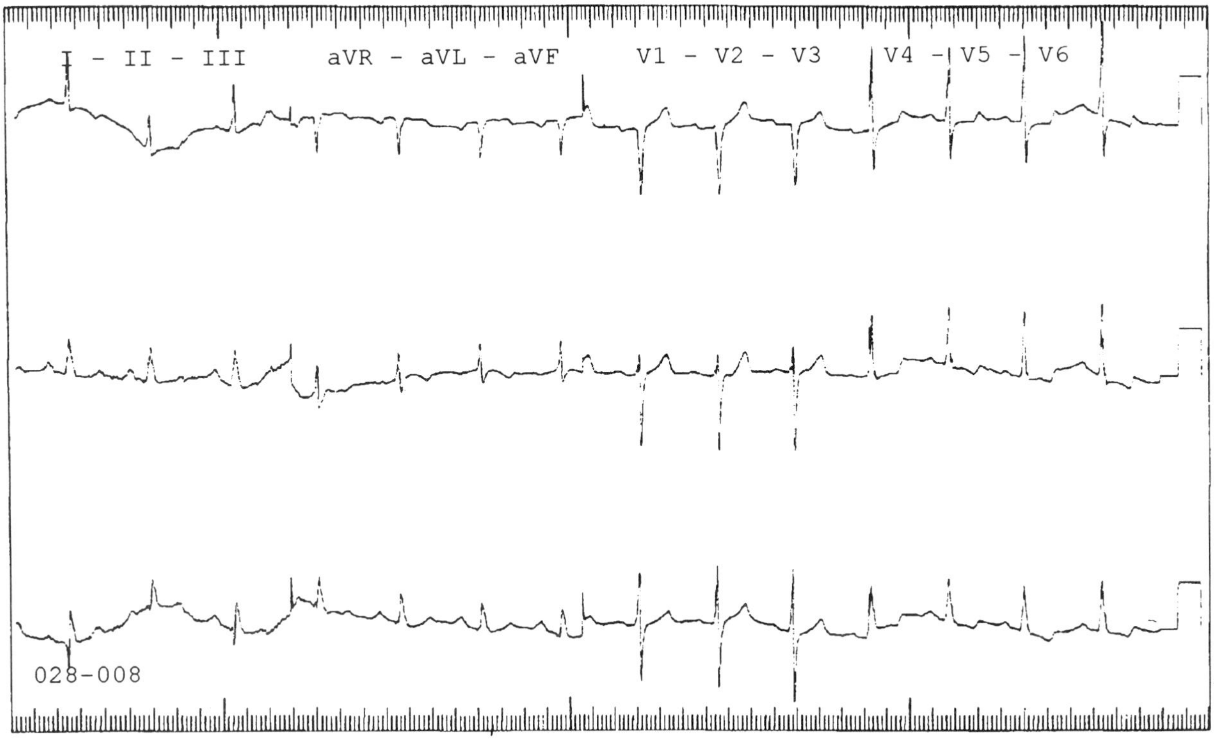


```
85     85    20     08    36      sinus
+45    0:15    V3    10:0       normal
                 none
            related to T
+135 low    +V1-3   ±V4   neg V5-6

(1) Sinus mechanism, rate 85
(2) ST-T abnormalities, sug-
    gestive of left ventricular
    overload
--Loose connection to left arm.
--The Q3 is not enough to call
--abnormal by itself.
```

Left Ventricular Overload, or Strain

No ST-T abnormalities are specific, but some fall into patterns that suggest explanations. Examples are those that point to one of the components of ischemia, increase in demand, as here, or lessening of supply (see Coronary insufficiency in the Index).

A strained muscle hurts before it hypertrophies. The EKG expression of this is that overload of a ventricle produces change in the most sensitive part of the tracing, the T wave, before the more stable part, the QRS. The typical pattern of left ventricular strain is orientation of T nearly opposite QRS without change in duration, amplitude, or contour. If QRS voltage suggests left ventricular hypertrophy, a consequence of overload, the probability that the left ventricle is the seat of disproportionate hemodynamic burden is increased. To call the ST-T picture secondary to hypertrophy, as done sometimes, puts the cart before the horse. The clinical setting and stability of the findings must be taken into account. The same EKG picture, transient and not associated with physical findings to explain hypertrophy, probably represents coronary insufficiency. Definition of the baseline is critical.

EKG 117

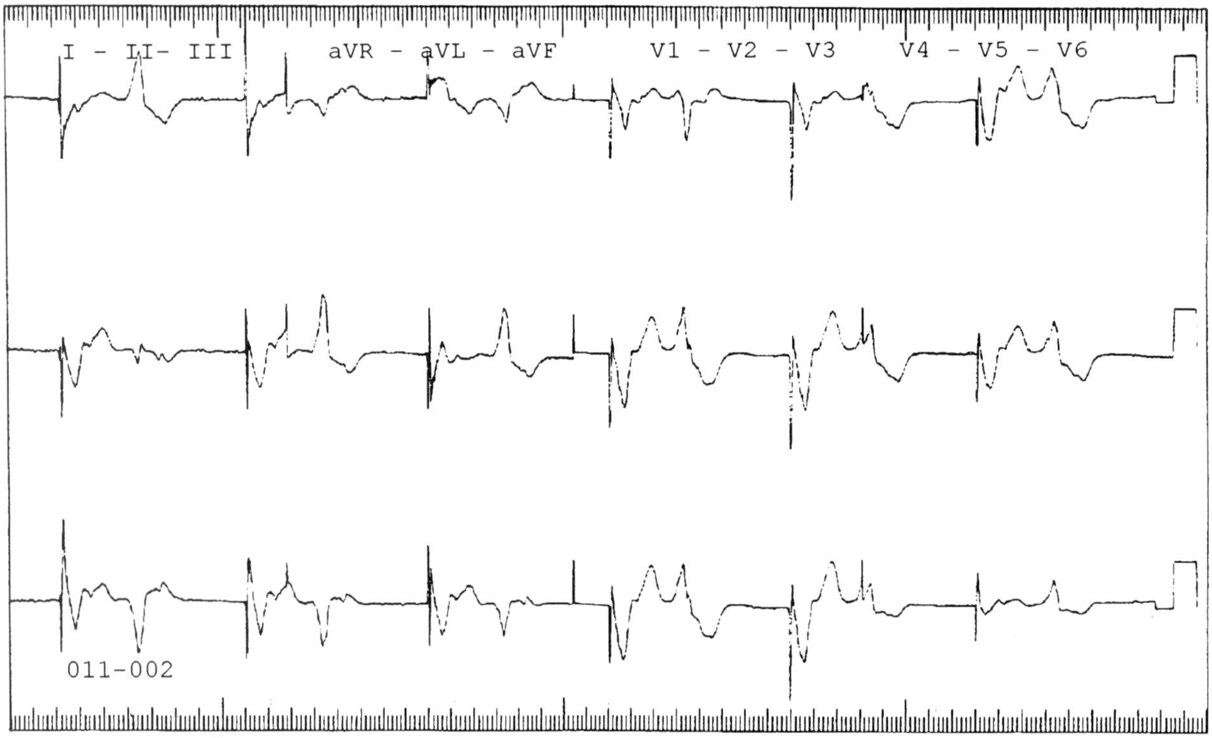

Bigeminy, PVCs, and Artificial Pacemaker

```
75  75  ??  16  44       see below
-30  2:8  V1½  5:0  diffuse slur
                         Q2, QS3.F
              none
          related to T
?+165   ±V1       negative V2-6(?)

(1) Atria depolarized from
    ventricles
(1) Artificial ventricular pace-
    maker, firing and capturing
    appropriately, rate about 60
(2) Bigeminy due to PVC's

--In the absence of conducted
  beats, ST-T cannot be inter-
  preted usefully.
```

"Bigeminy," two twins, identifies the rhythm, pairing of beats, but not the mechanism. In this case the only place atrial activity can be seen with confidence is in the P superimposed on ST, and negative in inferior leads, presumably representing retrograde activation of atria from ventricles. There are two ventricular foci; one is an artificial pacemaker, indicated by the spike introducing QRS in the first beat and every other beat after that, and the other intrinsic in a ventricle, probably the right (because the QRS pattern is like LBBB)(140).

More common forms of bigeminy include a PVC, or a PAC, following each conducted beat, and second degree AV block with 3:2 conduction. Escape-capture bigeminy describes a junctional, or idioventricular, beat followed by one of sinus origin, and there are other possibilities.

Groups of three beats are sometimes called "trigeminy," but the idea of three twins is complicated.

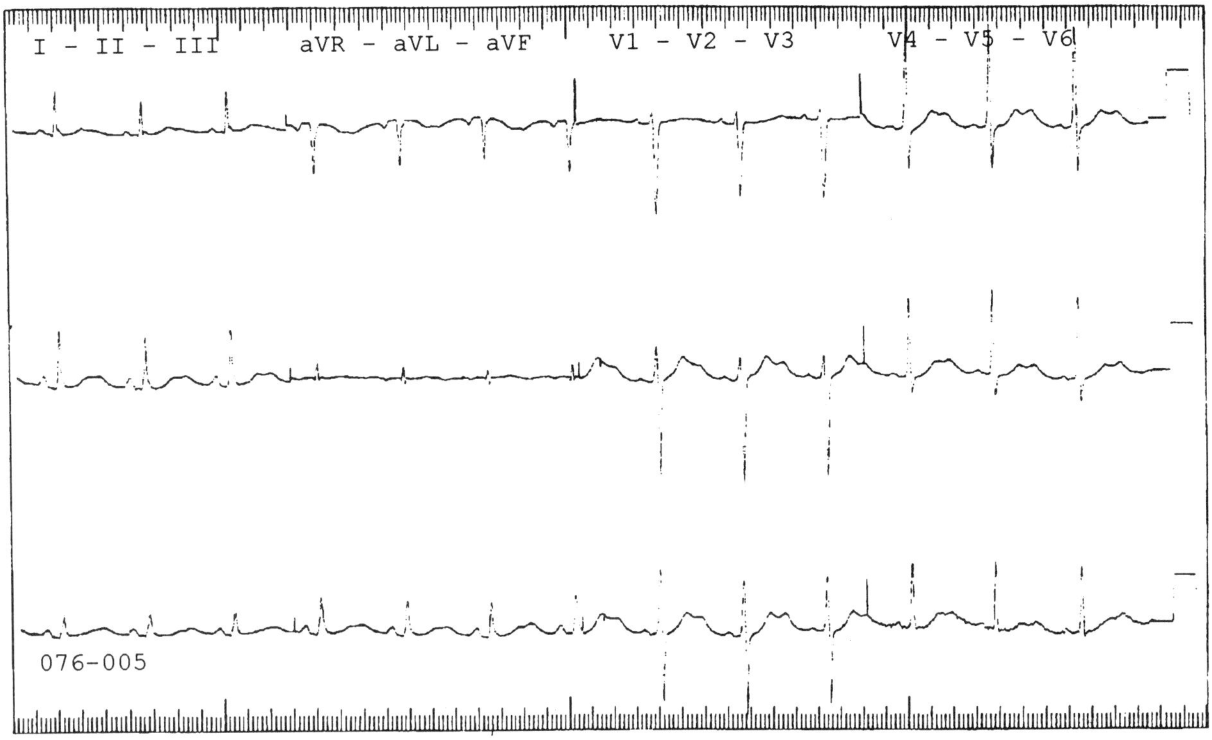

Notched T

```
80    80    16    08    36      sinus
+45   3:20   V3    15:0         normal
               none
               normal
low ?+60     ±V1    V2-5    ±V6
U: prominent

(1) Sinus mechanism, rate 80
(2) ST-T abnormality, nonspe-
    cific

--mostly just low T voltage, not
  far from normal.  The U wave
  is prominent, but not abnormal
  by itself
```

A notch is a transient reversal of direction of the trace within a wave. Notches are common in all components of the tracing, and definition of abnormal is arbitrary, a learned judgment. There is a notch in most unidirectional P waves, typically in Lead II, and small, sharp notches are common in QRS in one or more leads in most tracings, especially in transitional leads (see "A tutorial: Examination of one heartbeat" in Chapter 3). Notches in T are noted less commonly, and may cause some consternation (213). Most frequently, they are recognized for what they are, superimposed Ps. Remember that the position of the trace reflects the net of all the electrical activity in the body, and that atria and ventricles may be active at the same time. Often, as in this tracing, notches in the repolarization complex are explained by fusion of T with a prominent U, and they may represent simply an unusual contour, the limits of the method.

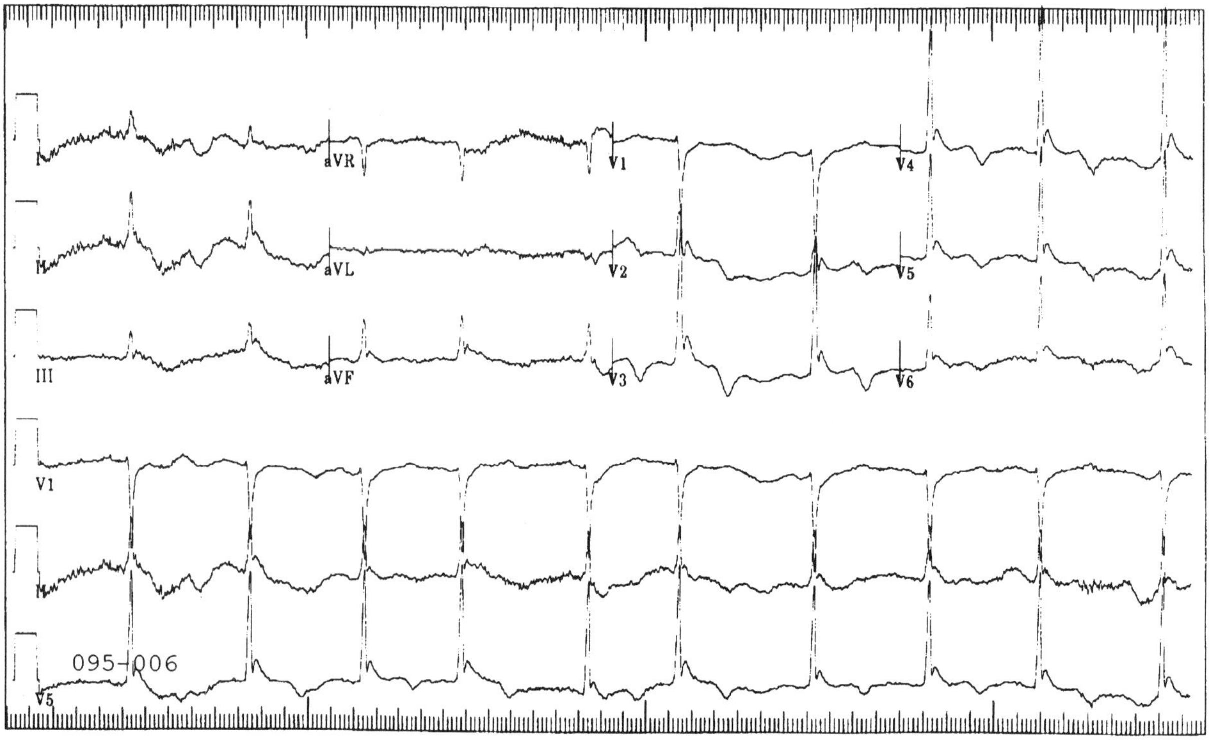

Hypothermia

This patient was an elderly man, discovered unconscious on the floor, in an unheated room after a very cold night, among signs of an alcoholic binge. He was unresponsive at the time of the tracing, with a rectal temperature of 80°F, but regained consciousness upon warming.

The tracing shows both QRS and ST-T evidence of hypothermia (42, 237). QRS is borderline wide, and its contour has the characteristic late notch. The combination of ST displacement and low T voltage produces the pattern of subepicardial injury.

These characteristics were recognized during animal experiments when induced hypothermia was in use to lower metabolic rate as an aid to cardiac surgery. Their significance was to warn that ventricular fibrillation was near.

EKGs 15 and 123 show other examples of hypothermia.

-- 60 -- ±10 ±50 see below
+60 1:20 V2 20:0 late notch
none
related to T
low ± V1-6

(1) Supraventricular mechanism, rate about 60, with irregular rhythm, probably sinus with PAC's. Atrial activity is not clear.
(2) Unusual QRS pattern (duration and contour) suggestive of hypothermia
(2) ST-T-U abnormalities suggestive of myocardial injury

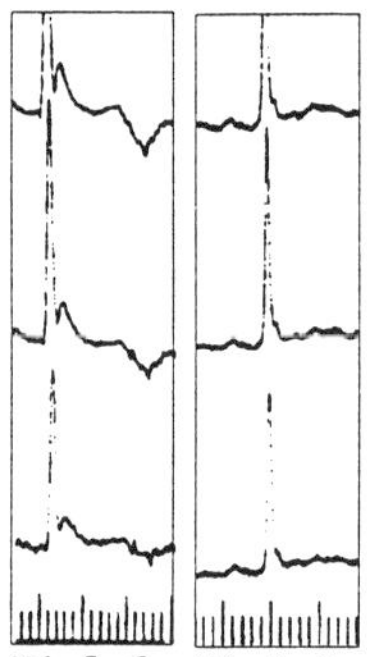

V4-5-6 80°F | V4-5-6 95°F

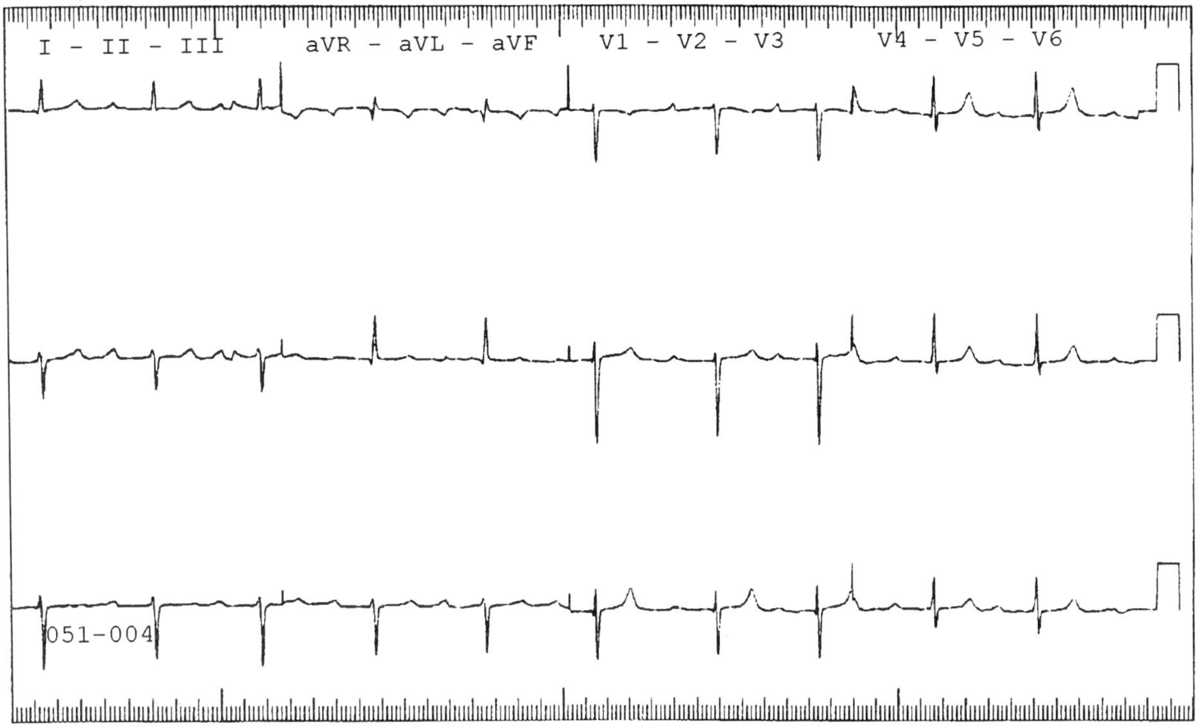

First Degree AV Block, Left Anterior Hemiblock

60 60 36 08 40 sinus
-60 1:10 V3½ 8:4 normal
none
some flattening
+30 ±V1, positive V2-6

(1) Sinus mechanism, rate 60
(2) First degree AV block
(3) Left anterior hemiblock
(4) Otherwise probably WNL, at worst only small ST-T abnormalities

The length of PR is always hard to measure precisely, and this limits the definition of normal. It depends on how close the beginning of P can be estimated, and which view of it, which lead, is used, and all intervals vary inversely with rate. The value most often assumed as the upper limit of normal, 0.20 s, would be described better as usual, not maximum. Computer programs apparently do not all use the same criteria for beginning and end, or for definition of prolongation; indiscriminate acceptance of a readout of first degree AV block is inappropriate. A conservative rule is not to call PR any closer than 0.04 sec. In general, if you have to wonder whether it is prolonged, it is not (27, 150).

Keep in mind that a long PR is a finding, not a disease. To refer to it as "heart block" is not to be as specific as possible. Bundle branch block is also heart block, and so is mitral stenosis. One patient, hearing "heart block" mentioned, and, knowing that the heart is a pump, feared that it was an indication for open heart surgery. The association of fascicular block and first degree AV block is probably of little importance.

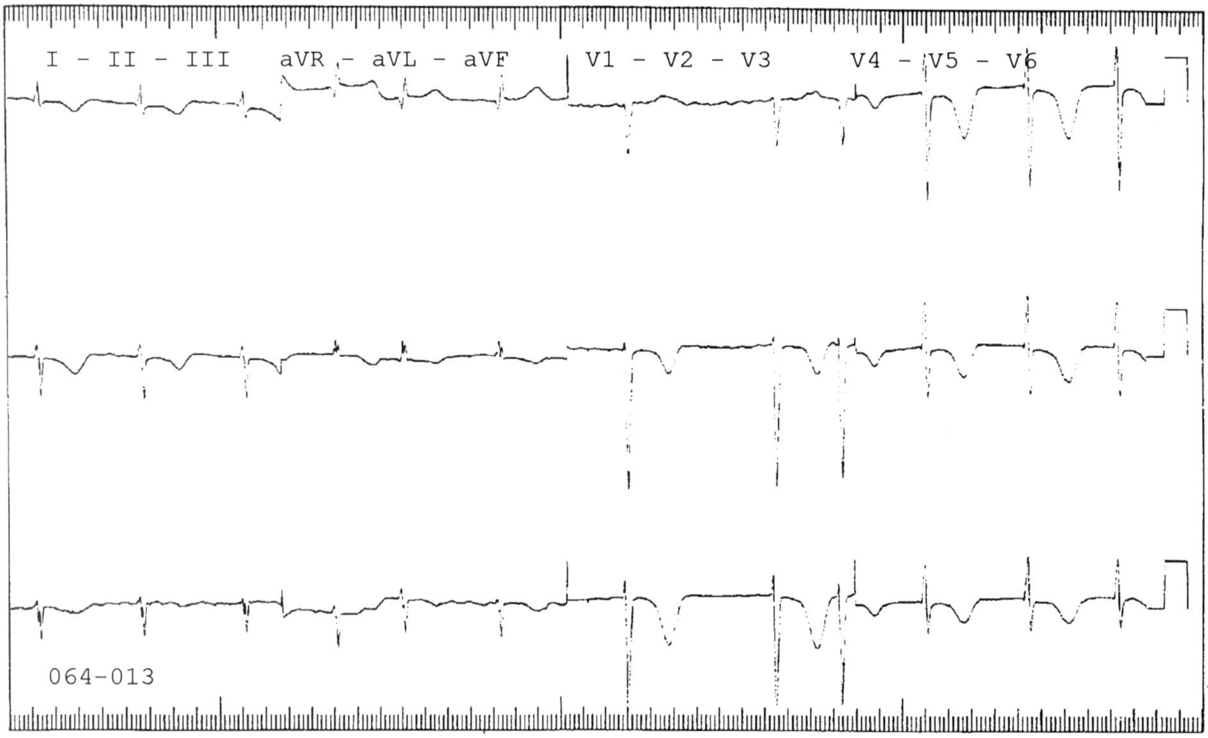

Atrial Fibrillation, Mid-Precordial ST-T-U of Coronary Insufficiency

```
 --    70    --   10    56        AF
 -75     0:10   V5    1:6        nl
                 none
            related to T
-165    pos V1 low      neg V2-6
                        deep V3-5,
                       symmetrical
U: prominent, continuous with T

(1) Atrial fibrillation, ven-
    tricular rate about 70
(2) Left anterior fascicular
    block
(3) ST-T-U abns suggestive of
    coronary insufficiency
```

Like the electrocardiogram itself, and findings on examination of the left lung, the U wave (51) does not usually contribute much, but sometimes it does, and its contribution cannot be judged until it has been evaluated. When prominent, it may be within normal limits, evidence of hypokalemia or something else. It may overlap T and be seen as a notch in T. It may be merged with T and read as a long QT...as it was in this case. Decision as to what is right depends on where T ends and U begins, and this is often not clear. The only evidence may be a small dimple in one lead, or just a very long measured QT that is really a QU. See EKGs 110 and 126

This tracing shows one of the few patterns in which the U wave is very important; negative U waves, especially when continuous with negative Ts in the midprecordial leads, correlate well with coronary insufficiency (217).

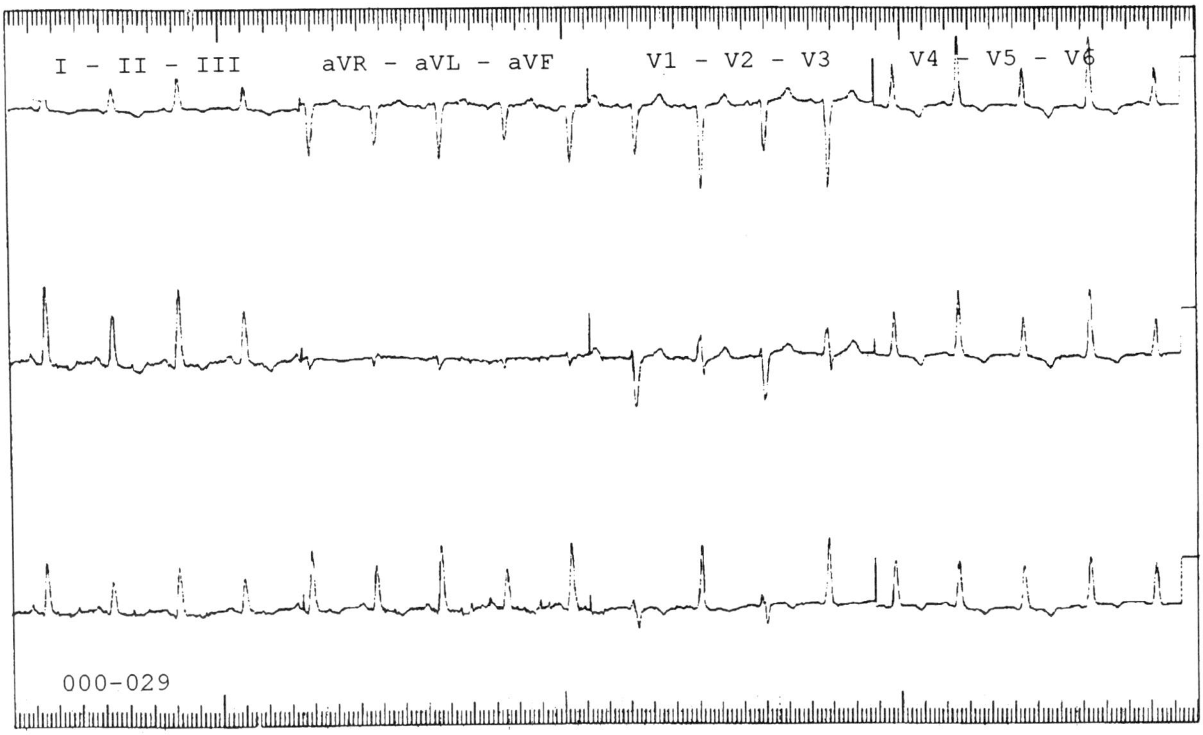

Electrical Alternans

105	105	12	08	36	sinus
+60	1:10?	V3?	10:0		normal
		none			
		related to T			
-120	pos V1-2			neg V3-6	

(1) Sinus mechanism, rate 105
(2) ST-T abns suggestive of left ventricular overload
(3) Electrical alternans

The name describes the findings: complexes alternate, large/small, positive/negative. Any or all components of the tracing may be involved, P, QRS, and/or ST-T (216, 233), but the QRS is the only one recognized in most instances. Alternation may be seen in ratios other than 2:1, and the alternate beats may be hard to distinguish from PVCs when the basic mechanism is sinus, which it usually is.

It is tempting to think in physical terms, equating electrical alternans with pulsus alternans, but this is probably specious reasoning. The phenomenon is not understood, but most likely represents events in cellular electrophysiology.

Electrical alternans has become associated in the minds of many clinicians with pericardial effusion, and there is some reason for this, especially when P, QRS, and ST-T are all involved, but it seems simplistic to assume pendulum-like swinging of the heart with each beat. Statistically valid proof is hard to come by.

In the present state of our understanding, the phenomenon has little clinical value; more interesting than applicable.

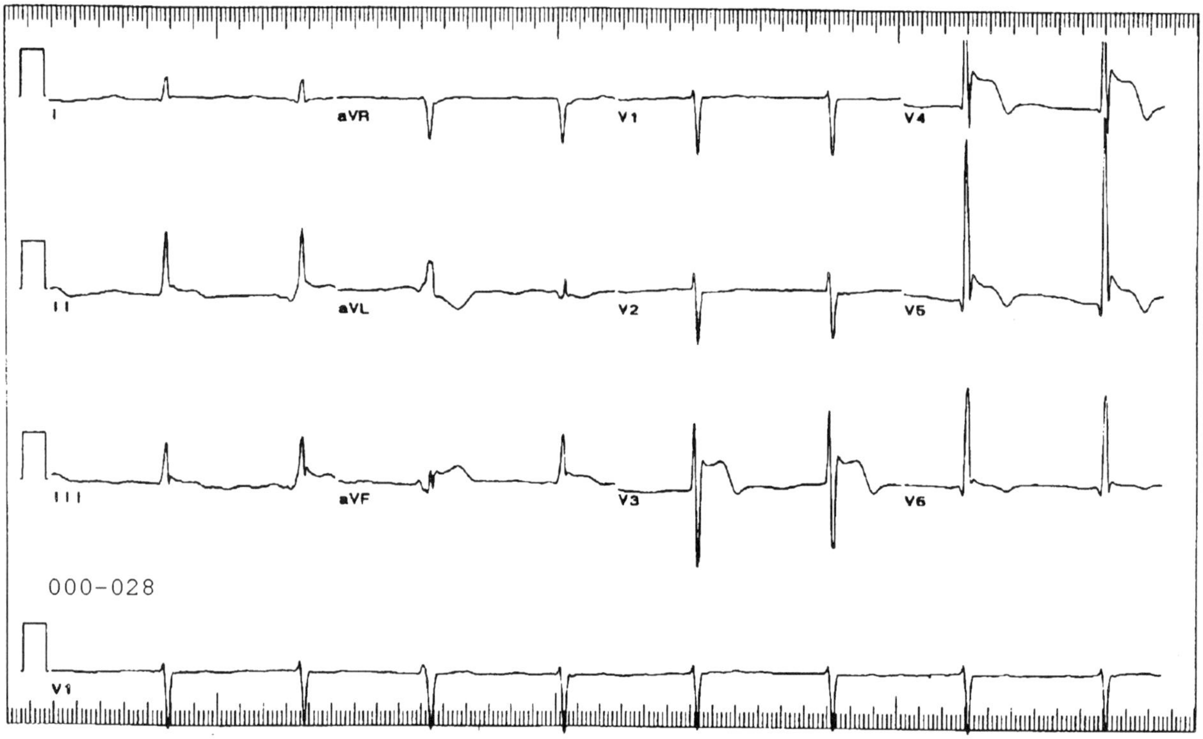

Hypothermia

The electrocardiographic pattern characteristic of hypothermia was described in 1953, by Dr. J. Osborn at a time when controlled hypothermia was the preferred way to diminish metabolic rate during cardiac surgery. Working with dogs, and concerned chiefly with arterial pH, he described a typical pattern (237). It had been recognized before, as he noted, but the characteristic deformity late in QRS has become known as an "Osborn wave." He described "a secondary wave closely following the S wave, so closely that it appears to be part of the QRS complex," making estimation of QRS duration difficult, and accompanied by prolongation of QT. It appeared "about 1/2-hour" before ventricular fibrillation and could be prevented by maintaining pH constant by manipulation of respiration.

This tracing is from a 50-year-old woman admitted to the ER from a psychiatric hospital. Her rectal temperature was 80°F.

```
--     50   --   10  56    see below
+60    2:12  V3   20:0  late notch
          up 2, 3, F, V3-5
              flattened
Low    ±V1-2, terminally neg V3-6

(1) Supraventricular mech, rate
    50, with regular rhythm,
    probably sinus, but as
    easily junctional.  Atrial
    activity is not identifi-
    able
(2) Unusual QRS pattern, sug-
    gestive of hypothermia.
(3) ST-T abn, typical of an-
    terior myocardial injury.
(4) The over-all QRS-T pat-
    tern probably means hypo-
    thermia.
```

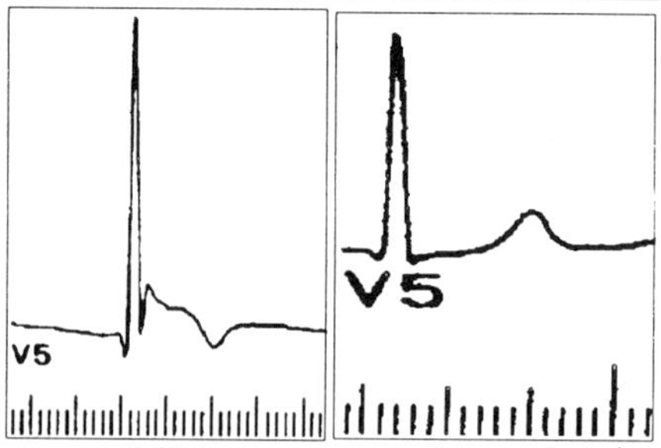

80°F   Control

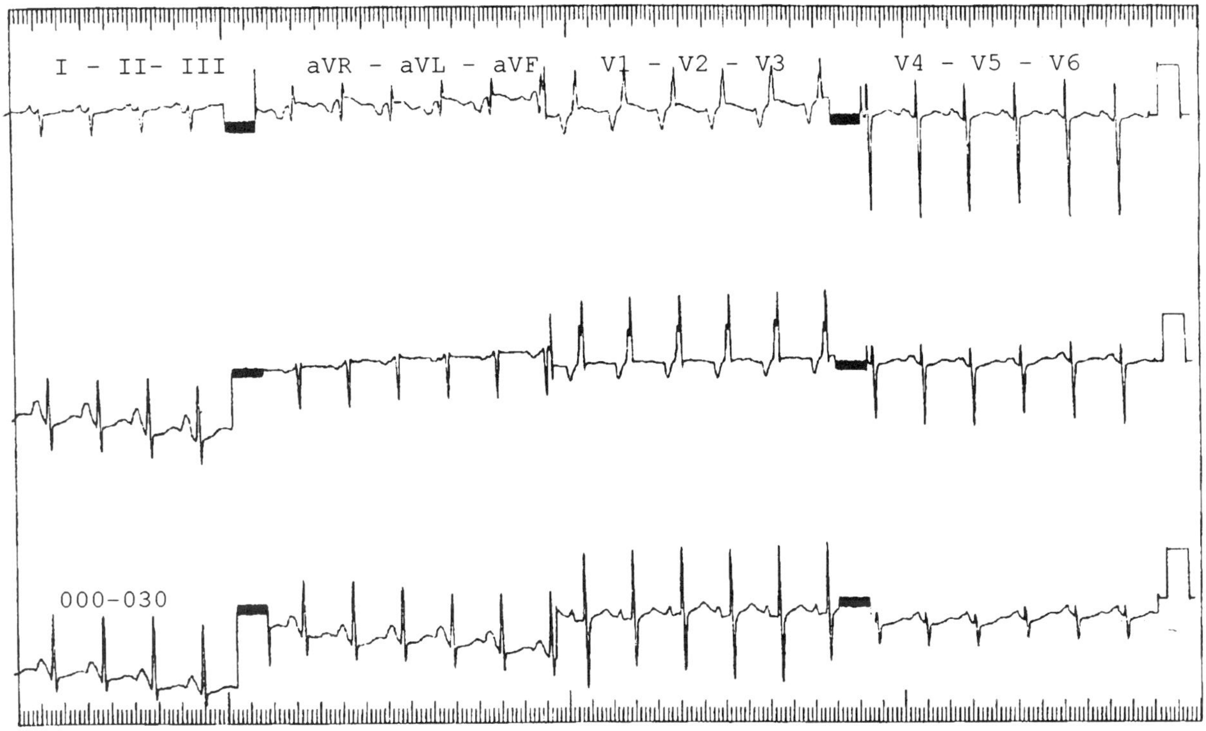

Mitral Stenosis

The tracing does not show mitral stenosis, of course, but the findings are enough to suggest it, and would offer strong support for the clinical suspicion. There is striking evidence of right atrial enlargement (29, 188), right ventricular hypertrophy (193), and left atrial enlargement (29, 188), a hemodynamic series that almost by itself identifies the mitral valve as the location of obstruction to flow. The absence of evidence of left ventricular overload, as might be expected if the lesion were to include regurgitation, is not evidence of its absence, but stenosis alone would explain everything nicely. Relating the findings to clinical medicine, they are almost enough to suggest age, gender, and hair color.

At a different level, the findings also demonstrate other fundamentals. The atria are activated sequentially in different directions, the right first, mostly left and down, in the frontal plane, followed by the left, mostly dorsad, perpendicular to the frontal plane. It is possible to identify abnormality in both (187). A force perpendicular to a plane (or a line) produces no projection on it; parallel to it, a maximum projection. The right atrium is identified in II, III, and aVF; the left, in V1.

```
135   135   16    08    --      sinus
+120    8:0    V3    3:3     normal
              nonc
          related to T
low     isoelectric V1-6
P: prominent, peaked 2, 3, F,
   prominent terminal negativ-
   ity V1

(1) Sinus mechanism, rate 135
(2) Right atrial enlargement
(3) Right ventricular enlarge-
    ment.
(4) Left atrial enlargement
(5) ST-T abnormality, non-
    specific
```

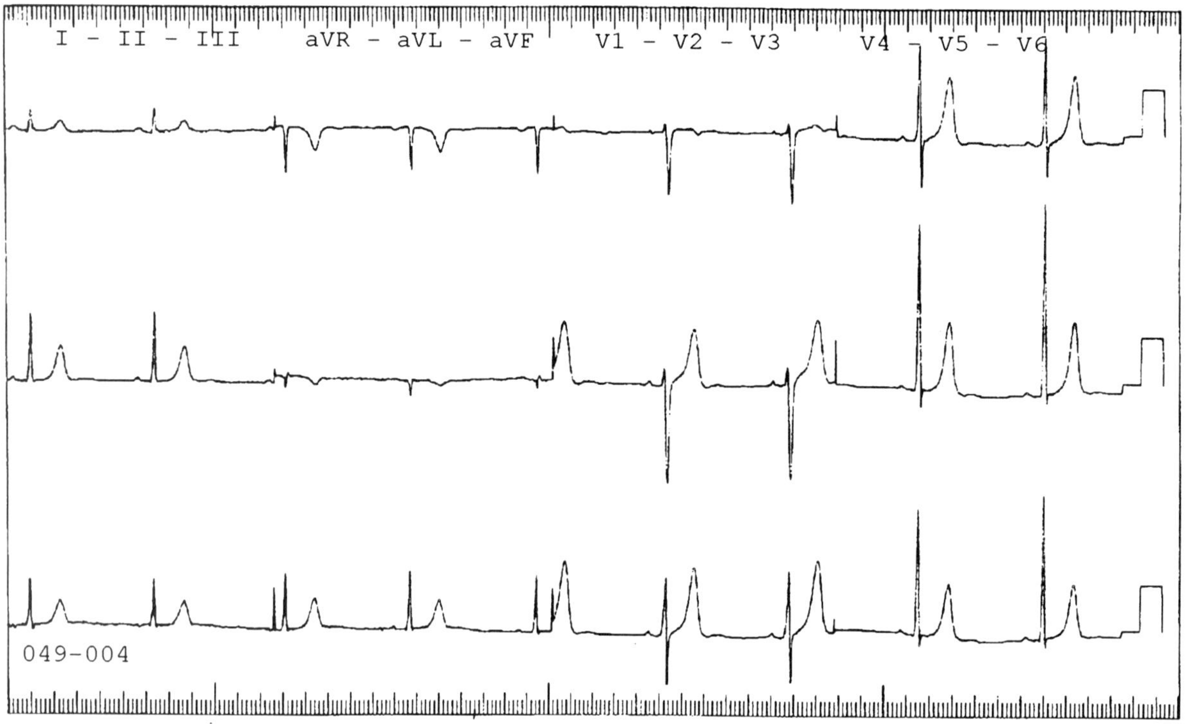

Tall, Peaked T

55	55	16	08	40	sinus
+75	2:15	V3	30:0		normal

none
some flattening
+75 ±V1, positive, tall, symmetrical V2-6

(1) Sinus mechanism, rate 55
(2) Suggests left ventricular hypertrophy
(3) Otherwise WNL

The differential diagnosis of tall T waves is complicated by the fact that the taller they are the less difference there is between the initial and terminal slopes, making "symmetrical" almost inevitable as part of the description, and both "tall" and "symmetrical" are relative. The pattern in this tracing could easily be evidence of hyperkalemia, coronary insufficiency, subarachnoid hemorrhage or some other intracranial lesion, or something else (29, 192), but with no clinical information and no control tracing, and remembering the admonition first to do no harm, it cannot be called abnormal. The primary physician has information other than that in the tracing on which to base a decision. The risk to the patient is that if one of these is suggested, and the doctor does not realize the differential, it may be taken as a statement of fact, confusing the picture and leading to unnecessary tests and procedures.

The sum of SV1 plus RV5 is great enough (no matter which beat is measured) to justify suggesting left ventricular hypertrophy (39, 192).

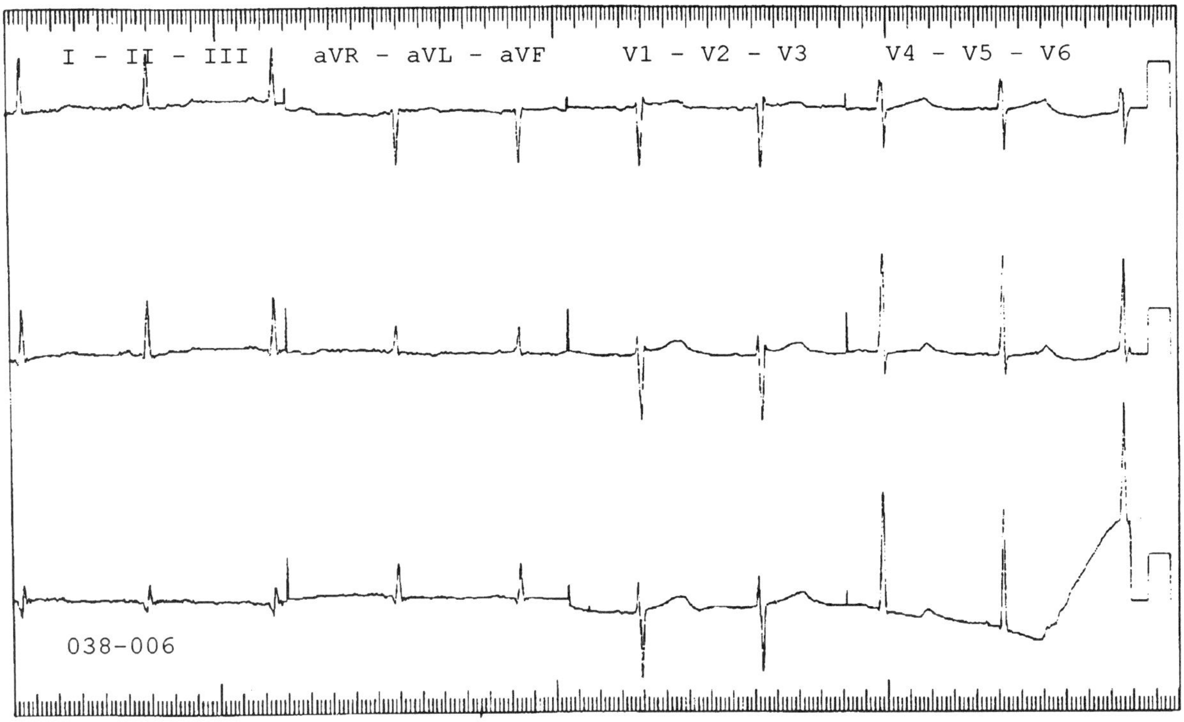

Low T, Prominent U, Long QT

```
55     55    20    08    ?40    sinus
+30   rSr 1:12:2, V4, 25:0     nml
                none
           related to T
low    ±V1     +V2-4 low     ±V5-6
U: Prominent

(1) Sinus mechanism, rate 55
(2) ST-T-U abnormalities,
    non-specific
```

One useful criterion for defining low voltage of T is that it is less than about 10% of QRS amplitude in a lead in which they are of the same sign and maximum amplitude, as in I, II, aVL, and aVF in this tracing (50). Low T voltage is a statistical abnormality, not a disease (5). As an isolated observation, it has no clinical application, but must be interpreted in context. The clinical picture, the stability of the pattern, and associated findings are all factors.

In this case, the prominence of the U wave continuous with T is one of those factors, and the time it takes for the ventricles to repolarize, the QT interval, is another, but no very meaningful figure for QT is available here. It was computed as 0.506 s, but this is really a measure of QU, and "correcting" it to 0.480 is specious.

One reasonable explanation for this ST-T-U pattern is hypokalemia, and hypocalcemia, or something else, may be a factor. Like low T voltage, prolongation of QT is a very nonspecific abnormality.

EKG 127

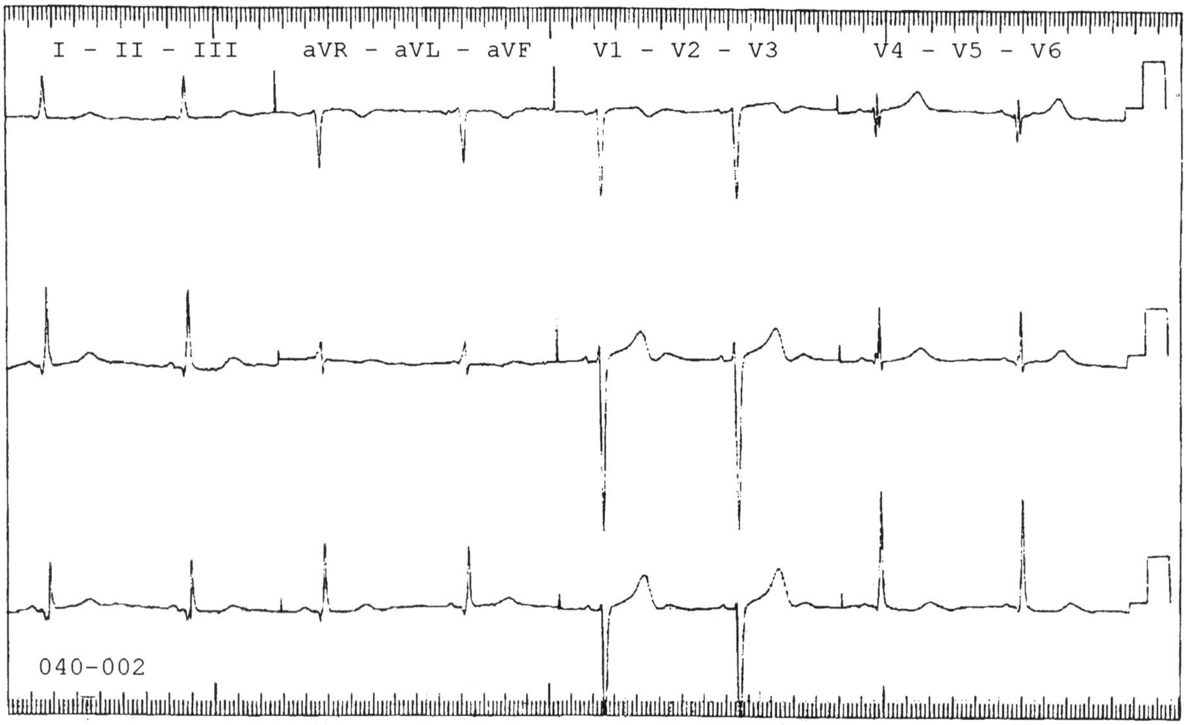

Prominent U

```
50    50    16    10    40       sinus
+60   1:20    V4     25:0     Q2,3,F
              none
             normal
+60     ?±V1,      positive V2-6
U: prominent

(1) Sinus mechanism, rate 50
(2) ST-T abns, nonspecific
```

The readout gave the QT interval as 0.526 sec, implying accuracy beyond the useful limits of the method, and including the U, really the QU interval. The computer is always right if right is defined as doing what it has been programmed to do, but the meaningfulness of the detail for which it can be programmed has to be evaluated. "Correction" of such an inherently ill-defined measure as the duration of QT, the "Qtc," is of little, if any, value (24, 202). The U wave (51, 217) is seldom of much importance at an actionable level. When negative, though, especially with negative T in midprecordial leads, it can be a strong signal for coronary insufficiency, and it may be accentuated by either hypokalemia or hypocalcemia. Merged with T, it may explain what is perceived as a notch, or dimple, in T, and failure to differentiate it from T, as in this tracing, may explain a very long "QT" interval.

The Q2,3 is prominent, and interpretation of it as suggesting an old infarct could be defended, but nothing at all looks new. Most computer programs are so sensitive to inferior Qs that they err on the side of calling inferior infarcts too often. This reflects the reality of wide overlap between normal and abnormal initial QRS forces. This one was not called abnormal.

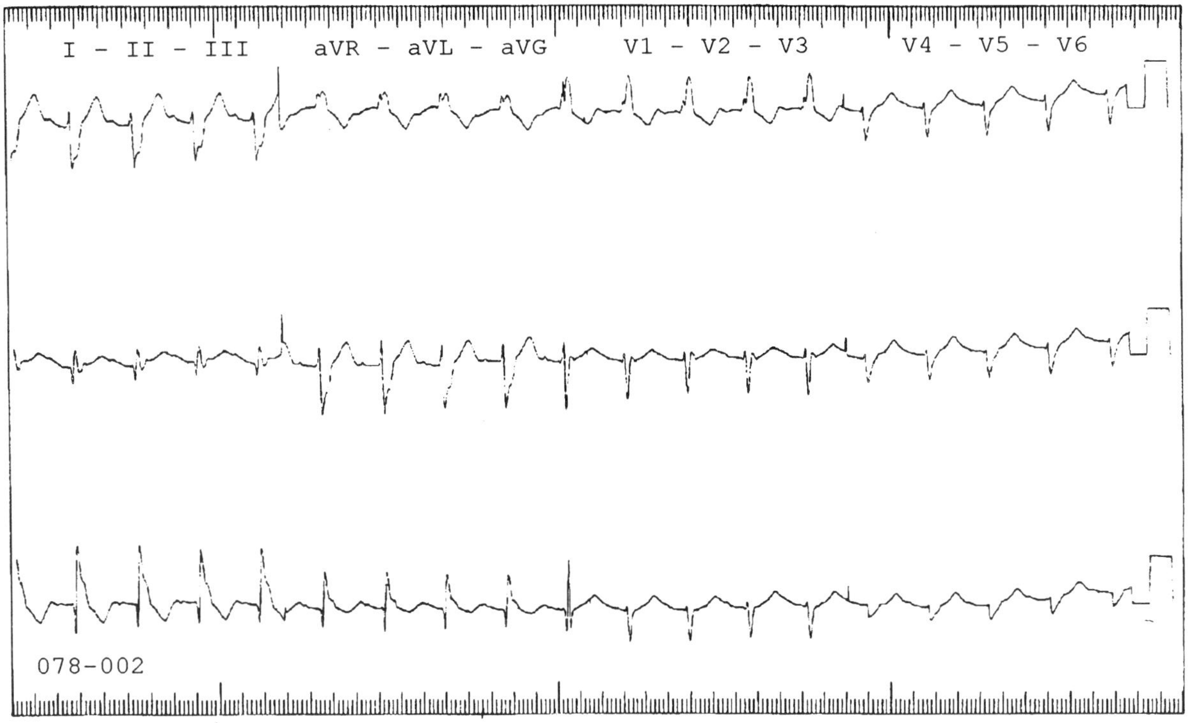

"Wide QRS Tachycardia"

The computer identified this as "wide QRS tachycardia," a term common in EKG reporting, but unacceptable because it is not as specific as possible, and likely to be equated with ventricular tachycardia (q.v,). The QRS here is indeed wide, and the rate fast, but there are several possible explanations for each of these independently (159, 168, 30). The key to why the QRS is wide is usually its contour, which, in this case, is typical of right bundle branch block.

"Tachycardia" says fast, but not how fast, and fails to recognize that atria and ventricles may function at different rates (120). "Fast" is an opinion; 110 is an objective finding. The doctor knew before the EKG was ordered that the ventricular (heart) rate was 110 with regular rhythm, and probably assumed it to be of sinus origin (123), but proof of the origin depends on the EKG. In this case, P is superimposed on T and seen best in Lead I (inset).

```
110    110    20    12    36      sinus
+150   8:0  ?V1½  1:5   BSTDRA,Q2,3,F
                  none
                 normal
?±0   neg V1,   ±V2   positive V3-6

(1) Sinus mechanism, rate 110
(2) Right bundle branch block
(3) Suggests old inferior mci
(4) Otherwise within normal limits

---Nothing at all looks new
```

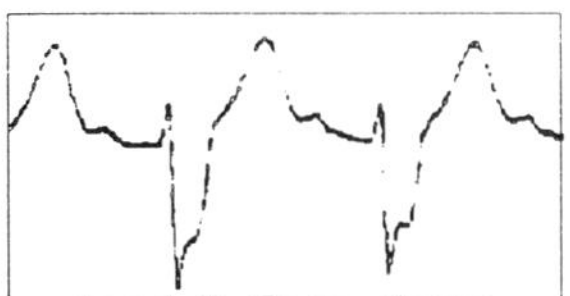
Lead I from above

The evidence for an infarct is equivocal: Q2,3,F is prominent, but clean and narrow.

EKG 129

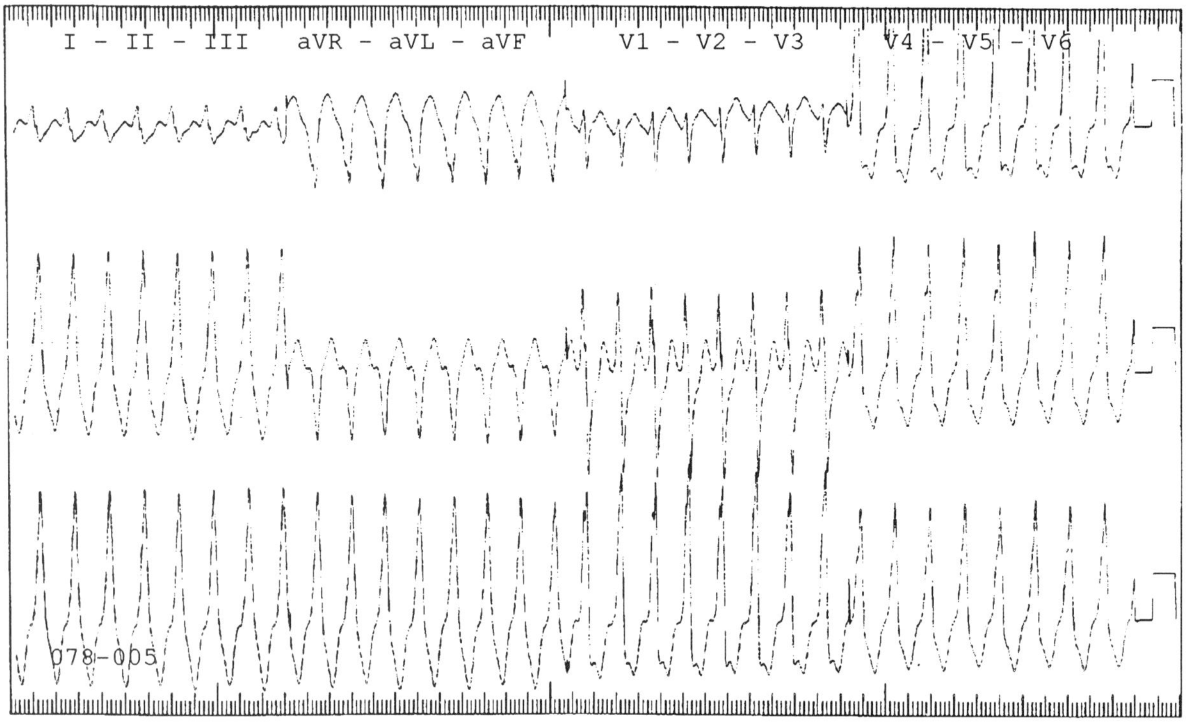

"Wide QRS Tachycardia"

```
--   200  --   12  ?28   see below
+90   3:8  V2   25:0     diff slur
    down 2,3,F, V2-6, up aVR
          related to T
-90      pos V1-2,        neg V3-6

(1) Ectopic mech, rate 200 with
    regular rhythm, prob of su-
    praventricular origin,
    junctional more likely than
    atrial.  Atrial activity is
    not identifiable.
(2) Atypical IV conduction  de-
    fect
(3) ST-T abns, prob cor insuf

--An alternative explanation
  for the whole picture is ven-
  tricular origin for QRS;
  i.e.,ventricular tachycardia
```

"Wide QRS (or wide complex) tachycardia" is a description of little clinical value, failing to satisfy the criteria for either mechanism or interpretation. "Tachycardia," a finding, does not require electrocardiography; "tachy" says fast, but not how fast, and "cardia" is assumed to refer to the ventricles. The absence of identifiable atrial activity does not prove that there is none, but regular ventricular rhythm at a rate greater than likely for sinus implies origin outside the sinus node, i.e., ectopic. With regular QRS rhythm, this could be atrial flutter, but an atrial rate of 400 is rare. If of supraventricular origin (125, 133), the AV junction is the most likely site by default, and that would leave the abnormality of QRS duration and contour to be handled separately (168). A ventricular origin ("ventricular tachycardia") could explain everything (144). The ST-T pattern of subendocardial injury would go well with either. Distinction between ventricular tachycardia, and supraventricular tachycardia with an IV conduction defect, is often not possible from the EKG alone. See also EKGs 12, 30, 61, 77, 91, 128.

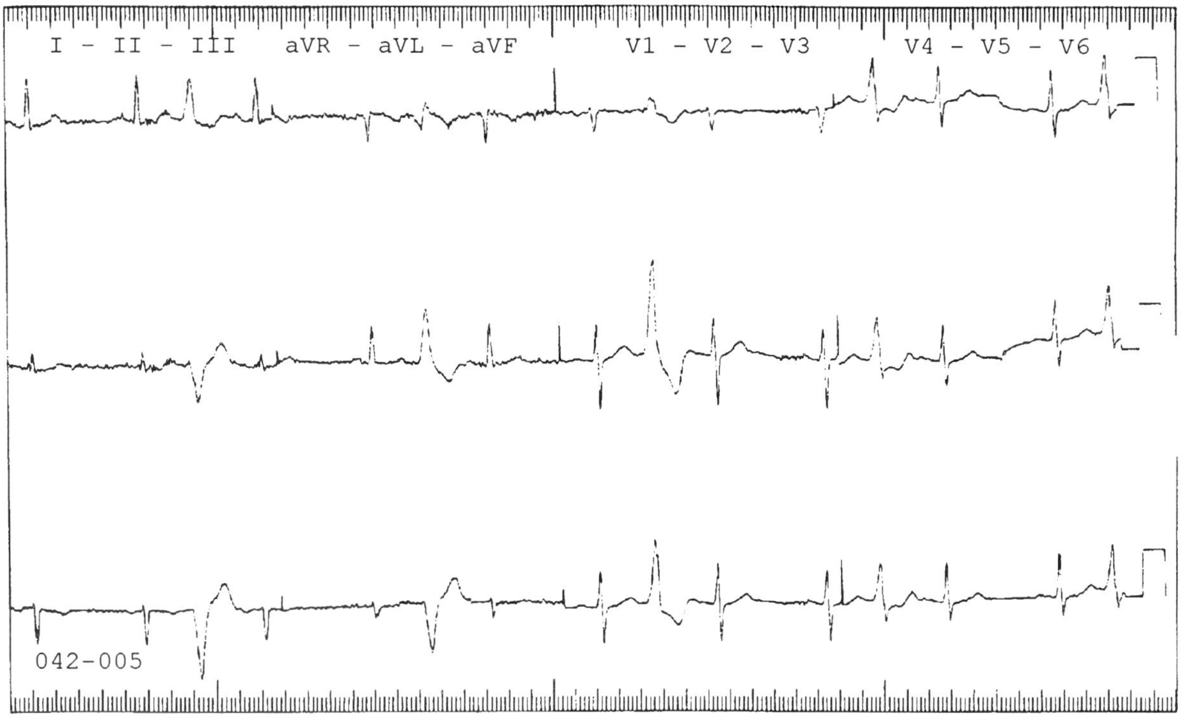

Interpolated PVCs

```
90   90   16   08   40     sinus with
                                 PVC's
-15   1:4,   V2-4,   10:3    normal
                  none
                 normal
±0     flat V1       positive V2-6

(1) Sinus mechanism, rate 90
(2) Interpolated PVC's
(3) Otherwise within normal
    limits
```

Premature contractions of ventricular origin (PVCs, PVBs, VPBs) used to be called extrasystoles. Most are not "extra," they just occur early so that the next impulse from above finds the ventricles refractory; the total number of beats per time remains the same. Occasionally, however, the relation among the intrinsic rate, timing of the premature beat, and the relevant refractory periods is such that this sequence does not take place; the PVC is "interpolated," truly extra (143).

Another variant of PVCs which sometimes warrants a special name is when the premature beat occurs after a P wave but before the atrial impulse has reached the ventricles, an "end-diastolic PVC." In this case the QRS may represent input from both the supraventricular focus and the ectopic one, a fusion beat (143). (See EKGs 63 and 109)

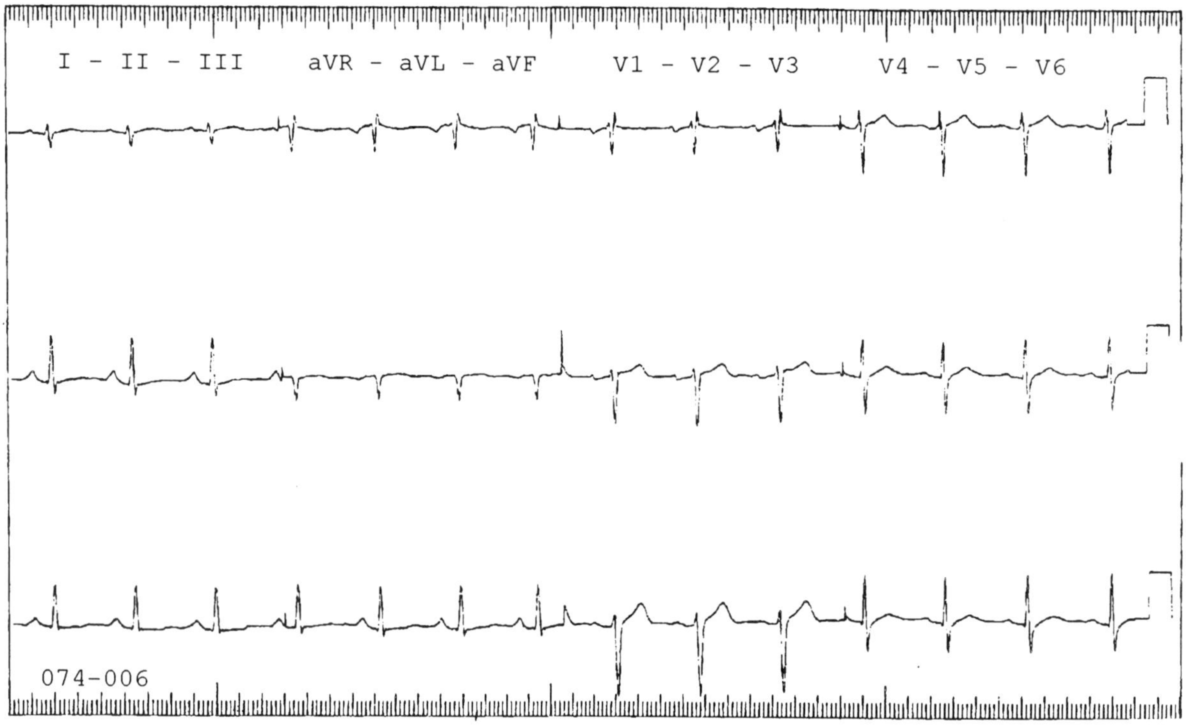

Incomplete Right Bundle Branch Block

```
85    85    20    08    40     sinus
+90   RSR 1:6:2  V5   10:6 normal
               none
           related to T
Low      ±V1        positive V2-6

(1) Sinus mechanism, rate 85
(2) ST-T abnormalities, non-
    specific

--Just low frontal T, not far
  from normal
```

The idea that bundle branch block, both left and right, should be subdivided into complete and incomplete has a long history. In the case of the left bundle, the practice has given way to naming subdivisions, left or right hemiblock (or fascicular block), but is still applied to the right bundle (159, 236). It satisfies the criteria for an interpretation (see "A tutorial: The mechanism..." in Chapter 3), but if "block" is perceived as an abnormality, may work to the patient's disadvantage. Sometimes the relevant finding, rSr V1, a description, is all that is reported. This does not qualify as an interpretation, but is not likely to put the patient at risk.

Given 0.10 sec as the upper limit of normal for QRS duration, and 0.12 s as the criterion for abnormal, incomplete block would have to fall between, and QRS duration cannot be estimated that close. An rSr in V1 may be evidence of right ventricular enlargement, especially when due of excessive flow, as with an atrial septal defect. Correlated with physical findings; e.g., a left basal systolic murmur in a child, it may contribute to understanding the problem, but the EKG pattern by itself should not be considered abnormal.

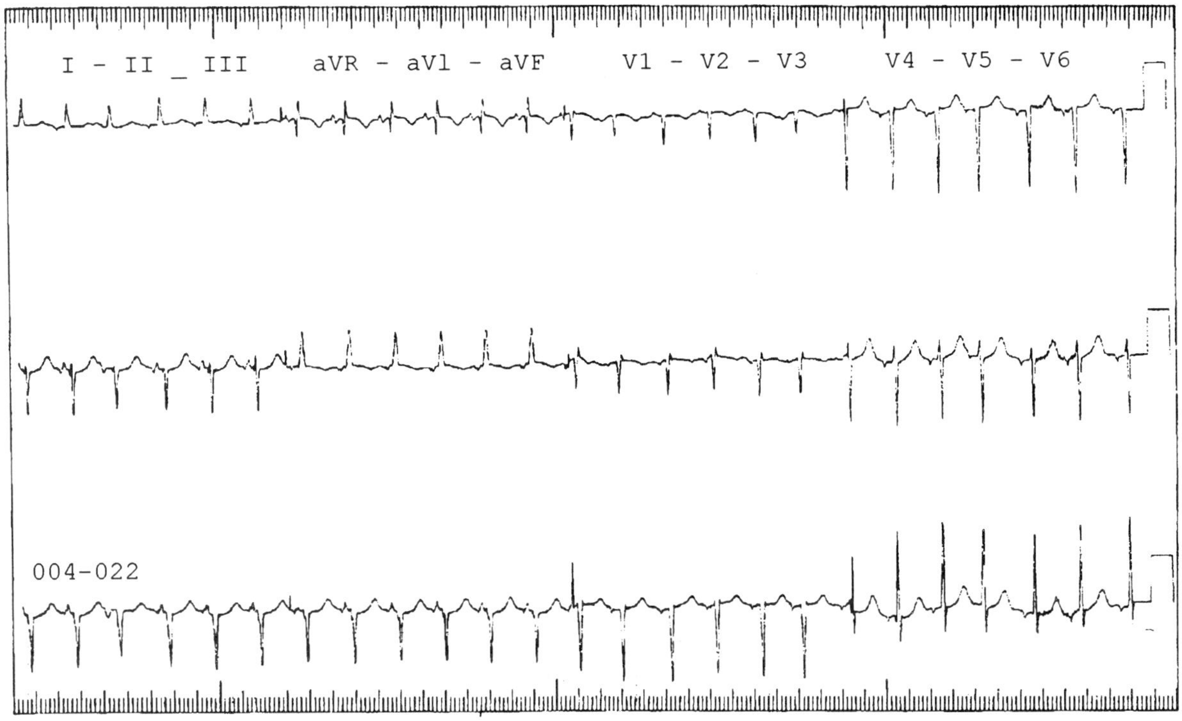

Usurping Atrial Ectopy

There is a problem in naming this mechanism. QRS is clearly of supraventricular origin, its rate, 150, is greater than usual for a sinus origin and slower than usual for 1:1 usurpation. It is typical of "flutter," but, given that atrial rate greater than ventricular is part of the definition of flutter (129), the 1:1 P:QRS ratio rules that out. "1:1 flutter" is accepted by some as meaningful, but compromises the definition of flutter. See EKG 91. Ventricular rhythm is not quite regular, but the presence of P waves eliminates atrial fibrillation. "Atrial tachycardia" has been all but replaced by the less precise "supraventricular tachycardia" as a name for benign paroxysms of rapid heart action with regular rhythm, but might fit here. Perhaps the combination of slight irregularity of rhythm, and varying contour of P, can qualify as "multifocal," or "chaotic" atrial tachycardia. In any case, the control (inset) with clearly sinus P waves, proves that it is usurping atrial ectopy, and beyond that the name is a matter of choice (122, 127).

150 150 ?08 06 28 see below
75 0:5 V5½ 20:3 normal
none
normal
+75 flat V1-2 positive V3-6

(1) Supraventricular mechanism, rate 150, with almost regular rhythm, prob of atrial origin; atrial activity is not altogether clear
(2) LAFB, prob, and/or old inferior myocardial infarct
(3) Otherwise within normal limits

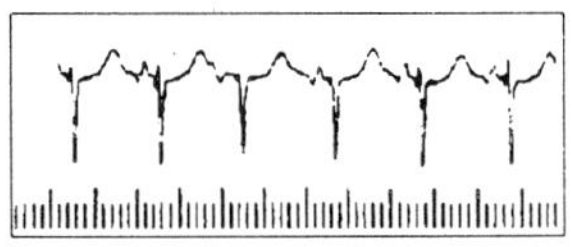
Lead II from above

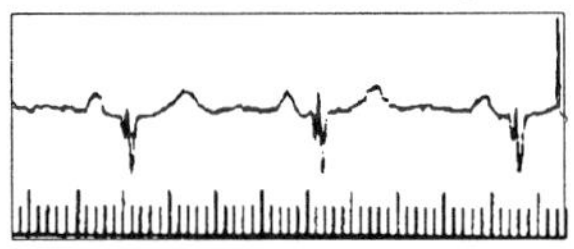
Lead II from a control

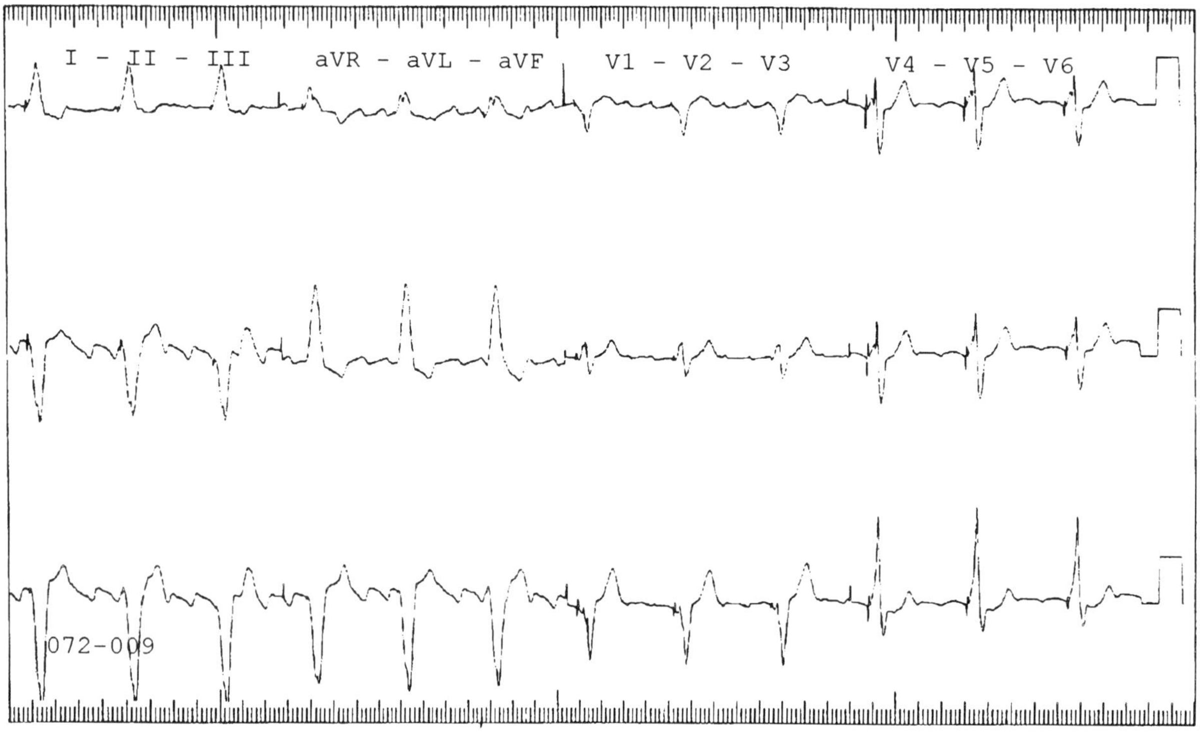

Atrial Tachycardia, Third Degree AV Block, Artificial Ventricular Pacemaker (VVI)

```
300   70   --   16   40    see below
-75   0:5  V4-5  20:5  diff slur
      slightly down V6
        related to T
+90   isoelectric V1, pos V2-6

(1) Atrial tachycardia, 300
(2) Third degree AV block
(3) Art vent pacemaker, cap-
    turning regularly, rate 70
```

The mechanism in this tracing is easy to describe in a way that tells exactly what is going on, but no single name covers it completely and adequately. The rate of the P waves, 300/min, practically rules out a sinus origin, and this is confirmed by their inscription cephalad. Some would combine these features and describe the atrial activity as flutter, but this depends on one's definition of flutter, and therein lies a problem. There is probably general agreement that the name implies usurpation of atrial activity by a process confined to the atria (reentry?, automaticity?), but not that the relation between atria and ventricles is part of the definition. One that includes both is that flutter is present when the rate of regular, repetitive atrial impulses exceeds the capacity of the AV node to conduct. With all QRSs of supraventricular origin, this defines second degree AV block, but due to overload of the system, not impairment of conduction. This means that in atrial flutter there are two abnormalities in the tracing, "tachyatria" and second degree AV block, but only one in the heart, usurping atrial ectopy (129, 137, 152, 140). In this case, AV block is complete, and the ventricles are driven by an artificial pacemaker, probably in the right ventricle

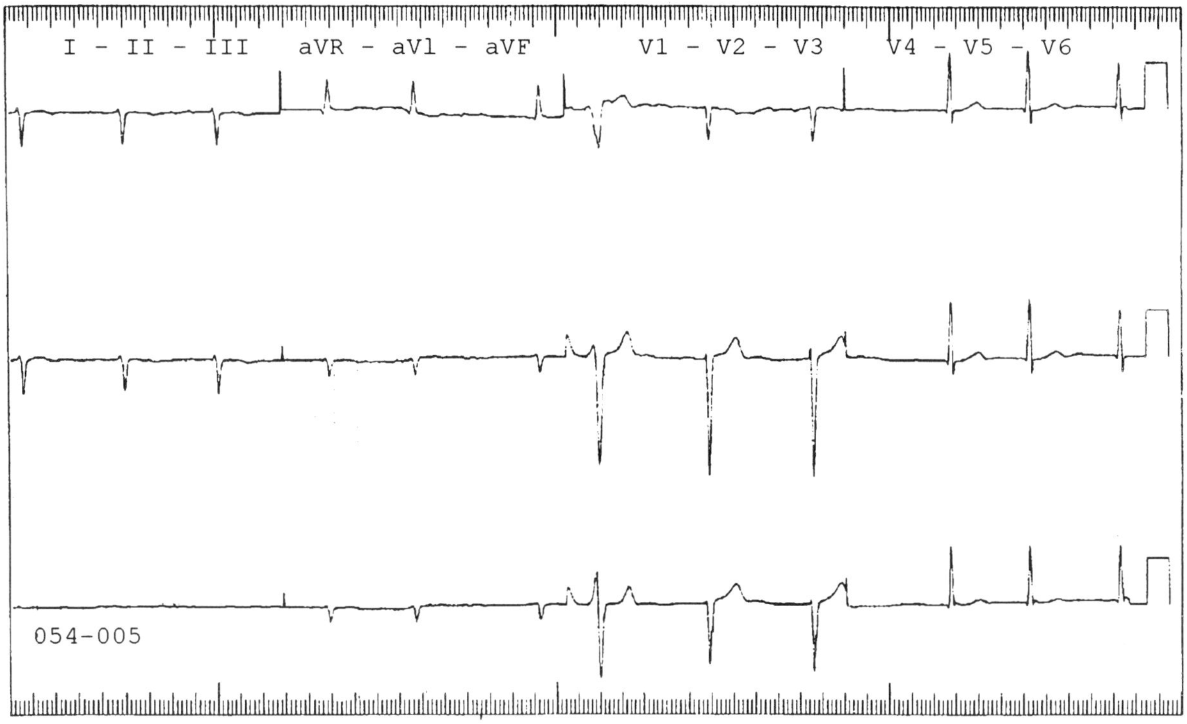

Flat Line, Lead III

A flat line in lead I, II, or III is a common artifact, serious chiefly in that it must be recognized as evidence that the tracing is incomplete, limiting its usefulness and introducing the possibility that it may be misinterpreted. What it implies is that the electrodes defining the lead involved are attached to the same apex of Einthoven's triangle; there is no difference in potential between them. For Lead III, this means transposition of left arm and right leg leads. The right leg electrode is used for grounding the body to the EKG machine and is effective for this purpose wherever it is attached, but the left arm electrode represents one of the apices, and when attached to the same apex as another, there is no triangle; one of the premises on which interpretation is based is not valid. aVR, aVL, and aVF are similarly limited in usefulness, but effect in V1-6 is minimal (95, 107).

The differential here includes very low voltage with MFQRS at +30.

-- 70 -- 08 40 see below
?? 0:5 V3½ 12:0 normal
none
related to T
low?? ±V1 pos V2-5 ±V6

(1) Atrial fibrillation, rate about 70
(2) Otherwise prob WNL or at worst only small ST-T abnormalities, but incomplete

--Recorded with left arm and right leg leads transposed

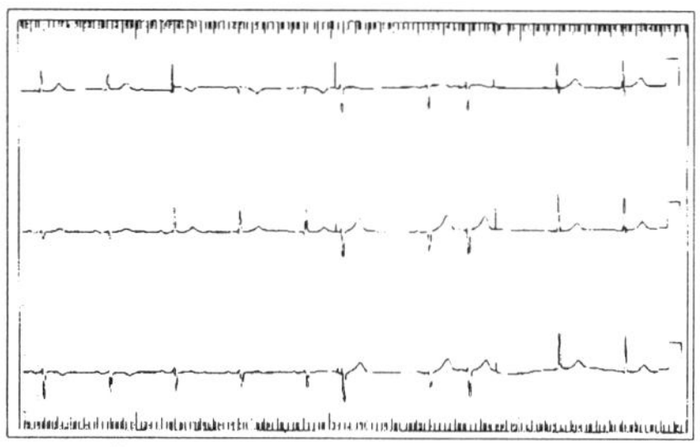
EKG #134 with proper connections

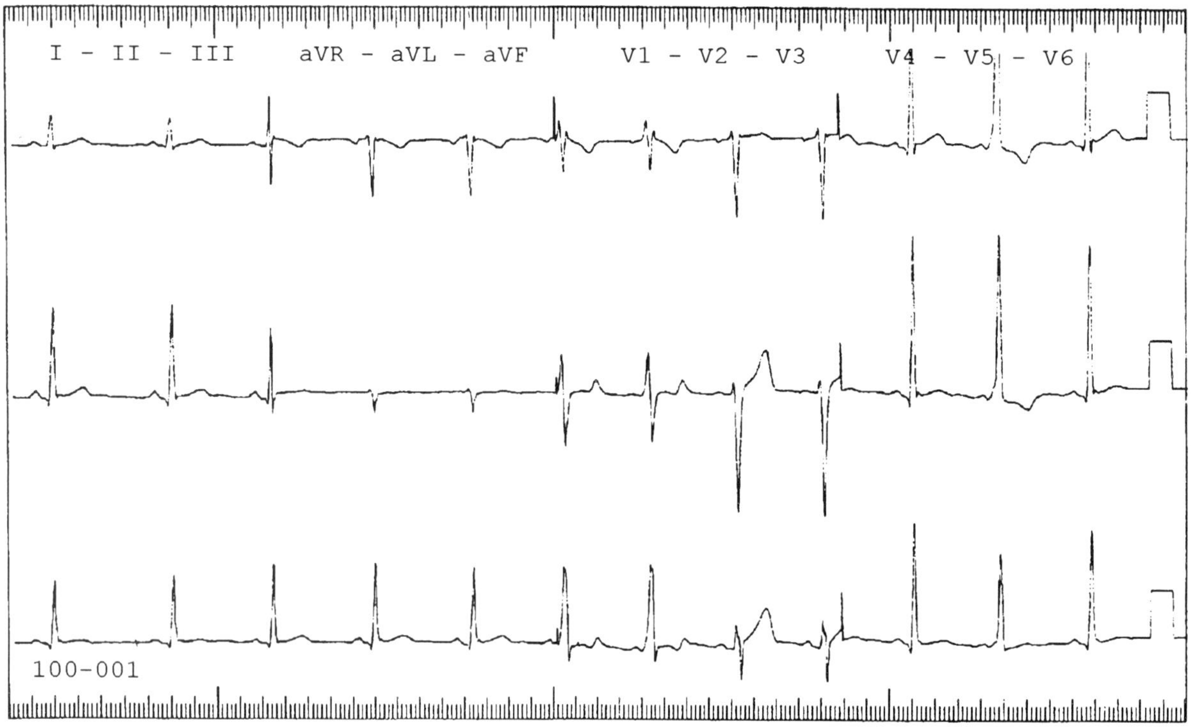

Ventricular Pre-Excitation, Intermittent

Ventricular pre-excitation (155), often equated with the WolffParkinson-White (WPW) Syndrome, is one of those things that can be established by EKG findings when they are present, but, because it may be inconstant, cannot be "ruled out" by their absence; it may be found in some beats and not others, or in some tracings and not others. The wide beats may be mistaken for PVCs, as the computer program did here, and, in a sense they are; QRS begins prematurely, but because of "pre" excitation, not discharge of an ectopic focus. The impulse from the atria reaches the ventricles via an anomalous pathway, bypassing the slower normal one and explaining shortening of PR, and, because QRS ends on time, widening of the complex; the PJ interval does not change. With bundle branch block, PJ is long and PR is unchanged. Change in the route of depolarization necessarily changes the route of repolarization; note the difference between the ST-T pattern in normally conducted and anomalous beats. The anomaly cancels the normal Q in this case, but in others may produce a Q that can be misinterpreted as evidence of an infarct.

70 70 16 10 40 sinus
+75 1:15 V3 25:0 initial slur
none related to T
+45 ±V1 pos V2-6, low V5-6

(1) Sinus mechanism, rate 70
(2) Ventricular pre-excitation, intermittent
(3) Otherwise prob WNL, at worst only small ST-T abnormalities

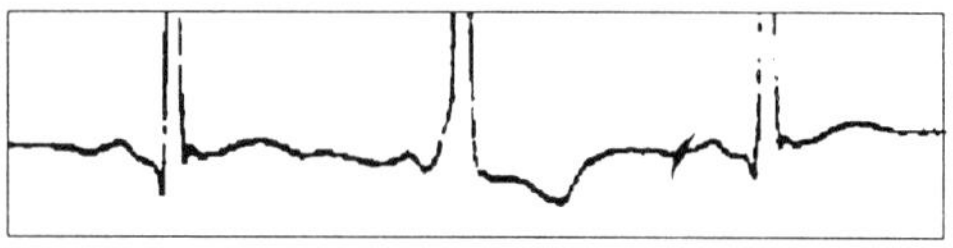

V5 from above

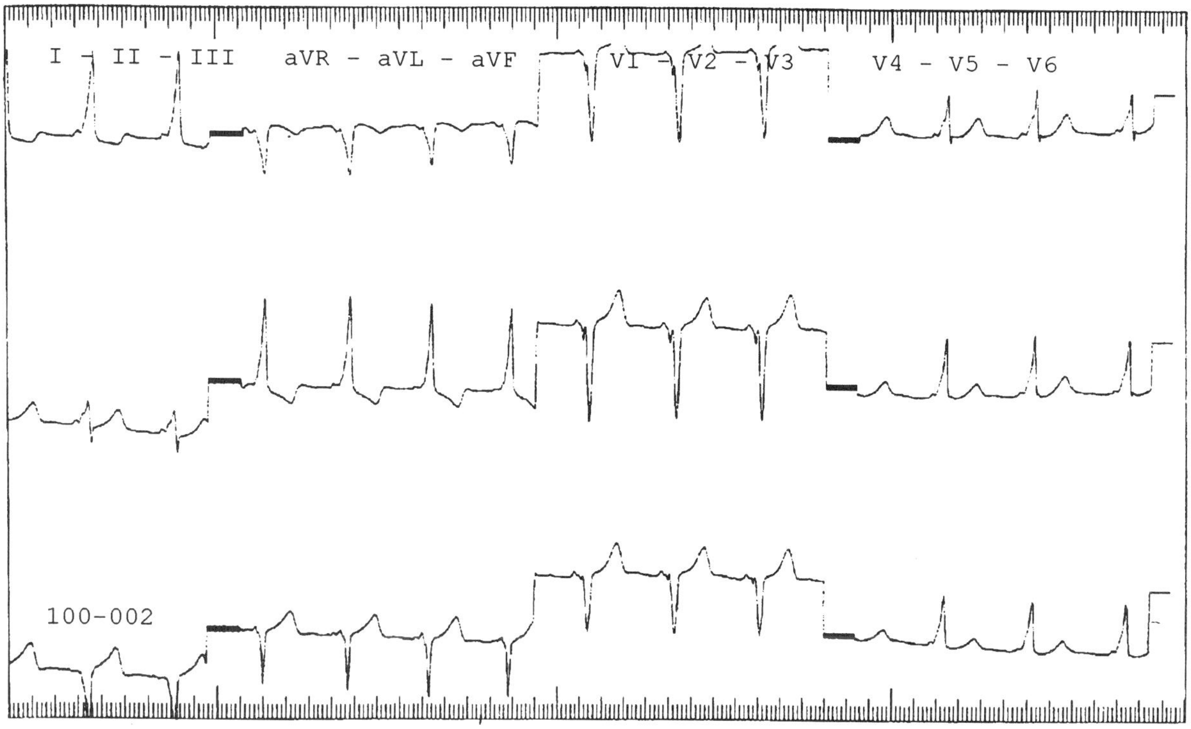

Ventricular Pre-Excitation, Type B (vs Myocardial Infarction)

80 80 08 12+ ?44 sinus
-30 0:20 V3½ 10:0 early
slur
none
normal
+90 positive V1 - 6

(1) Sinus mechanism, rate 80
(2) Ventricular pre-excitation, Type B

Specific features of the evidence of pre-excitation depend on the location and structural and functional characteristics of the anomalous pathway. The pattern sometimes resembles right bundle branch block, Type A (EKG 137) and sometimes left (Type B) (155).

Myocardial infarction is a much more common explanation for abnormality of initial QRS forces, and distinction fro preexcitation is not always possible from the EKG alone. It would be easy to see the pattern in this tracing as evidence of an old infarct, either anterior and/or inferior. With an infarct, though, PR need not be short, and the ST-T pattern is often typical.

Pre-excitation also may mask evidence of an infarct. This is rare, and most likely to be recognized when pre-excitation is transient.

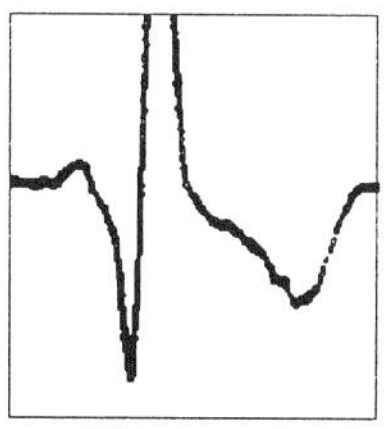
Q3 pre-ex
EKG #17

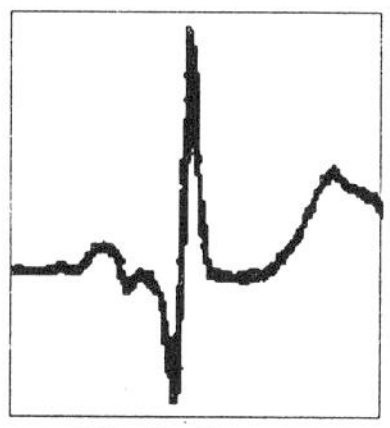
Q3 infarct
EKG #76

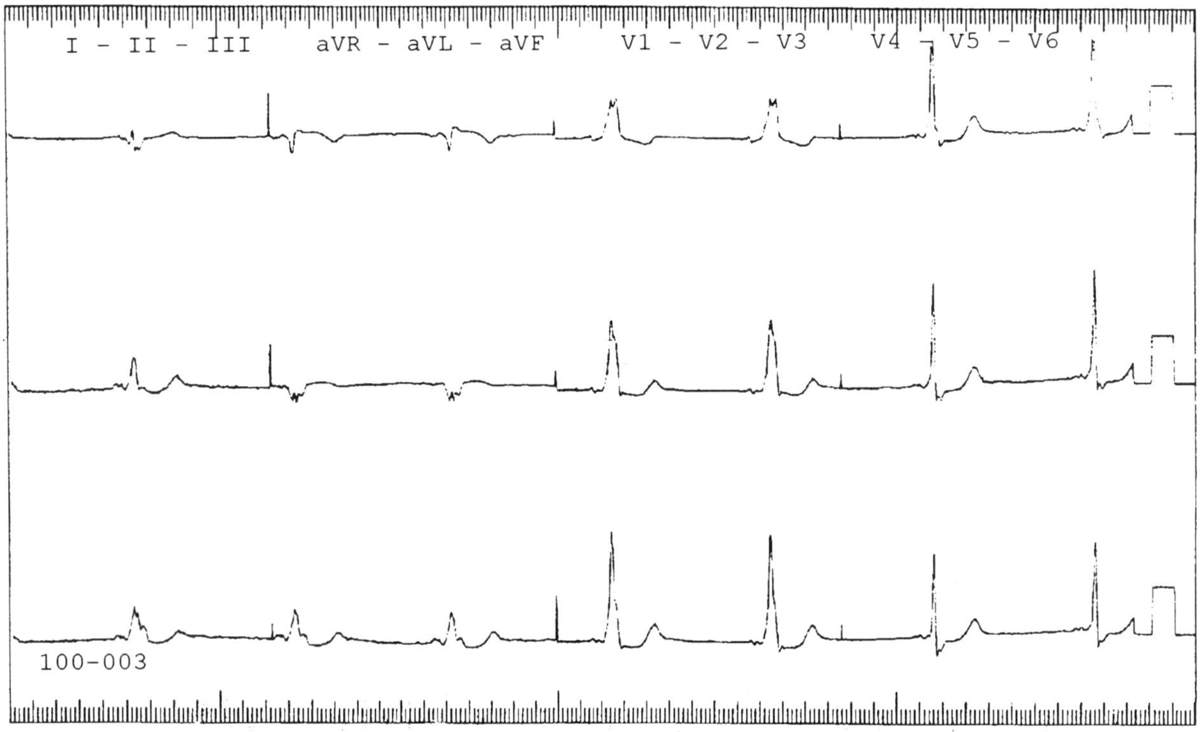

Ventricular Pre-Excitation, Type A

45 45 12 16 48 sinus
+105 10:0 -- 15:3 BSTDRA
slightly down V3-6
flattened
+60 low neg V1, pos V2-6

(1) Sinus mechanism, rate 45
(2) Ventricular pre-excitation, Type A
(3) Equivocal ST-T pattern suggestive of coronary insufficiency

When the pattern of pre-excitation was first recognized by Drs. Wolff, Parkinson, and White (155), it was seen as an unusual form of bundle branch block, an interpretation easy to understand. As experience grew, it was apparent that in many cases the abnormal forces were directed chiefly to the right and ventrad, as here, simulating right bundle branch block, while in others (EKG 136) the pattern was more nearly that of left bundle branch block. These became known as Type A and Type B, suggesting the location of the anomalous pathway, but most cases do not fit neatly into either type. Type A is more likely to be associated with atrial fibrillation or flutter than Type B, but, now that precise location of the pathway, and its ablation, is possible, the distinction is of little value.

Pre-excitation is recognized best in leads with unidirectional QRS, and may be consistent or intermittent (EKG 135). Differential diagnosis involves mostly bundle branch block and myocardial infarction.

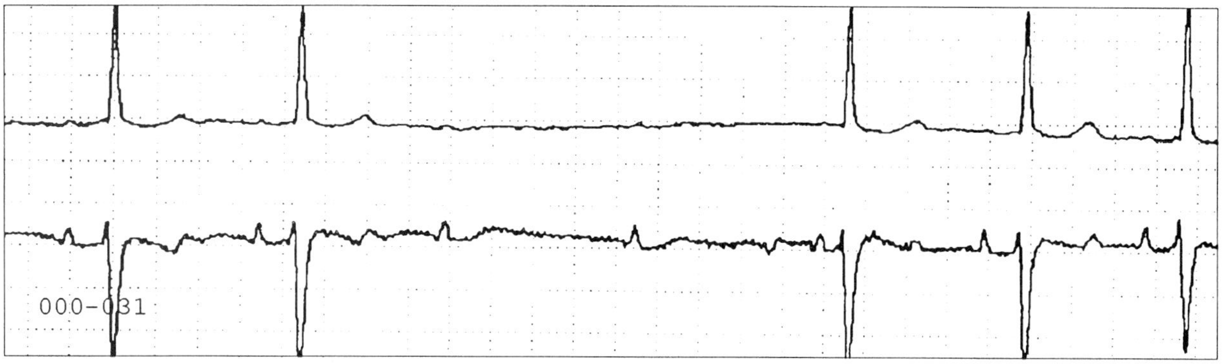

Second Degree AV Block, Type II (Mobitz)

```
65   ±50   --   08  40    see below

(1) Sinus mechanism, rate 65
(2) Second degree AV block,
    Type II, ventricular rate
    about 50
(3) Otherwise within normal
    limits, but there are only
    two leads
```

In a practice that reviews approximately seventy thousand EKGs a year, almost all from adults, from about fifty hospitals and clinic groups, Type II second degree AV block (Mobitz) is recognized perhaps once or twice.

This one is from a Holter monitor (10) from a patient who had been referred to an electrophysiologist. PR is normal in the first two and last three beats, but the two P waves in the middle are not followed by QRSs. In Type I (Wenckebach), the common variety, PR increases with succeeding beats until one is dropped (152).

It is interesting that Dr. Wenckebach, also the first to recognize the antiarrhythmic properties of quinine (which led to the use of quinidine), described this phenomenon from observations of the jugular and apical pulses, not the EKG; Dr. Mobitz described the same findings using the EKG. Both men described both types (68, 152).

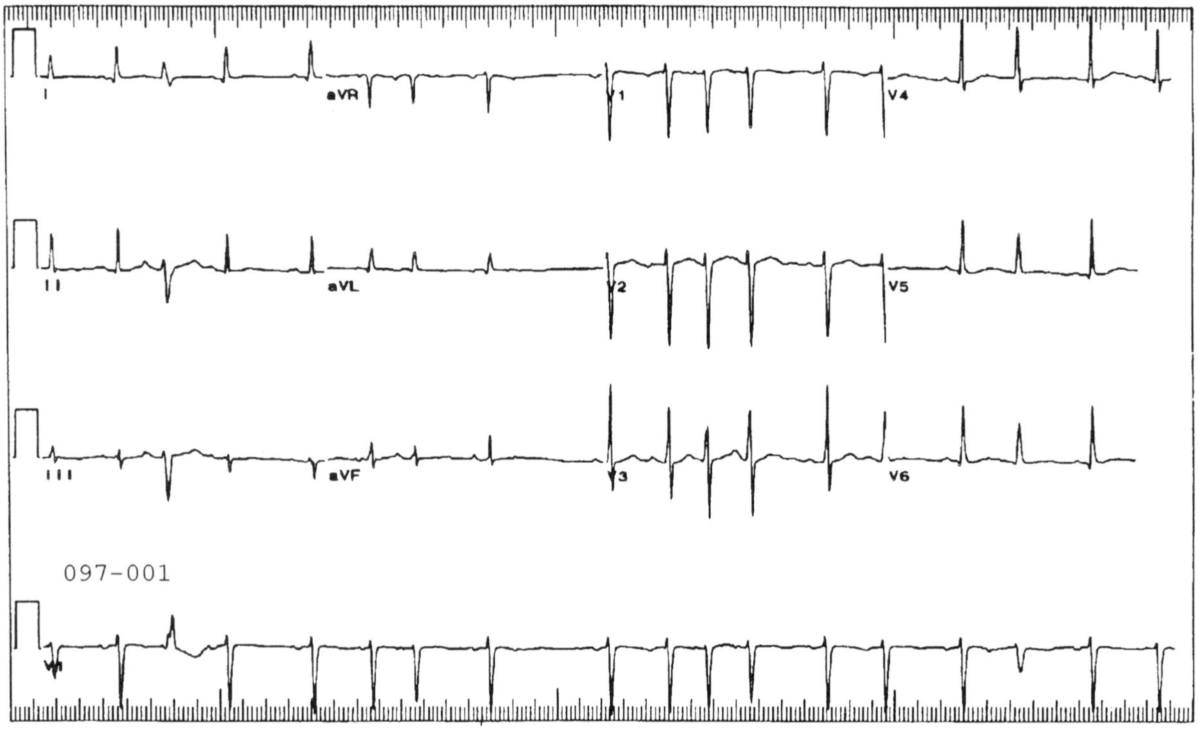

Frequent PACs

```
90   90   16   08   ?32    See below
+15   1:12   V3   12:0   normal
              none
          related to T
low   ±V1    +V2-3 low    ±V4-6

(1) Sinus mechanism, rate 90
(2) Frequent PAC's
(3) ST-T abnormalities,
    nonspecific
```

This mechanism calls for no name more precise than sinus with frequent PACs. It might qualify as "multifocal atrial tachycardia" in the judgment of some, but that term is not altogether standard, probably identifying only a level of usurping atrial ectopy beyond the presence of a few PACs, as seen commonly in normals, but not fulfilling anyone's criteria for either flutter or fibrillation. Computer programs often recognize the problem, but call it atrial fibrillation, and, given the ill-defined taxonomy of usurping atrial ectopy, this is a reasonable interpretation. If the rhythm, of both atria and ventricles, were regular, and the configuration of the P waves constant, it might be called atrial tachycardia.

Though not likely to be pointed out as part of the problem, a major factor is how to define a P wave (27, 70). This can lead to awareness of the limitation of the method for estimating the length of PR, a feature of every tracing, but not given much thought when it is not obviously in question.

Compare this tracing to those indexed as atrial fibrillation, atrial flutter, "supraventricular tachycardia," and junctional.

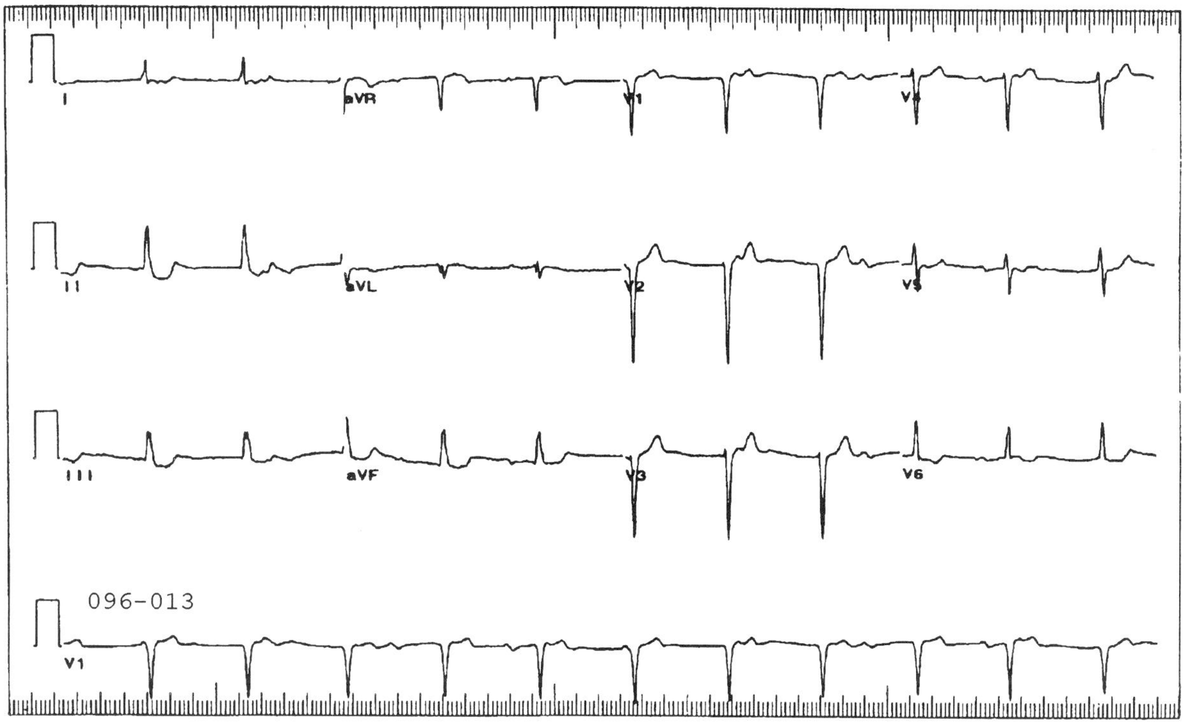

Accelerated Junctional Mechanism

```
60   70   --   09  40      see below
+75     0:12    V5    6:0     normal
   sl depressed II, III, aVF
              sagging
low    pos V1-4,    ±V5,     neg V6

(1) Sinus mechanism, rate 60
(2) Junctional pacemaker, rate
    70
(3) ST-T abnormalities,
    nonspecific
```

The findings in this tracing present the challenge of choosing a useful name for the mechanism. It is basically sinus with normal AV conduction, but there is also a junctional pacemaker firing at a rate greater than sinus. Instead of being passive, suppressed by the faster one but ready to escape if needed, the junctional focus has become active and usurped pacemaker function for the ventricles. If its signal arrives when they are still refractory from a conducted sinus beat, though, they cannot respond. All QRSs may arise from the junctional focus, and ventricular rhythm will be regular, but if the rates of the two foci are not fixed, some sinus beats get through and it is irregular. Accelerated junctional mechanism, isorhythmic dissociation, and interference dissociation are variants of the same thing. In this tracing, QRS rhythm is very nearly regular, but there are Ps at a slower rate. Another name for the combination is "AV dissociation," accurate, but not as specific as possible; atria and ventricles are also dissociated when there is second or third degree AV block.

A control from the patient above with sinus mechanism, first degree AV block, and no ectopy.

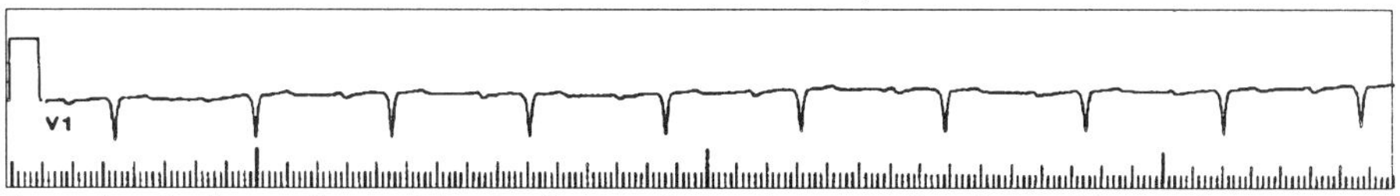

A control from the patient above with sinus mechanism, first degree AV block, and no ectopy

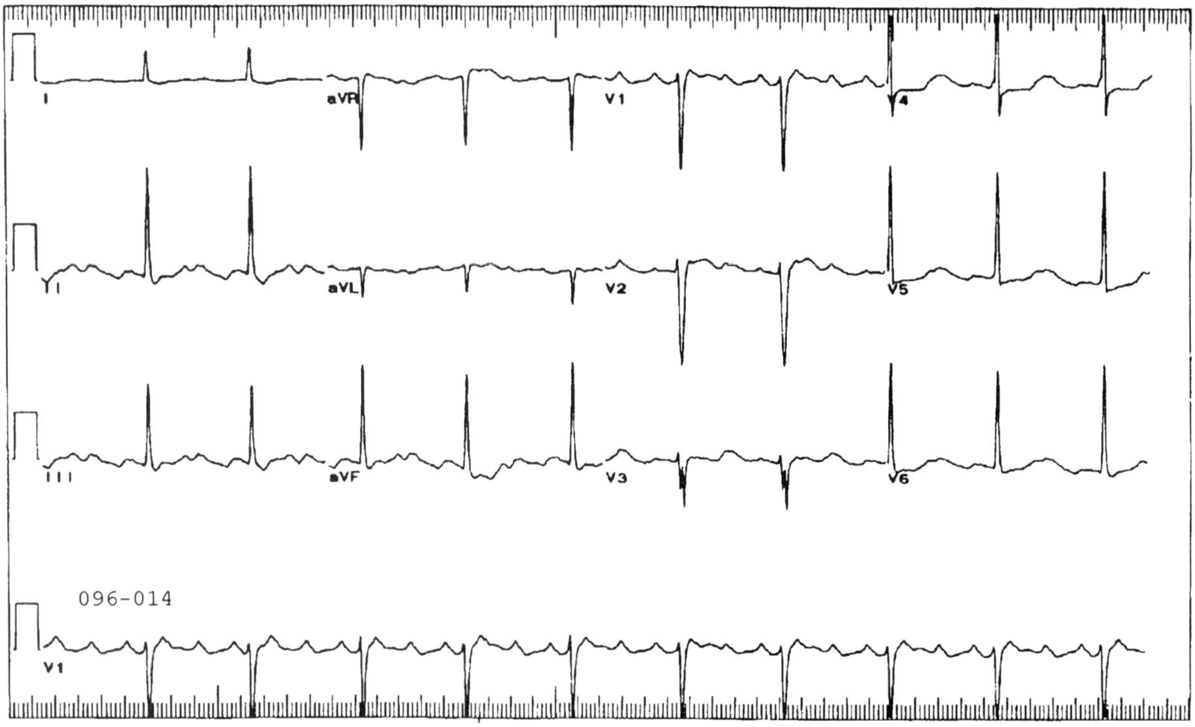

PAT with Block (or Flutter?)

```
195   65   --   08   ?40   see below
+75   1:20  V3½  20:0       normal
        slightly down V4-5
             flattened
Low          isoelectric V1-6

(1) Atrial tachycardia with
    block (flutter?), 195/65
(2) ST-T abnormalities suggest-
    ive of coronary insuffi-
    ciency, but small
```

As with other examples of usurping atrial ectopy, a name for this mechanism is arbitrary. There are obvious P waves (10, 27) that are positive in aVF, identifying them as arising high in an atrium, and they are separated by periods of no electrical activity, suggesting automaticity rather than reentry as an explanation for how the action is sustained. Their rate is strong evidence against a sinus origin (123), and a control tracing (inset) with a typically sinus rate supports this interpretation. Atrial activity, considered alone, could be described as "tachyatria," but the nearest to a standard term for it is atrial tachycardia. All QRSs are of atrial origin but not all atrial beats are conducted to the ventricles, defining second degree AV block; thus, "atrial tachycardia with block" or, the traditional term, "PAT with block." Distinction from atrial flutter depends on whether an explanation for the means by which activity is sustained, reentry or repetitive firing of an atrial focus, is included in the definition.

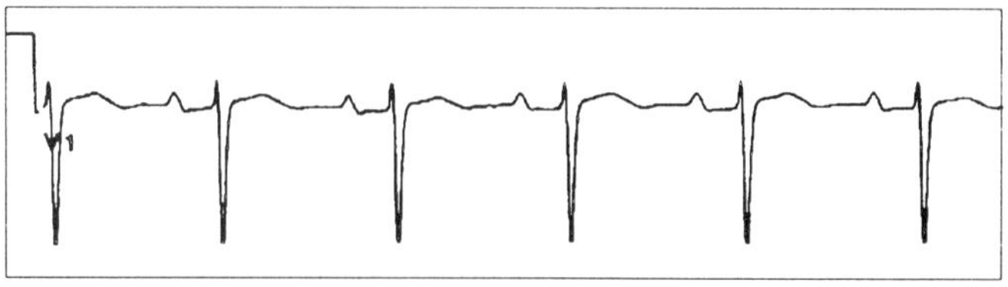

Same patient as above, twenty-four hours later

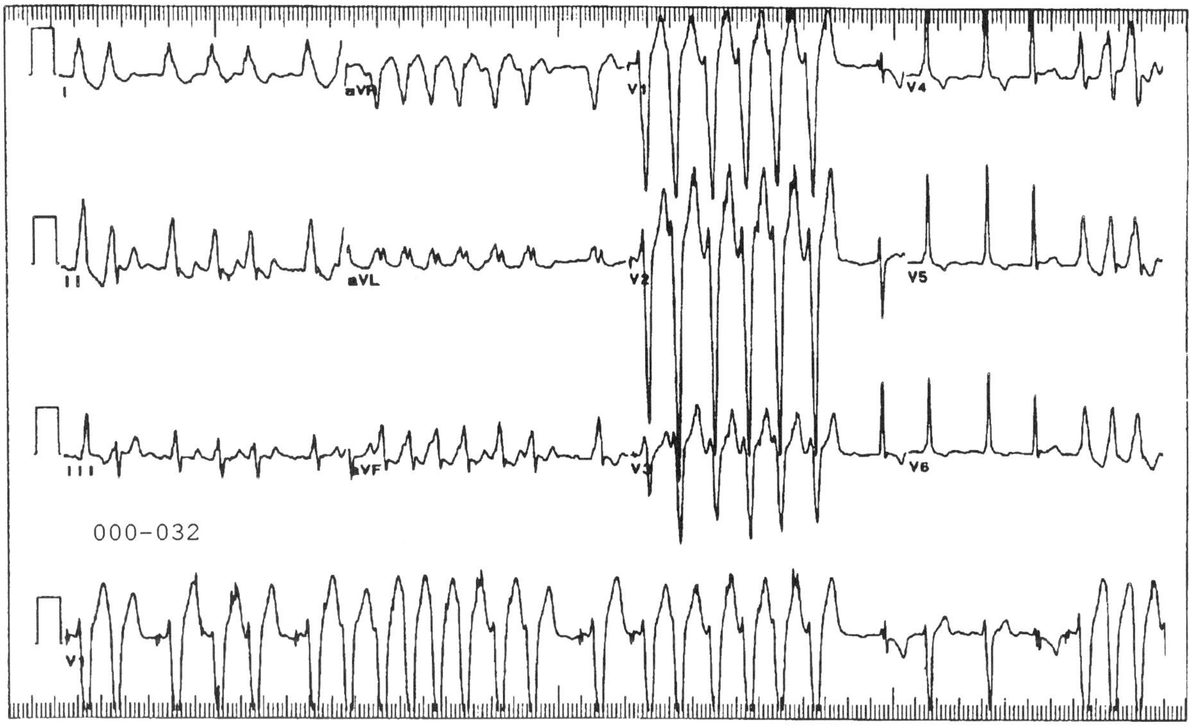

Ventricular Pre-excitation, Uncertain Mechanism

In most instances the paroxysms of rapid heart action associated with pre-excitation are benign, often of no more than nuisance value, but, rarely, may be life-threatening, especially if there is atrial fibrillation. The means by which the tachycardia is sustained, a circus via both normal and anomalous pathways (AV reentry), may cancel both the short PR and the early QRS slur, obscuring the nature of the problem, and making it indistinguishable from ventricular tachycardia. When it can be recognized, the location of the principal abnormality of QRS at the beginning of the complex may be the only lead (157). The clinical setting, especially if there is a control tracing showing pre-excitation, is critical. Coexistence of left or right bundle branch block, and/or a myocardial infarct, complicates the problem.

```
--   ?100   -- ?10 ?32   see below
+30  03:25  V3½ 15:0 early slur
              none
sagging/flattened/related to T
low ?+105   pos V1-3,   neg V4-6

(1) The basic mech is of supra-
    ventricular origin, rate
    about 100, with irregular
    rhythm, prob AF, but
    atrial activity is not
    clear
(2) Intermittent tachycardia,
    rate about 170, also with
    irregular rhythm, and QRS
    widening, probably of su-
    praventricular origin with
    aberration or pre-excita-
    tion, but almost as easily
    ventricular; i.e.,ventricu-
    lar tachycardia
(3) ST-T abnormalities, non-
    specific
```

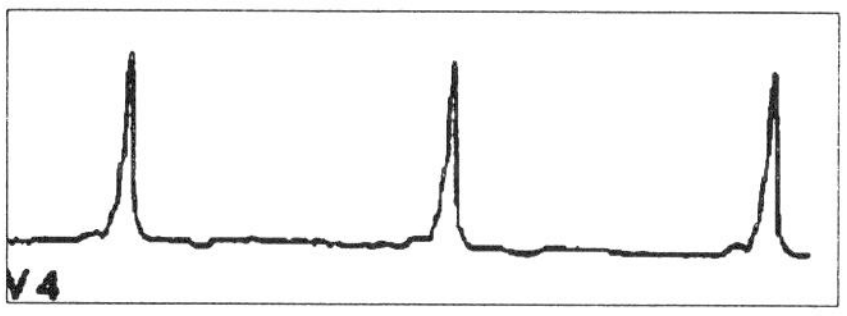

Control, showing pre-excitation

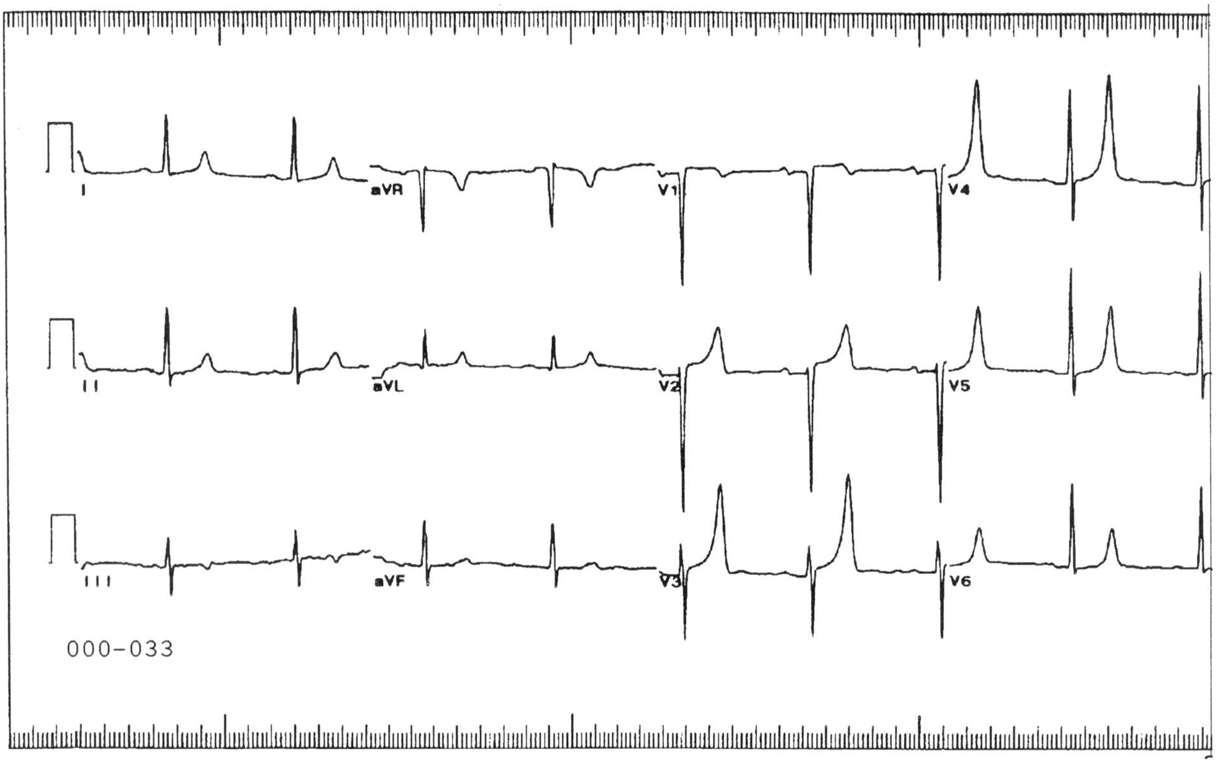

Hyperkalemia

This is the classic picture of hyperkalemia (231). T is tall (210), narrow, and symmetrical. ST is flattened.

This patient was a 35-five-year-old man in renal failure. His serum potassium level at the time of the tracing was 8.3 meq/L.

In more advanced stages of poisoning with potassium, QRS becomes wider, PR longer, and there may be ST displacement as with myocardial injury. Ultimately, the whole P-QRS-T complex may appear as a single sine wave.

In view of the current practice of determining serum electrolytes almost routinely, the probability that the EKG picture will be the first evidence pointing specifically to hyperkalemia, or useful for monitoring the level during treatment, is small. Both were important, however, when the relation between the EKG picture and the serum potassium level was first apparent, and spectrophotometers were rare.

The differential diagnosis includes coronary insufficiency.

```
55    55    20    08    40      sinus
+30   0:25    V3½    15:1 . normal
            none
          flattened
+30  ±V1, tall, symmetrical V2-6

(1) Sinus mechanism, rate 55
(2) ST-T abnormalities sugges-
    tive of hyperkalemia
```

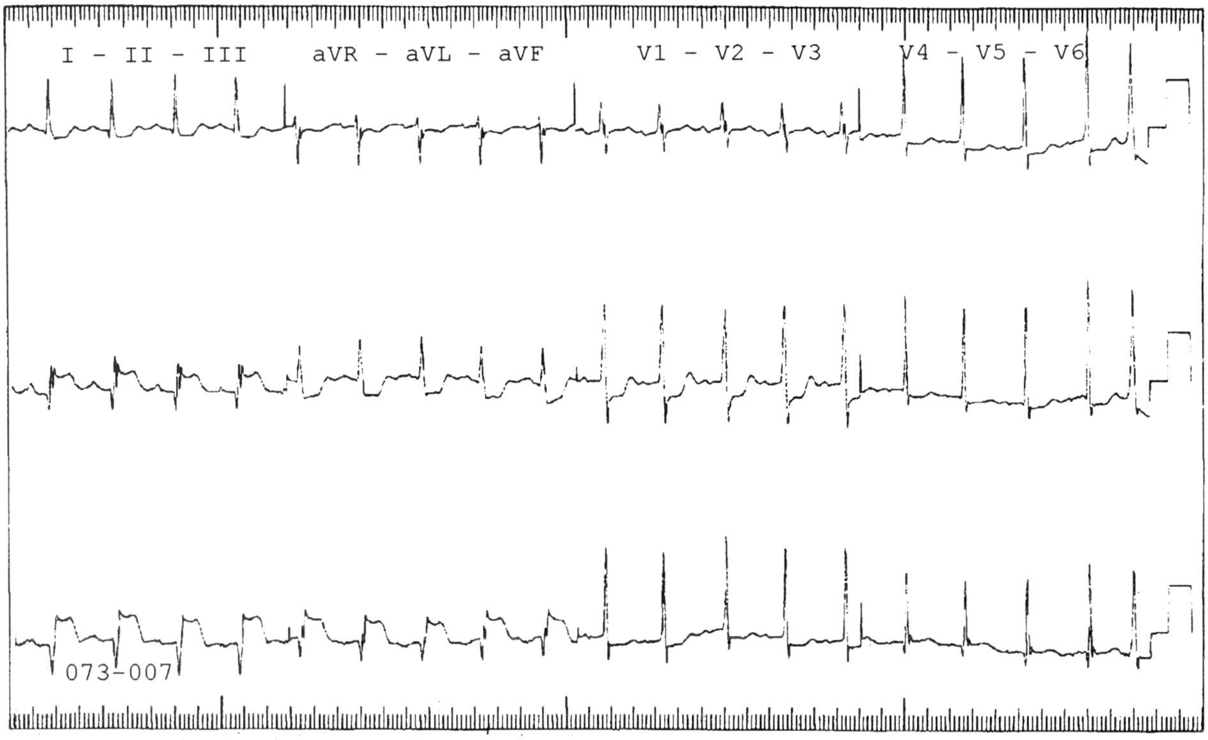

Acute Inferior Myocardial Infarct

```
115   115   20   08   36        sinus
?±0   6:3    V1½    15:0     Q2,3,F
        up 2,3,F, down L,V2-3
?+90  ±V1      +V2 low      ±V3-6

(1) Sinus mechanism, rate 115
(2) Acute inferior myocardial
    infarct
```

The *sine qua non* of the EKG diagnosis of myocardial infarction is abnormality of the initial part of QRS, signifying a circumscribed area of electrically inactive tissue deep in the myocardium, and this usually takes the form of an *abnormal* Q (174), but it is not the only feature that counts. Everything in the tracing must be considered, and not every finding has to be typical to justify a confident diagnosis. When an infarct is suspected, for instance, the ST-T picture of injury (180) offers strong support even though the anatomic lesion is not demonstrable. Q is equivocal here, but evidence of injury is impressive from both anterior and inferior views. This "reciprocal" ST-T pattern is common with inferior infarcts but relatively uncommon with anterior ones (see EKG 62), and to see it as evidence of two lesions rejects the fact that the trace represents the position of only one point. Note inconstancy of QRS voltage, especially in V4-6. LVH is not in question here, and the computer did not call it, but noting every feature of every tracing is the only way to become aware of the limitations of the method and avoid attaching too much significance to computer readouts or equivocal findings; e.g., QRS voltage when the computer calls LVH. Inferior infarcts may have a dorsal component just as anterior ones have a lateral component, and the initial RV1 may reflect that.

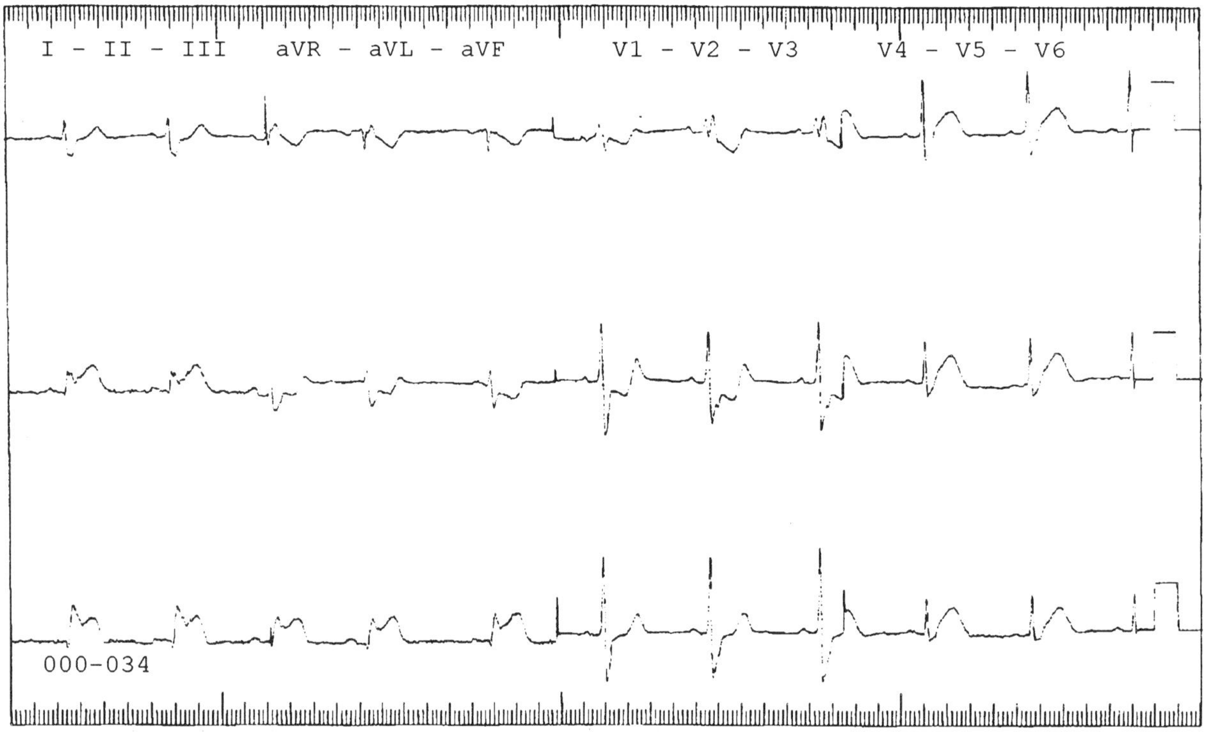

Right Bundle Branch Block, Acute Inferior Myocardial Injury

This tracing illustrates three things: right bundle branch block (159), the ST-T pattern of myocardial injury (47, 202), and the importance of identifying both time and space in analyzing the findings.

Right bundle branch block, a structural lesion, produces change in the last part of ventricular excitation selectively, and the picture here is typical.

The marked ST displacement, characteristic of myocardial injury, a functional abnormality, is clear in both frontal and horizontal planes, emphasizing the three-dimensional nature of the method, the same phenomenon seen in two views. This orientation implies an inferior lesion, and cannot be attributed to RBBB. It suggests an early phase of an infarct.

```
65   65   20   12   40     sinus
??   RsR 2:1:4  ??  8:1   BSTDRA
       up 2,3,F   down L,V2
       flattened/straightened
+60  negative V1, positive V2-6

(1) Sinus mechanism, rate 65
(2) Right bundle branch block
(3) ST-T abnormalities typical
    of acute inferior myocard-
    ial injury as with at least
    coronary insufficiency

--probably an early phase of an
  infarct
```

There is no identifiable evidence of an infarct, but this is not because there is RBBB. QRS evidence of an infarct is in the initial forces, and is not affected by the presence of right bundle branch block. Perhaps 30% of acute infarcts do not produce typical EKG abnormalities.

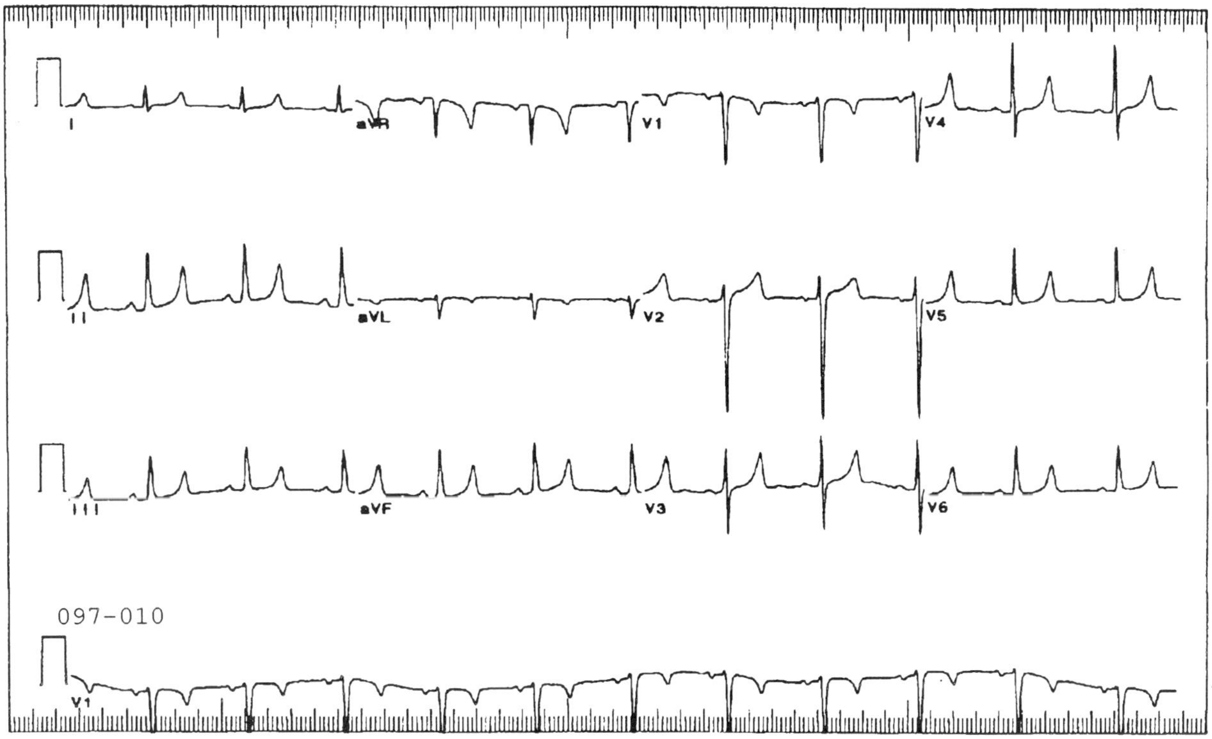

Hyperkalemia (vs Within Normal Limits)

The doctor writing an EKG report serves as an interpreter, converting the information recorded by the galvanometer to doctor talk; speculation beyond what is implicit in the tracing must be limited. No ST-T abnormalities are specific by themselves, but some do suggest explanations. In this case, with no knowledge of the clinical setting, not even the patient's age, the borderline amplitude and contour of T cannot be called abnormal with confidence (210), and to list all possible explanations, if they are abnormal, is beyond the limits of the method. The primary doctor has information that will put the findings in context, but the EKG interpreter has only the tracing and the information, if any, supplied with the requisition. Sometimes EKG reports, even those modified by "possible" or "cannot rule out," are assumed to be directly relevant to the patient's complaints, even when they are not. The one who writes the report must remember, first, to do no harm. In this case, it turned out that the potassium level was 7.7 meq/L on the day of the tracing, and this, with a control made later (inset), showed that the pattern probably was evidence of hyperkalemia.

```
70    70    16    08    40      sinus
+75   1:15     V3     10:0       WNL
              none
         some flattening
+60 neg V1,pos V2-6 symmetrical

(1) Sinus mechanism, rate 70
(2) WNL, probably

--The ST-T pattern may mean
hyperkalemia but is not clearly
abnormal.  The clinical setting
and stability of the findings
are important unknowns.  Other
interpretations are possible.
```

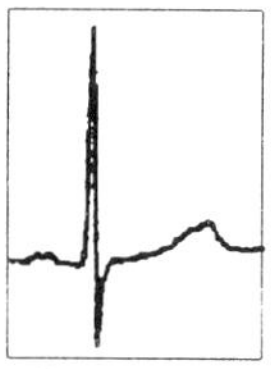

V5 control
for above

Junctional Mechanisms, Default

These segments have been selected from the tracings indicated in the captions for demonstration of the second most important feature of a P (its presence is the first), its orientation, an indication of the locus of the focus from which it proceeds.

A and B are from the same patient. In A, the atria are depolarized caudad (P is positive in aVF) indicating origin of the impulse in the cephalic end, presumably the sinus node). The absence of identifiable atrial activity in B suggests, but does not prove, origin in the center of the "junction," with spread of the impulse in both directions at once so that P is obscured by QRS.

Retrograde depolarization of the atria is indicated by the negative P in C and D. That P follows QRS in C is taken as evidence that the impulse reached the ventricles before the atria, implying that it originated "low" in the junction, probably in the His bundle. In D, it reached the atria first, implying a "high" origin (also called low atrial).

All of these are slow rates, representing escape of a lower, slower focus by default when, for whatever reason, the sinus node fails to fire, a compensatory, backup, defensive device, but these ectopic foci can function over a wide range of rates. When faster than sinus, they usurp pacemaker function and can be indicated by a choice of names that range from "accelerated" (see EKG 140) to various mixtures of description and putative explanations, e.g., "SVT," "AVNR." See the index for examples of several of these.

Understanding of what is going on is encouraged by differentiating among the three components of the mechanism; the locus of the focus driving the atria, its rate, and its rhythm, the same for the ventricles, and the causal relation between atria and ventricles.

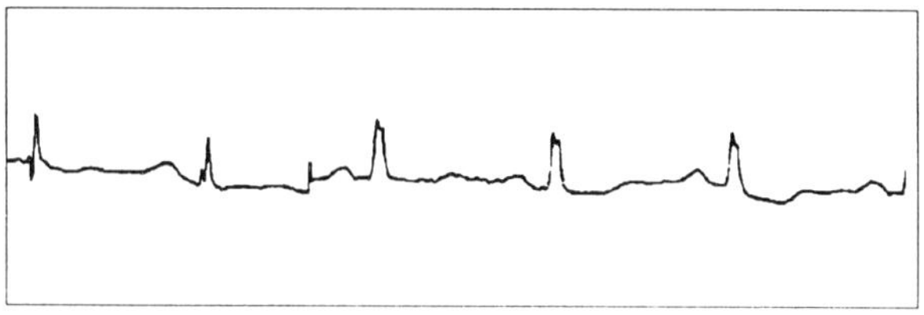

A III and aVF, EKG #84 Sinus mechanism

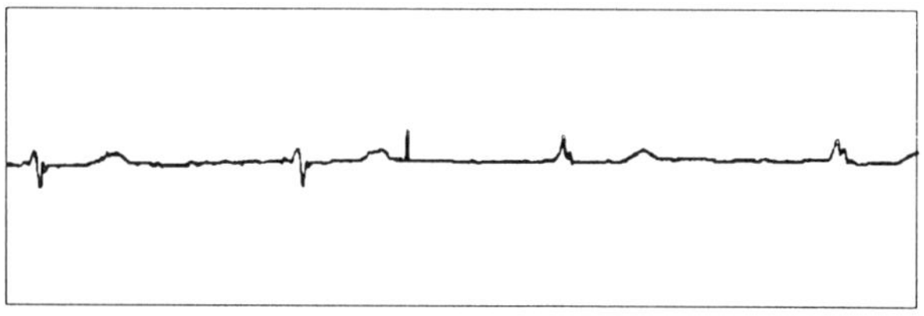

B III and aVF EKG #84 Mid-junctional mech

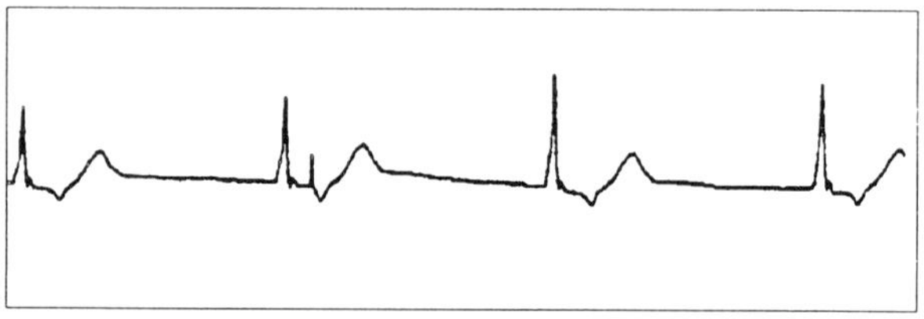

C III and aVF EKG #66 Low junctional mech

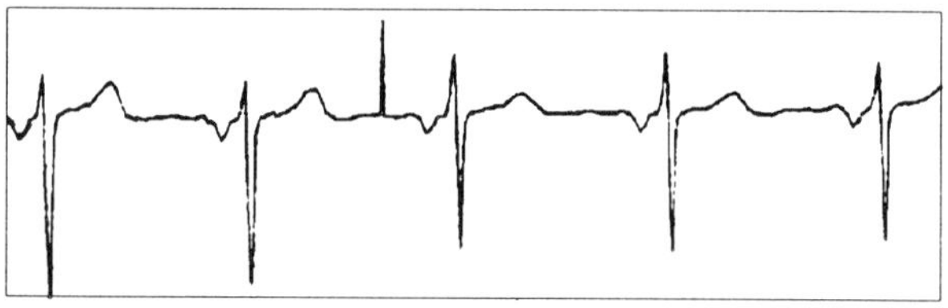

D III and aVF EKG #79 High junctional mech

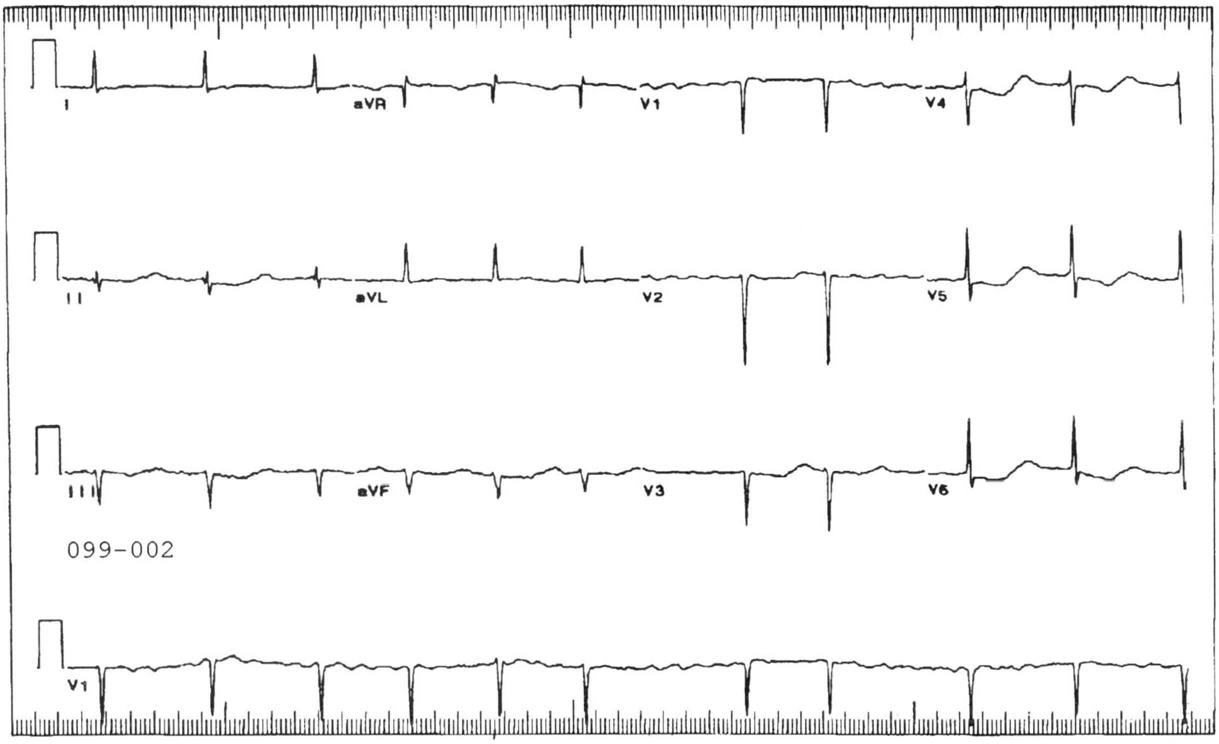

Atrial Fibrillation, Hypokalemia

```
--    65    --    08    ??       AF
-30   0:10    V4½   10:2    normal
              none
          related to T
low      isoelectric V1-6
U: prominent

(1) AF, rate about 65
(2) ST-T-U abnormalities, non-
    specific, but suggestive of
    hypokalemia
```

The tracing represents the motion of only one point, and the position of that point at any instant is the result of many potential variables. Three of which, mutually exclusive but not unrelated, are mechanism, structure, and function. Often, as in this case, more than one can be identified with confidence. Here, the mechanism is atrial fibrillation (131), identifying atrial function and precluding recognition of atrial structure (since there are no P waves). Neither orientation nor duration, amplitude, or contour of QRS is abnormal. The computer called both anterior and inferior infarcts, age indeterminate, but that is overdoing it. Neither can be "ruled out" but evidence for the diagnosis of either is very small.

The striking feature here is the combination of low T voltage and prominence of the U wave, producing a pattern typical of hypokalemia, but not specific for anything. The serum potassium level was 2.4 meq/L. The computer called the QT interval 0.58 s, really the QU, a very ill-defined value at best. When QT is seen as much greater than about 0.44 s, it probably includes the U wave.

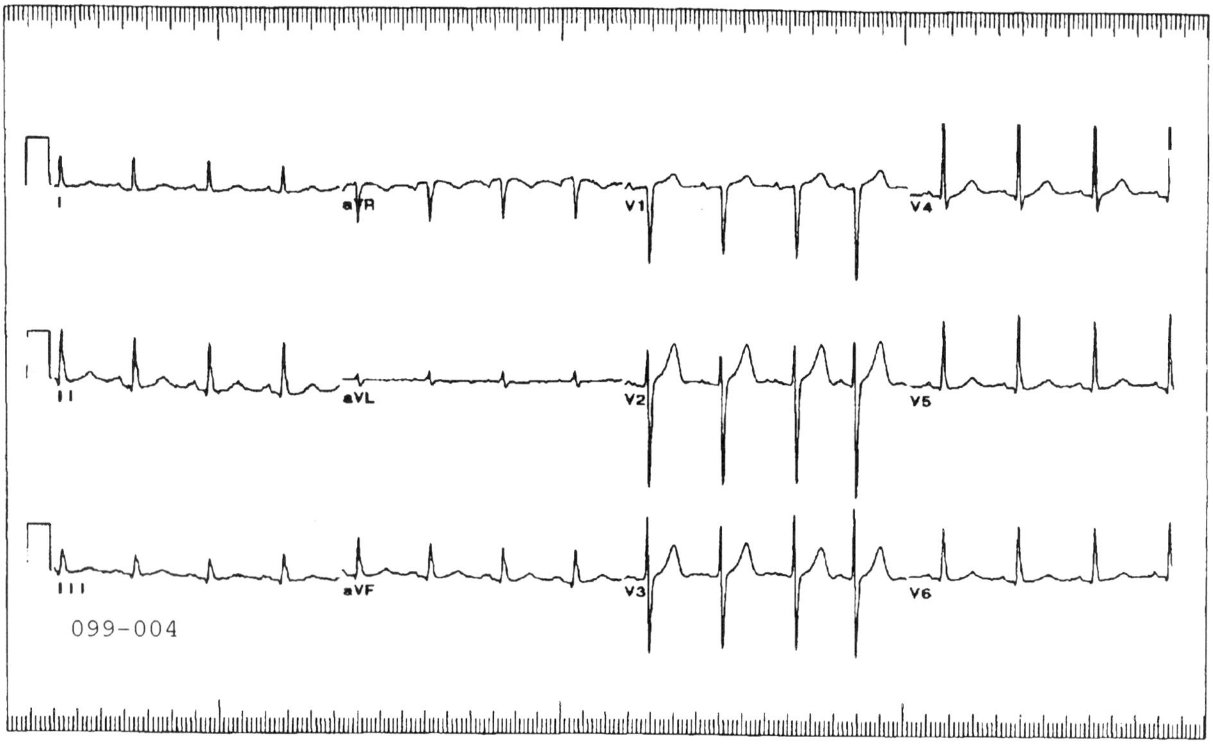

Vectorcardiogram (VCG)

The electrical activity of the heart can be recorded as a scalar value, documenting the position of a point on a line, or as a vector value, documenting its projection on two lines at the same time, a plane. The scalar version is what we know as an electrocardiogram. The vector version, a vectorcardiogram, presents exactly the same information, but in a different form (inset)(90). Vectorcardiography has been available since shortly after Einthoven's time, but has never become very popular as a routine study. It contains no information not found in the conventional presentation, and is much less suitable for study of timing, the spatial relation between QRS and T, and intrinsic characteristics of P and ST-T.

By far its most useful application is as a method for understanding the relationship among leads, and of the components of a beat (70).

90 90 16 08 36 sinus
+60 0:15 V3 10:0 normal
none
normal
+60 positive V1-6

(1) Sinus mechanism, rate 90, with PAC
(2) Within normal limits

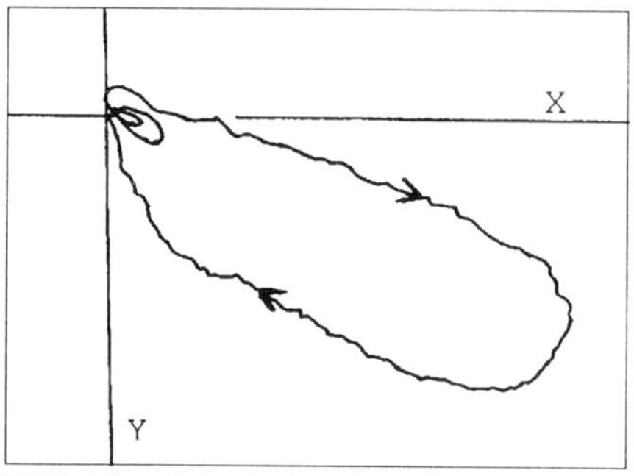

VCG derived from the scalar tracing above

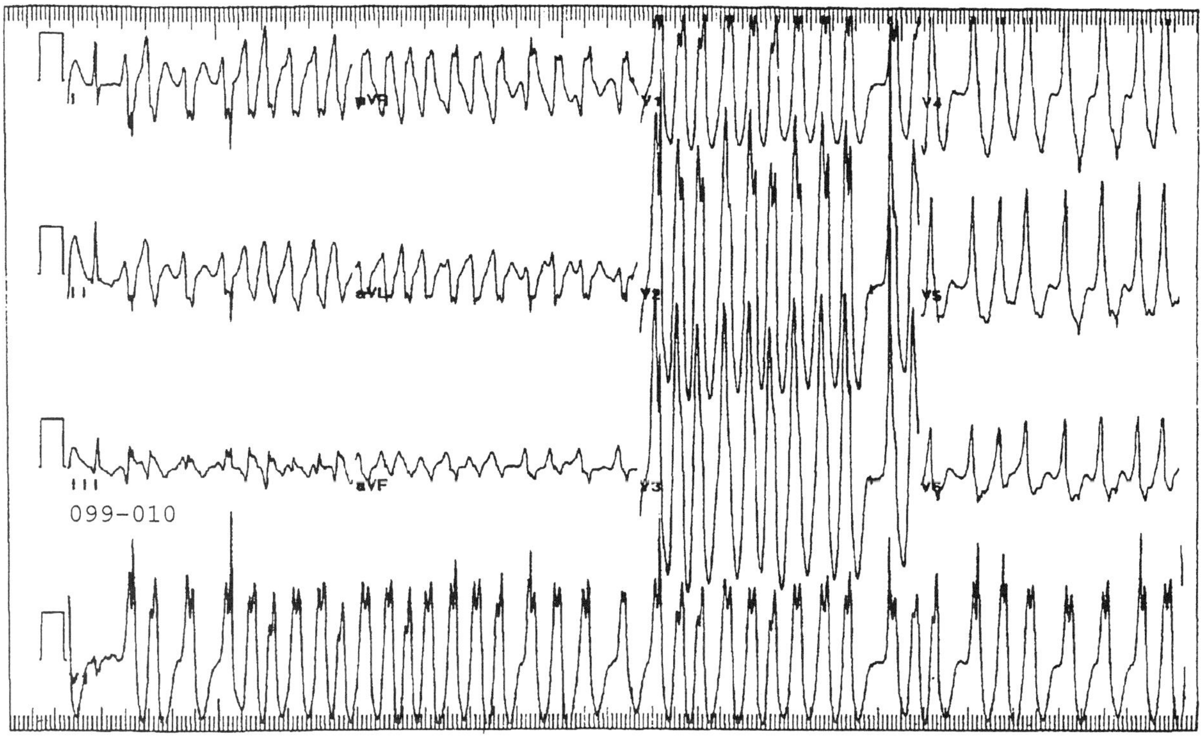

Ventricular Tachycardia/Fibrillation

The difference between ventricular tachycardia and ventricular fibrillation is often arbitrary at best, and rarely critical. Given only the information in the tracing above, even the clinical setting is unimportant, the indication for interruption of the life-threatening ectopy is clear, but later management depends on what initiated the problem. When atrial fibrillation occurs in a patient with an anomalous AV pathway that conducts faster than the AV node, as in this 13-year-old known to have ventricular preexcitation (see insets), the "electrical funnel" of the AV node (121) is bypassed, and the result is ventricular fibrillation (155). Another way to describe it is atrial fibrillation with pre-excitation.

```
--  215  --  16  ??   see below
??  20:0 --  10:?  diff slur
                   rt and ant
            ??
      related to T
??    negative V1-6

(1) Ventricular tachycardia/
    fibrillation-
```

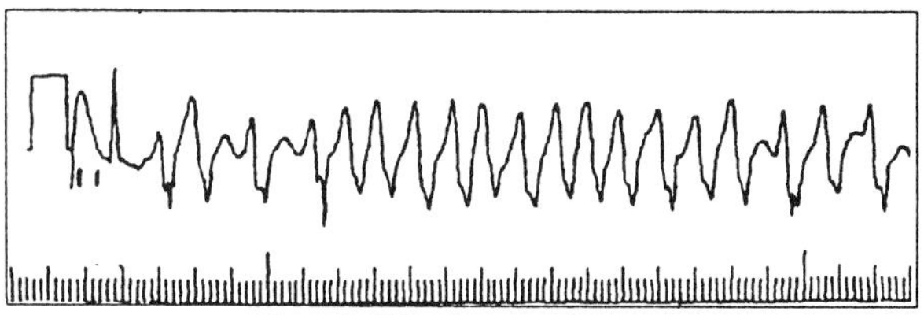
Lead II from above

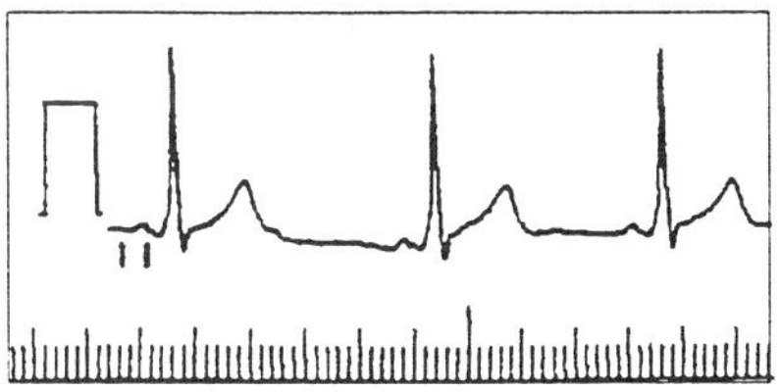
Old tracing

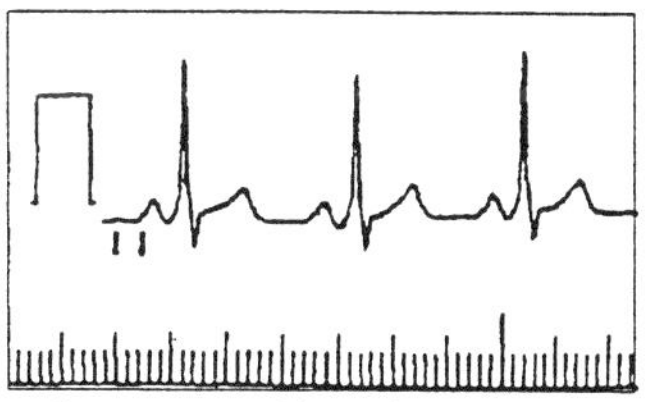
After defibrillation

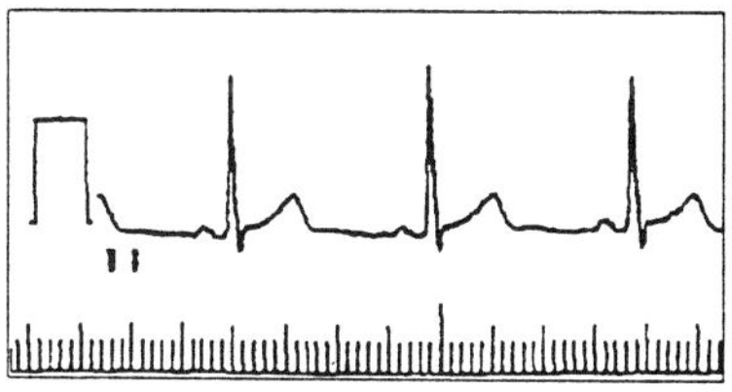
After ablation

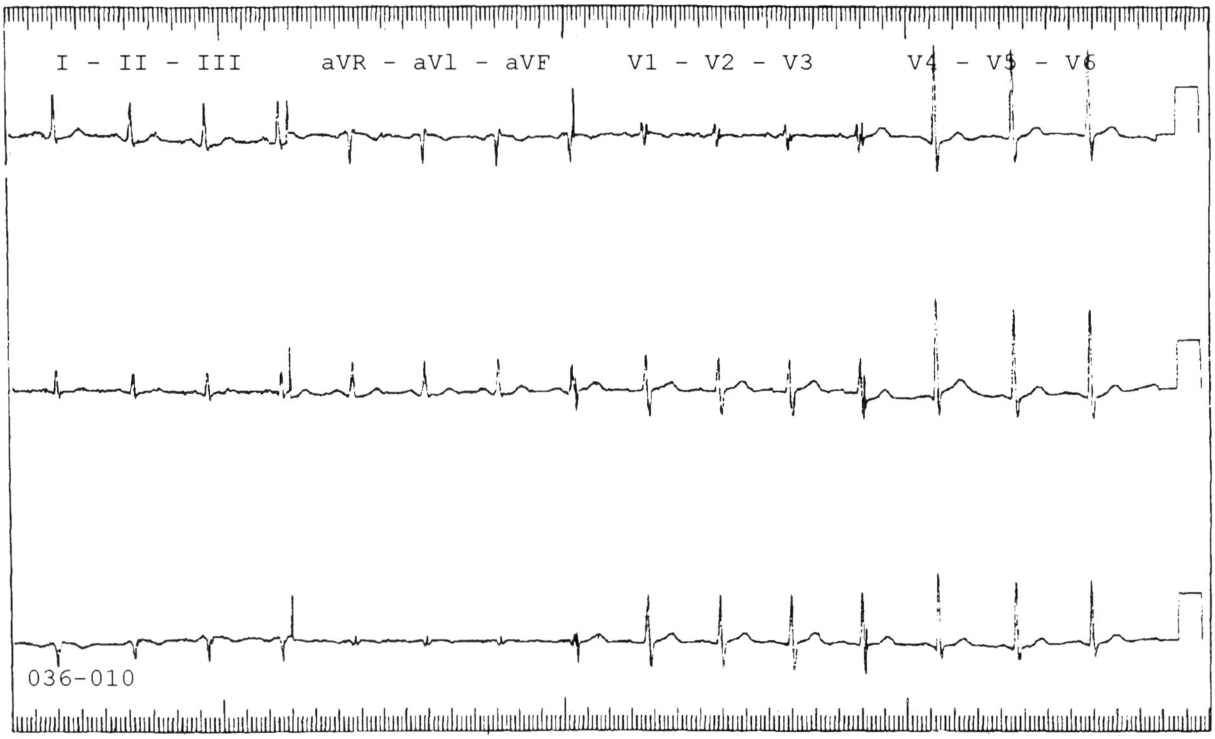

Crossed Left Arm And Leg Leads

95 95 16 06 36 sinus
+60 RSR 2:2:2 V2 12:2 normal
none
normal
+60 ±V1 positive V2-6

(1) Sinus mechanism, rate 95
(2) Within normal limits

--Interpretation corrects for recording with left arm and leg leads transposed.

This is a very common artifact, and with only one tracing, and no clinical information, it can only be suspected. All three corners of Einthoven's triangle are represented; the tracing is complete, but mislabeled (104). Once the problem is recognized, compensation for it is easy. The key is the negative P in lead III, a good example of the potentially large impact of a tiny feature of the tracing, usually hardly noticed, a "pebble." A negative P3 is not necessarily abnormal, but one explanation for it is reversal of polarity of Lead III. In this case, the computer provided another hint to one who knows the patient; it called an inferior infarct, the only caveat being that its age was "undetermined" (indeterminate), a reasonable interpretation of the findings as labeled. *Point: when the readout does not fit the clinical picture, suspect technical error.* Corrected, I is II, II is I, aVL is aVF, aVF is aVL, the polarity of II is reversed, and aVR and the V leads are not affected. See inset. Nothing at all looks like an infarct (108).

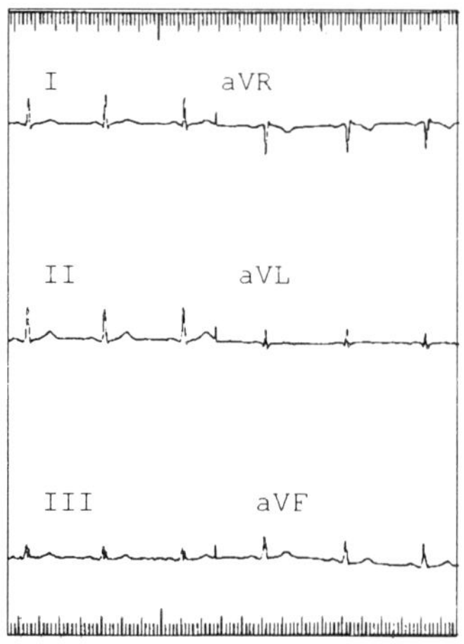

Tracing above recorded correctly

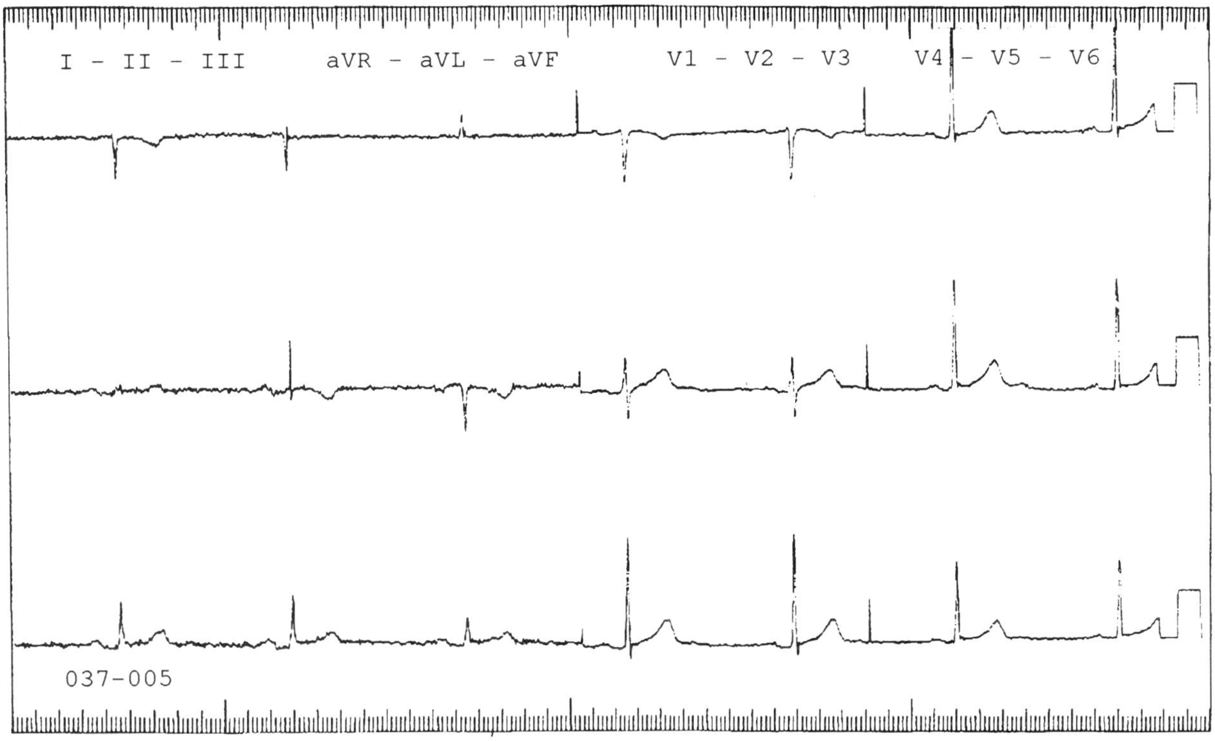

Crossed Arm Leads Interpreted as Infarct

```
40    40    20    08    44      sinus
+30    0:10    V2    15:0    normal
            none
           normal
+60  Neg V1 low    positive V2-6

(1) Sinus mechanism, rate 40,
    with normal AV conduction
(2) Within normal limits

--Interpretation corrects for
  crossed arm leads.
```

This is a very common problem, and its potential importance depends on the characteristics of the heart involved. In this case, the computer recognized the QS in I and aVL and called a lateral infarct. Perhaps the most obvious indication that something is awry is that the MFQRS points both right and left; negative in Lead I and positive in V6 (85). The P wave is a big help. A P wave is small, and often hardly noticed, but, like a pebble, it may be very important in context. P is almost always negative in aVR, and in this tracing the negative PaVL and flat PaVR suggest that the leads are transposed.

When there is atrial fibrillation, the contribution of P is lost, and the answer is not so clear Also, if QRS is nearly biphasic in all leads, "S1,2,3" (35), its orientation does not help.

This tracing is complete, and correction is easy (104). Lead I is upside down, II is III, III is II, aVR and aVL are reversed, and aVF and the V leads are not affected. Dextrocardia (EKGs 82 and 85) produces the same pattern in the frontal leads, but a different one in the precordial leads.

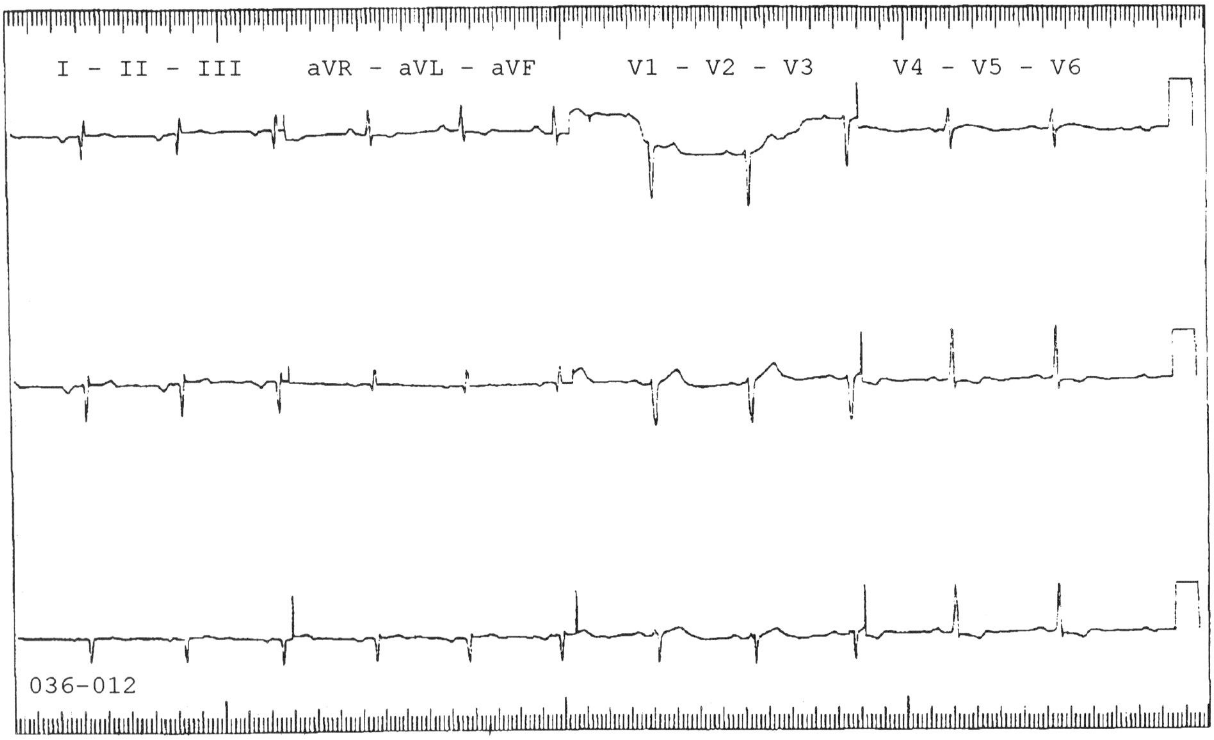

Crossed Right Arm and Left Leg Leads

This is one of those settings in which the P wave, usually not very important, a "pebble," becomes critical. Its negativity in Lead I and aVL makes one think immediately of crossed arm leads. If that were the case, correcting for it would make an inferior infarct likely, and not recognizing it would make a lateral infarct reasonable. The computer called both in this case. The thing to remember is that the atria almost always depolarize away from aVR. AVR almost always has a negative P, usually a negative QRS, and, unless there is an abnormality of repolarization, a negative T, i.e., aVR almost always looks like aVR, no matter where it is found (105). In this tracing, it is the position for aVF.

```
70    70    20    08    36     sinus
+45   1:10    V4    10:1.    normal
              none
         related to T
?-105, +V1-3, ±V4, neg V5-6 low

(1) Sinus mechanism, rate 70
(2) ST-T abns suggestive of
    LVO, but small

--Interpretation corrects for
  recording with right arm and
  left leg leads transposed.
```

Assume that if the right arm lead is on the left leg, the left leg lead is on the right arm, and work from there. That makes Lead I really III upside down, II is II but with reversed polarity, III is I upside down, aVR and aVF are transposed, and aVL and the V leads are unaffected. The tracing is complete and interpretable, but the patient is at some risk.

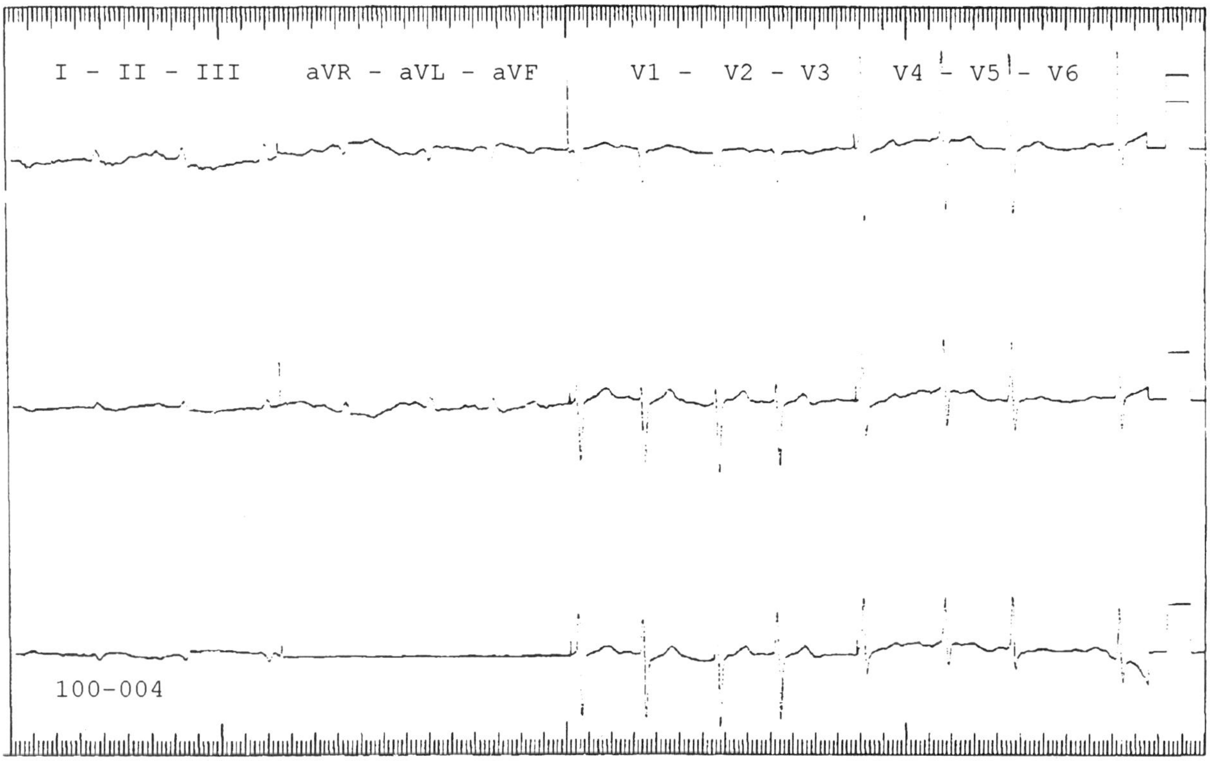

Defective Patient Cable, Flat Line aVF; Atrial Fibrillation

Absence of information, a flat line, in an augmented unipolar (aV) lead, aVF in this case, means that the patient cable to the arm or leg concerned is defective. Note that leads II and III, and aVR and aVL, are mirror images. This is different from a flat line in I, II, or III because of the way the data are acquired (85, 94). I, II, and III are "bipolar" leads, each pole represents only one apex of the triangle; the positive pole of an aV lead represents the apex named, but the negative pole is attached to both the others. All leads are affected by this technical problem, but the effect in the V leads is small. There is a lot of information in the tracing, but it is not complete, and, if this is not recognized, the findings may be interpreted as evidence of cardiac abnormality. Frontal leads from a control tracing are shown in the inset.

-- 85 --, -- ?40 see below
?? 0:5 V3 103 normal
none
related to T
??low ±V1, pos V2-4 low, ±V6

(1) Atrial fibrillation, ventricular rate about 85
(2) ST-T abns, nonspecific

--Incomplete, defective patient cable to left leg

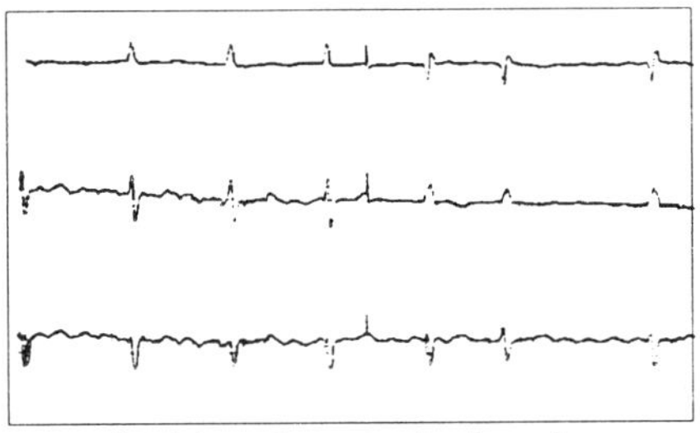

EKG #154 frontal leads recorded properly in the same order as above

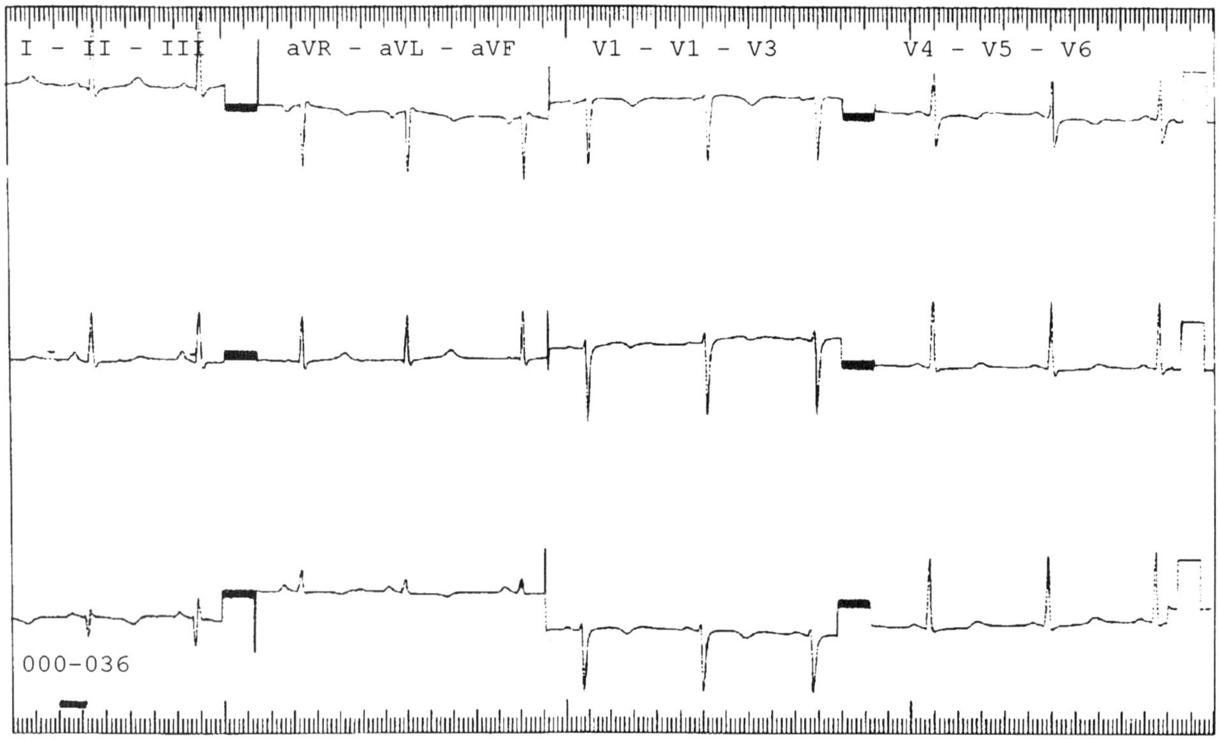

ST-T Abnormalities, Nonspecific; Hypocalcemia?

```
65    65    16    08    ?48    sinus
+15   1:12   V4    15:0       normal
             none
             flat
-30 low   neg V1-4 low      ±V5-6
U: Prominent

(1) Sinus mechanism, rate 65
(2) ST-T abnormalities, not
    specific, but suggestive of
    hypocalcemia
```

The only abnormal finding in this tracing that can be identified with confidence is not far from normal, and completely nonspecific. ST is flatter than usual in most leads, but that is hard to quantify. U is not very large, but, because T is so small, it is prominent. The combination of these findings fits the traditional picture of hypocalcemia (231). The computer readout suggested "electrolyte imbalance," and this is probably as nearly specific as it can be called. Potassium and calcium imbalance often coexist, and this pattern would go almost as well with hypokalemia as hypocalcemia. There is not a very close relation between serum level of either and the EKG picture.

The computer called the QT interval 0.492 s, implying a degree of accuracy that is beyond the limits of clinical usefulness. When QT is measured longer than about 0.44 s, there is a good chance that is really a QU interval.

Note that in this format time is continuous in the first half of the tracing, and in the last half, but not between halves.

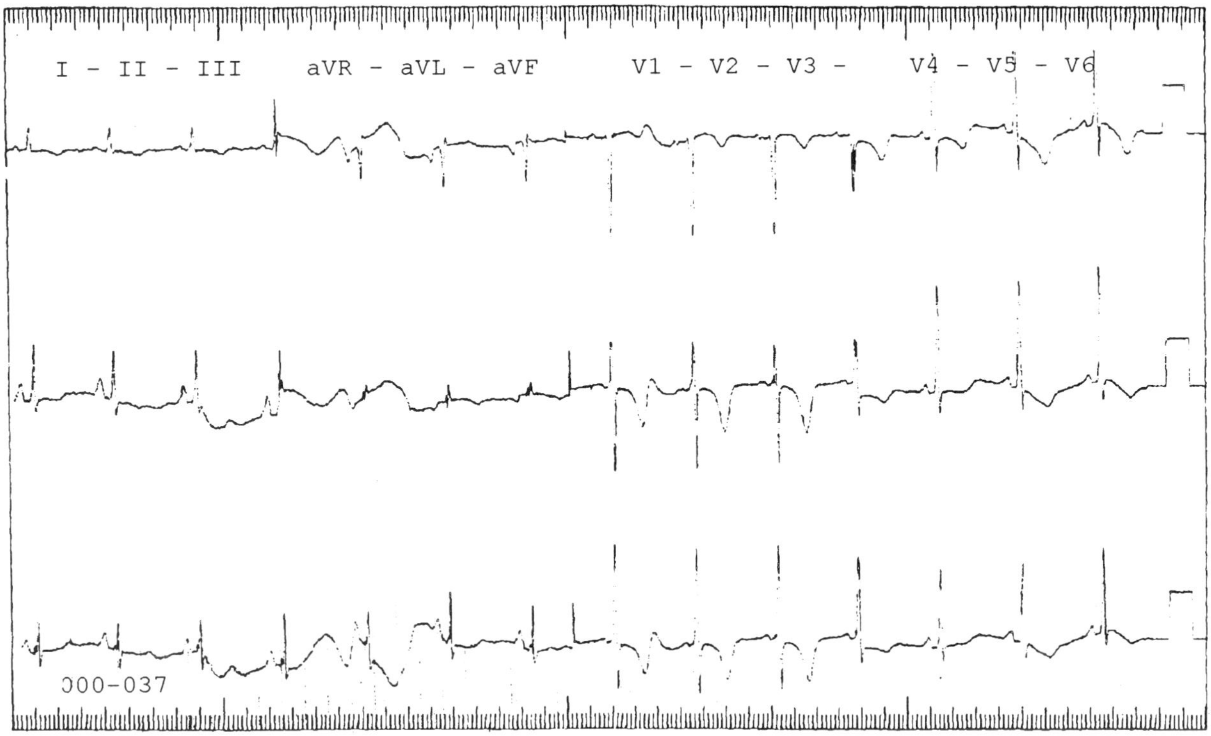

Midprecordial T Negativity
(Typical of coronary insufficiency),
Right Atrial Enlargement

85 85 12 08 40 sinus
+60 0:20 V2½ 15:2 normal
none
related to T
?+120 low neg V1-6, deep V2-4
symmetrical
P: prominent II, III, aVF

(1) Sinus mechanism, rate 85
(3) Right atrial enlargement
(2) ST-T abnormalities, probably evidence of coronary insufficiency

The most striking feature of this tracing is described easily; T is negative all the way from V1 through V6 (counting the last two beats in V5-6), deeper in V2-4 than in leads to the left or right of them, *and* symmetrical. The interpretation of this combination of abnormalities of orientation, amplitude, and contour usually includes the word "ischemia." It is typical of ischemia (136) to be sure, but the pattern permits a closer call than that; it is much more likely to represent impairment of flow than overload of the left ventricle (189) (EKG 72). Differential includes normal (in an asymptomatic child) and local myocardial hypertrophy (EKG 14). Not all coronary insufficiency is due to atherosclerosis; sickle cell disease sometimes explains it.

One can wonder whether lung disease, suggested by the picture of "P pulmonale" (the symmetrical, peaked P in leads II, III, and aVF) (188), may have some clinically useful relation to the ST-T evidence of impairment of oxygen supply to the myocardium.

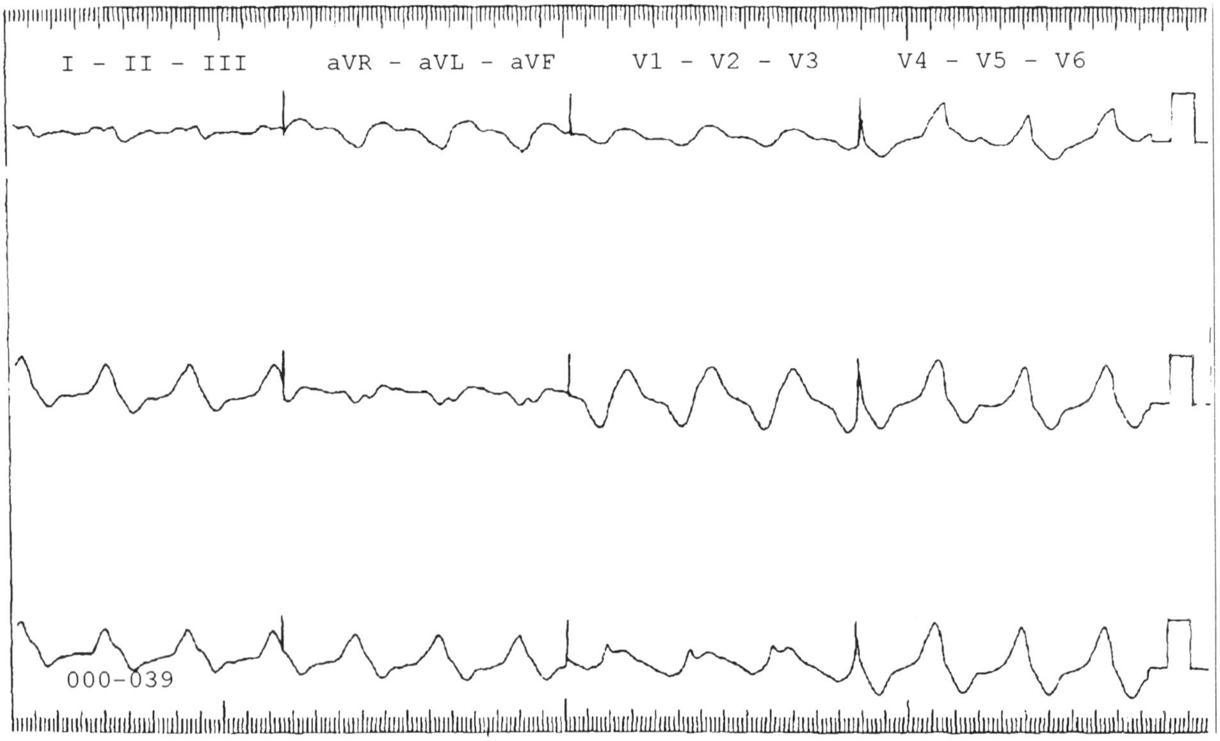

Hyperkalemia

```
80?   80   ?   ±24   ±50   see below
+90   0:?2   V2½   8:0...diff slur
            up V2-3
          related to T
-75   ±V1   pos V2   ±V3   neg V4-6

(1) Ventricular rate 80 with
    regular rhythm, prob sinus;
    Atrial activity  not clear
(2) Atypical IV cond defect,
    probably LBBB
(3) ST-T abnormalities

--The picture as a whole is
  strongly suggestive of
  hyperkalemia
```

The serum potassium level is not known, but the requisition identified the patient as a 47-year-old-man pre-op for a renal transplant, and the picture of advanced potassium intoxication is classic. Atrial activity is not clear, but with a regular ventricular rhythm at a rate of 80 (the computer called it 134) sinus is the best choice. QRS is wide, diffusely slurred, and directed caudad, posteriorly, and a little leftward, a pattern more like LBBB than anything else. QT is long. ST-T is directed opposite QRS but otherwise not very remarkable. Taken individually, the findings might be explained by first degree AV block with a small P continuous with T, left bundle branch block, and nonspecific ST-T abnormalities. Considered as a group, however, they describe the "sine wave" configuration of P-QRS-T that has been recognized as typical of advanced potassium intoxication, and the report must call attention to this (231).

The differential includes a ventricular origin of QRS, and other explanations for its prolongation (168).

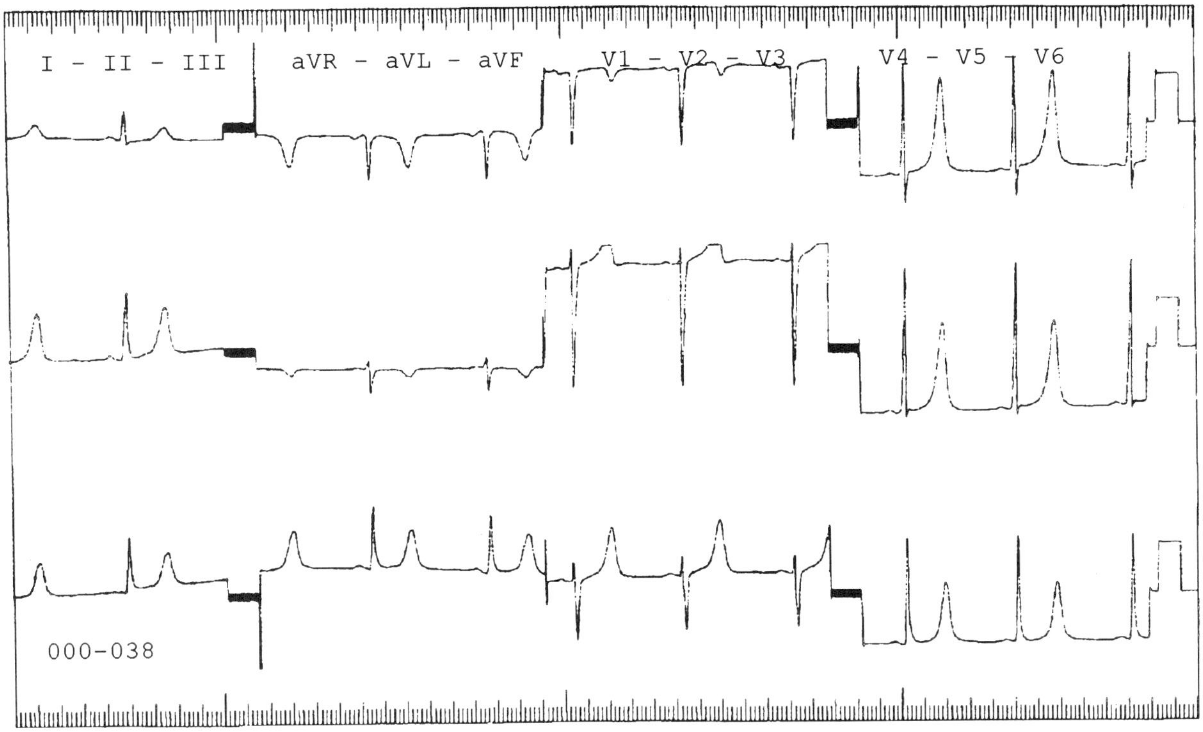

Hyperkalemia

60	60	16	08	44	sinus
+75	0:15	V3½	20:0	normal	

none
flattened
+75 neg V1, pos V2-6, tall and peaked V3-6

(1) Sinus mechanism, rate 60
(2).ST-T abnormalities, probably evidence of hyperkalemia

The features of this tracing that are probably abnormal are the ST-T contour, and the amplitude and symmetry of T. The pattern is seen best in leads in which the spatial orientation of T is close to that of QRS: i.e., QRS and T are of the same sign, the ventricular gradient is small (51, 80, 210). It is seen best in II, III, aVF, and V3-6 in this case. At just what amplitude a T wave becomes "tall" (or deep) is a matter of judgment based on experience (50, 210). A good observation to use as a starting place is that most T waves in normals are not more than about half the height (or depth) of QRS in leads in which QRS and T are of the same sign.

The evidence here for an excessive concentration of potassium can be described as flattening of ST and very tall T. The combination makes for little difference between the rate of inscription of the initial and terminal limbs of T, producing symmetry, or peaking. Another way to describe it is that the tall T has a narrow base. This pattern has been associated with hyperkalemia so long that it must be noted as at least suggestive (not "compatible," "consistent with," or "possible"). The differential includes normal, intracranial lesions, and coronary insufficiency (212).

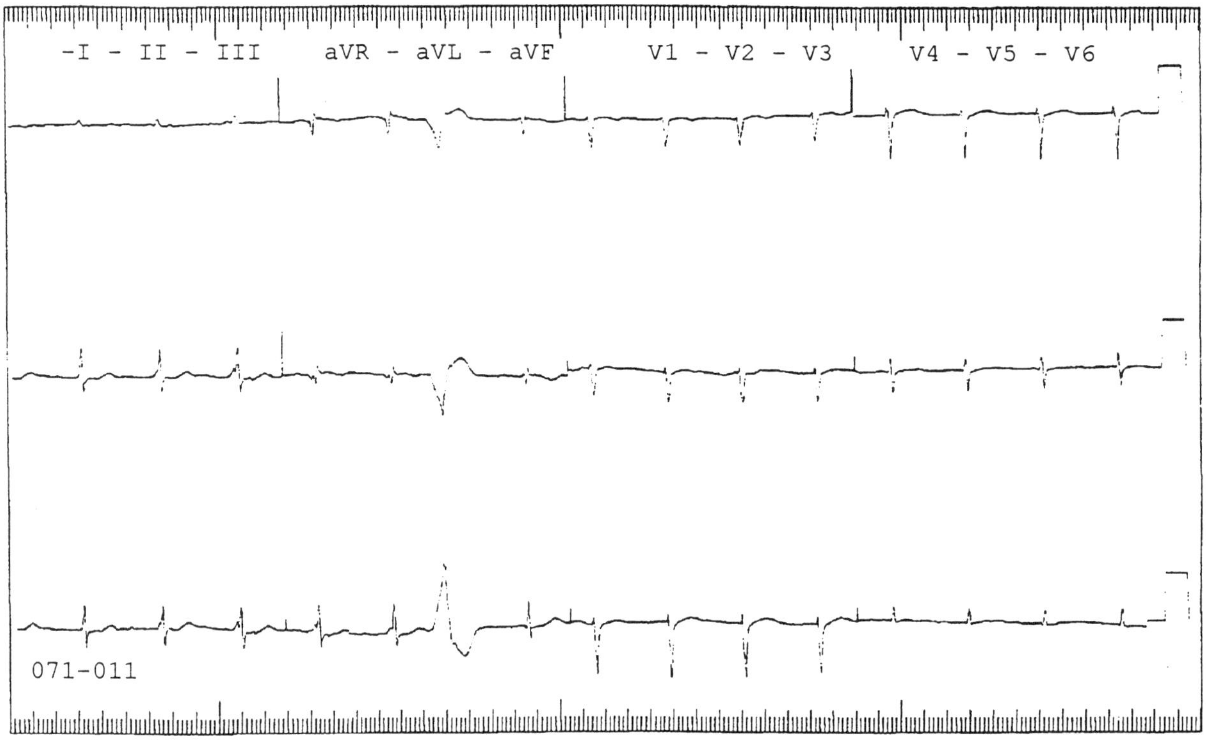

Isorhythmic Dissociation

There is no satisfactory single name for the mechanism in this tracing. Of the ones in common use, "isorhythmic dissociation," "accelerated junctional rhythm," and "interference dissociation" come closest. Keeping in mind the criteria for defining the mechanism, though, it can be described meaningfully. Sinus activity is apparent in the Ps visible in Lead II at a typical sinus rate. They are merged with QRSs to varying degrees, and cannot be said to give rise to them, but a junctional pacemaker will explain them nicely, except for the one following the PVC and preceded by a P, a sinus beat. There are two supraventricular foci firing at substantially the same rate, but independent of each other, isorhythmic dissociation. The junctional rate is faster than its default, or passive, escape rate. It is accelerated, active, usurping. There is only one abnormality, junctional automaticity at a rate greater than usual. The availability of a control, inset, is helpful (134).

```
90   90   --   08   ?40     see below
+75   1:5    V5½    3:0       normal
                none
           related to T
low ?+90     isoelectric V1-6

(1) Sinus mechanism, rate 90
    with one PVC
(2) Junctional pacemaker, rate
    also 90, with "isorhyth-
    dissociation"
(3) ST-T abnormalities, non-
    specific
```

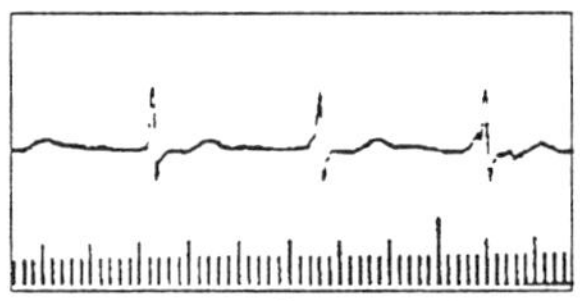

Lead II from above

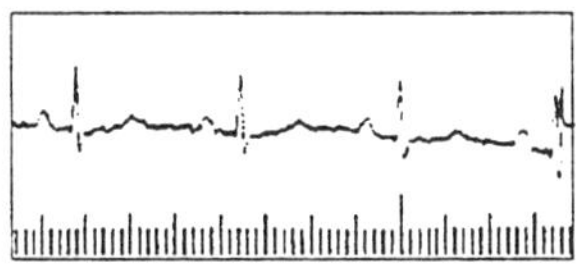

Lead II control

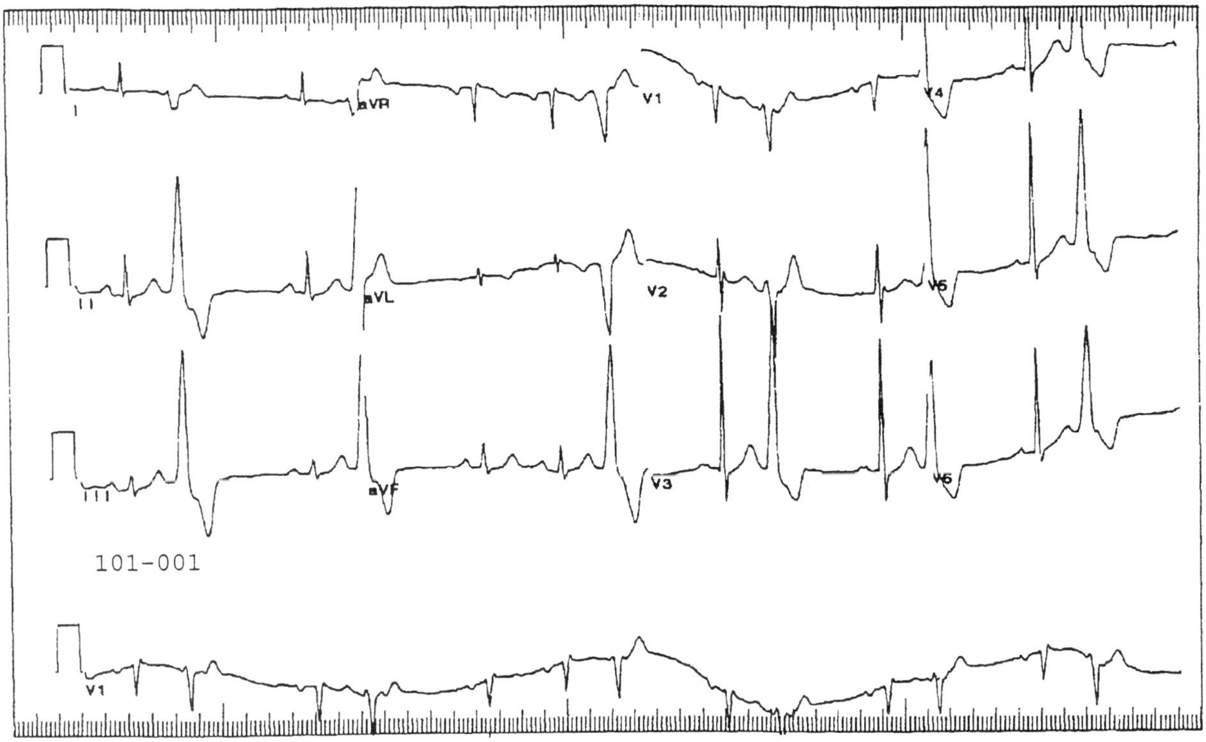

Frequent PVCs

The only abnormality here is frequency of PVCs at unpredictable intervals. The number required to be called "frequent" is arbitrary, but one or two in the standard 12-lead tracing, 10 s, are so common that they do not always merit comment in the report; three or more probably should be noted. The importance of PVCs depends on the clinical setting, varying from insignificant, or of only nuisance value, in the healthy heart to potentially serious in the patient with myocardial inflammation such as a recent infarct. The more frequent they are the more likely they are to be significant. Other features that increase their importance are multifocal origin and occurrence in groups. Predictability, every other beat (bigeminy) or every third one, for instance, probably means little (142).

```
90   90   16   08   36      see below
+60    0:5    V2    22:2      normal
              none
             normal
+90      ±V1..positive V2-6

(1) Sinus mechanism, rate 90,
    with normal AV conduction
(2) Frequent PVC's
(3) Otherwise within normal
    limits
```

The computer called this one exactly right, including the statement that completes the interpretation after an abnormality has been noted, "otherwise within normal limits." The reason for the comment about normal AV conduction in the description above is just reassurance that AV conduction was evaluated. It is not known why the tracing was ordered; atrial fibrillation or AV block may have been suspected.

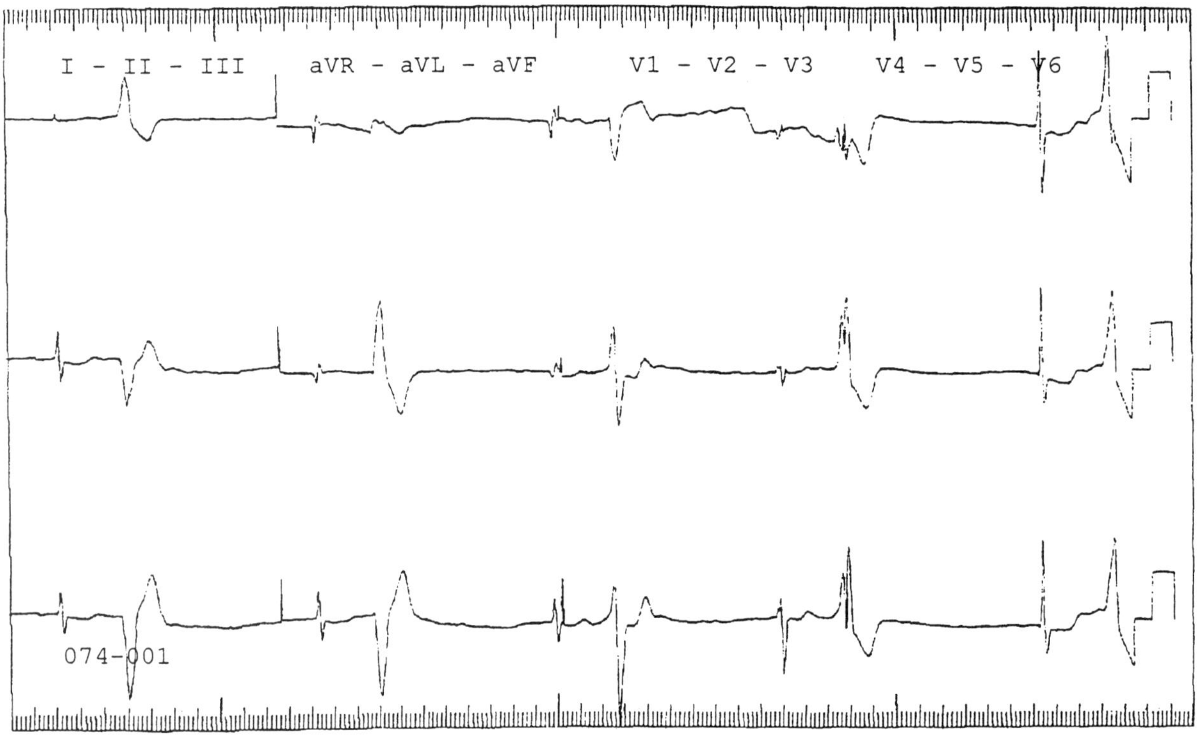

Atrial Fibrillation, Bigeminy due to PVCs

```
--   55   --08   40   see below
??   QR/1:1  V4  15:5    normal
       slightly down V4-6
        sagging/flattened
low  ±V1-4     negative V5-6 low

(1) Atrial fibrillation
(2) Bigeminy due to PVC's
(3) ST-T abns suggestive of
    coronary insufficiency,
    but small
```

Fibrillary waves are seen best in V1. "Bigeminy" means that beats occur in pairs (146), and irregularity of the basic ventricular rhythm does not preclude this; definition of prematurity when the ventricular rhythm is irregular is a small point; they are called PVCs.

The requisition gave no hint as to why the tracing was ordered, but did identify the patient as a 66-year-old man. In such a setting it is almost certain that the findings, both usurping ectopy and at least a suggestion of inadequacy of blood flow to the deep layers of the myocardium, are a result of coronary atherosclerosis. The computer suggested "ischemia" *or* digitalis effect ("and/or" would have been better; they are not mutually exclusive). It also read the QT interval as long, and offered "myocardial disease, electrolyte imbalance, *or* drug effects" as explanations to be considered. None of these suggestions are mutually exclusive, and they cover a very wide spectrum of possibilities. It did describe the mechanism accurately, and noted that there is an ST-T abnormality. The computer readout is always useful, but never the answer by itself.

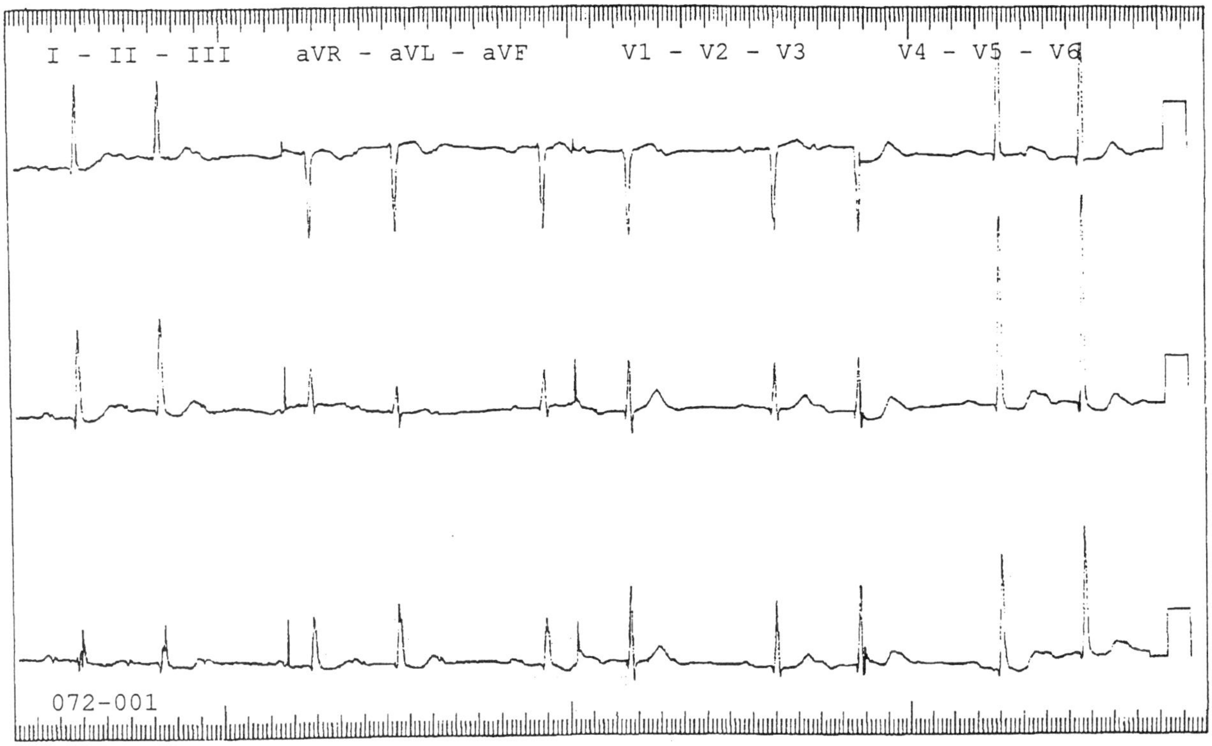

Bigeminy due to Second Degree AV Block

This is a fairly common form of bigeminy, and it would be very difficult to identify on physical examination. PR is only slightly prolonged in the first beat of each pair, longer in the second (Type I, or Wenckebach), and P is not followed by a QRS in the third (146). The report identifies all components of the mechanism as facts, but does not suggest an explanation. It notes that there are ST-T abnormalities (fact), and speculates beyond that to the degree considered appropriate. No ST-T abnormalities are specific, but this contour, sagging of ST with low T voltage, does make one think of digitalis effect, i.e., suggests it, not just that it is "possible" or "consistent with" it. The clinical significance of these findings has to be interpreted by the patient's doctor, who knows that digitalis can produce AV block, and will consider whether the dose should be reduced, if the patient is taking it.

```
90   60   --    08    40    see below
145  0:15  V1½  25:0       normal
             none
            sagging
low    ±V1       +V2-3        ±V4-6

(1) Sinus mechanism, rate 90
(2) Bigeminy due to 2° AV block
    Type I, with 3:2 conduction
(3) ST-T abnormalities suggest-
    ive of digitalis effect
(4) Suggests left ventricular
    hypertrophy.
```

Left ventricular hypertrophy is often suggested in computer readouts as "by voltage criteria," leaving one wondering what other criteria were considered and why they were not applied. The evidence here depends to some extent on which QRS in V5 is used (192).

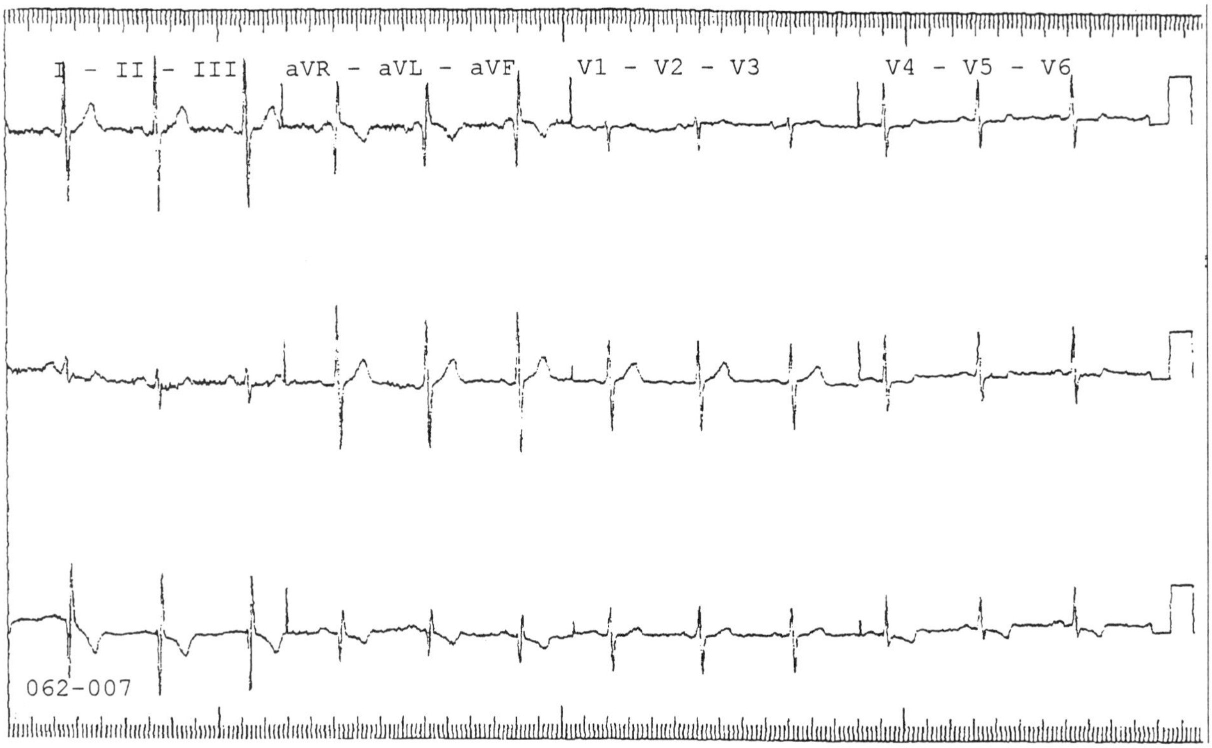

Axis Indeterminate, Within Normal Limits

75	75	16	08	36	sinus
??	1:5	V2-5	8:1		normal
		none			
		normal			
-30	±V1	posV2-3	±V4-5		negV6

(1) Sinus mechanism, rate 75
(2) Within normal limits

"The axis" (34) is always noted in describing an electrocardiogram, and often accorded the status of a diagnosis, but, by itself, means little (334, 226); it is a finding to be considered with all the others. Its counterpart on physical examination, the position of the patient, is kept in perspective, not always even mentioned. The axis, expressed as an arrow, or vector, extending outward from the center of the system toward a specific point in space, is determined by the net area of QRS. In effect, presenting the complex as an instantaneous event. It has value, just as the position of the patient does, but ignores changes in amplitude, rate, and direction of excitation that occur during its course from endocardium to epicardium. These important features are evaluated in the orientation, duration, amplitude, and contour of the components of the complex, the Q, R, and S waves individually. When the course of the point that QRS represents is nearly circular, it projects a more or less biphasic curve, an "S1,2,3" pattern, on all the leads; the axis is reported as "indeterminate," or "none." When QRS duration and contour are normal, S1,2,3 is simply an interesting pattern (227).

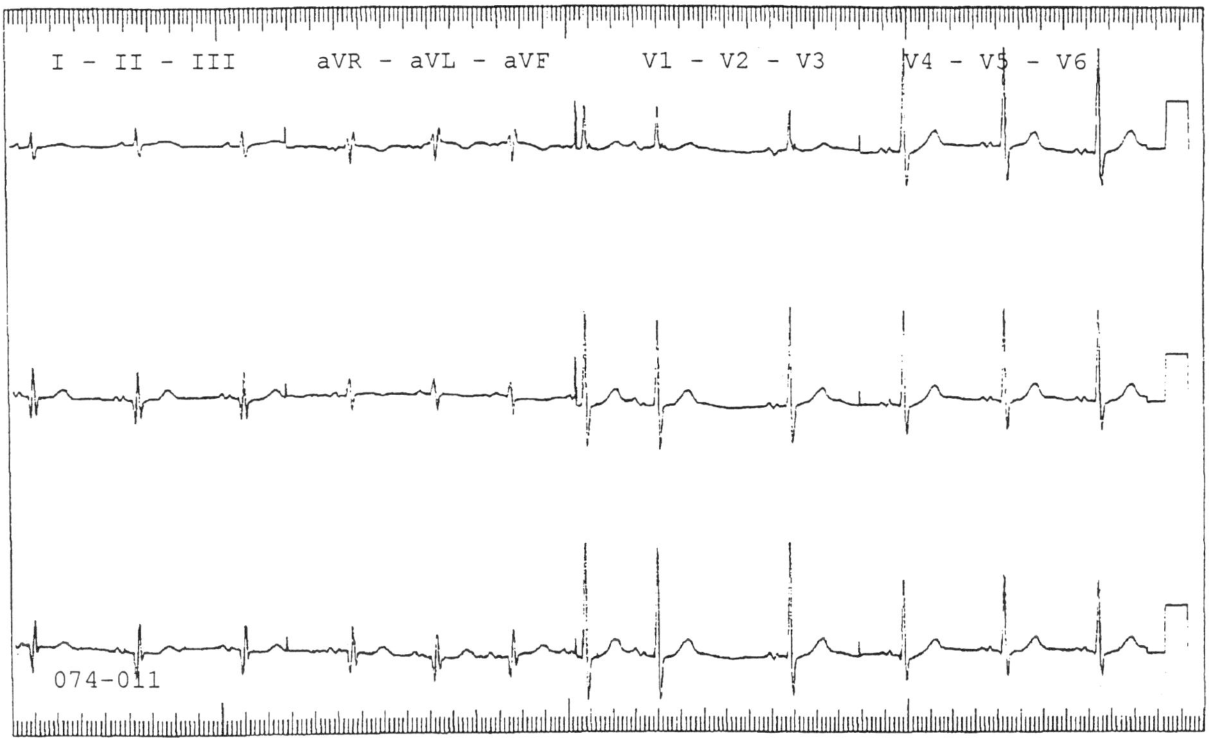

Inferodorsal Myocardial Infarct

```
70    70    16    08    40      sinus
??    8:0   --    15:5        Q2,3,F
              nonc
             normal
+60        ±V1    positive V1-6

(1) Sinus mechanism, rate 70,
    with PAC
(2) Old infero-dorsal MCI
(3) Otherwise WNL
```

The feature of an EKG that indicates scarring deep in the myocardium characteristic of an infarct (173) is abnormality of initial QRS forces. Every lead shows all the electrical activity in the heart, but they show it from different views. In most people, the complex generated by simultaneous excitation of the ventricles is directed leftward, downward, and dorsad. This is why the positive poles of the 12 standard leads are where they are, providing a good view of both normal and most abnormal variants. Infarcts that produce abnormalities perpendicular to the frontal plane are seen best in anterior leads; parallel to it, in frontal leads. Infarcts may occur anywhere in the myocardium, and nothing about the heart is limited by rectilinear coordinates. Anterior lesions, for instance, often have a (left) lateral component manifest in Leads I, aVL, II, and V6. Inferior lesions may have a dorsal component, and, since there are no leads from the back, this will be recognized by change in QRSV1, an abnormal initial R. There is little myocardium depolarized strictly dorsad, and little evidence in the literature that a truly dorsal infarct can be recognized (178). Inferior infarcts were once called posterior, but "posterior" now probably means dorsal.

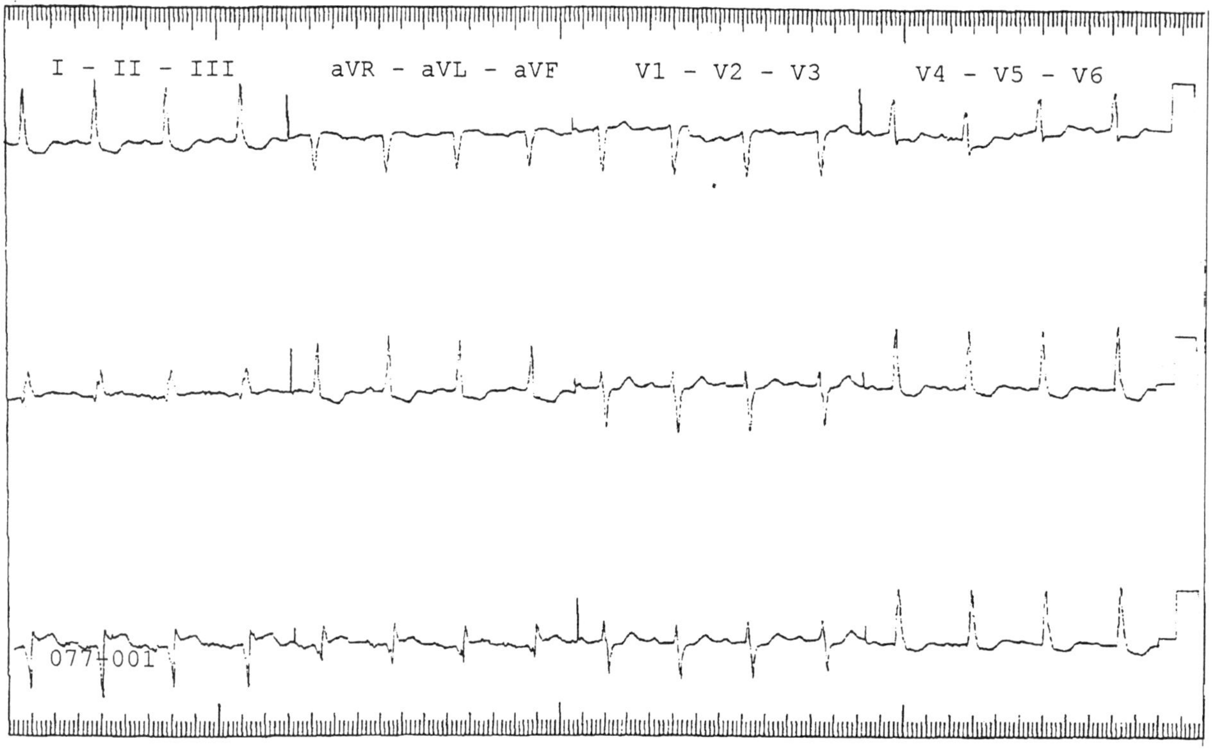

Inferior Myocardial Infarct (Acute?, Old with Ventricular Aneurysm?)

The tracing above was made August 5th; the one in the inset (with enlarged Leads III and aVF), the preceding March 19. Given only the August tracing, with no clinical information, and no earlier tracing for comparison, the diagnosis of an acute infarct is actionable, but this is changed when the control is introduced. With only the EKGs to go on, another possibility to be considered is that there is new damage in the vicinity of an old infarct.

The explanation is not known, but it is an established fact that, though injury is transient by definition, its EKG picture may not be. When stable in a tracing that shows an infarct, ST displacement is at least suggestive of a ventricular aneurysm (180, 185). Stability cannot be assumed when there is only one tracing, but it can be suspected.

95 95 20 10 36 sinus
±0 0:8 V3½ 12:0 Q2,3,F
up 3,aVF, sl down V3-4
sagging/arched
low +120 ±V1 +V2-3 low ±V4
neg V5-6 low

(1) Sinus mechanism, rate 95
(2) Acute inferior myocardial infarct

--An alternative is an old infarct with a ventricular aneurysm. The clinical setting and stability of the findings are important unknowns.

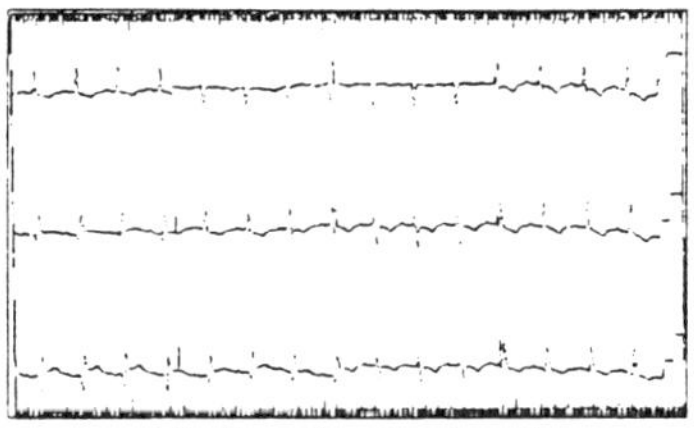

12-lead, Control

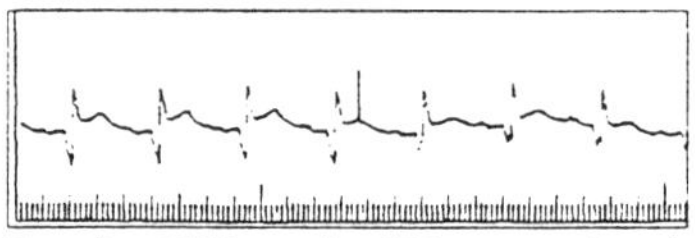

Leads III and aVF, control

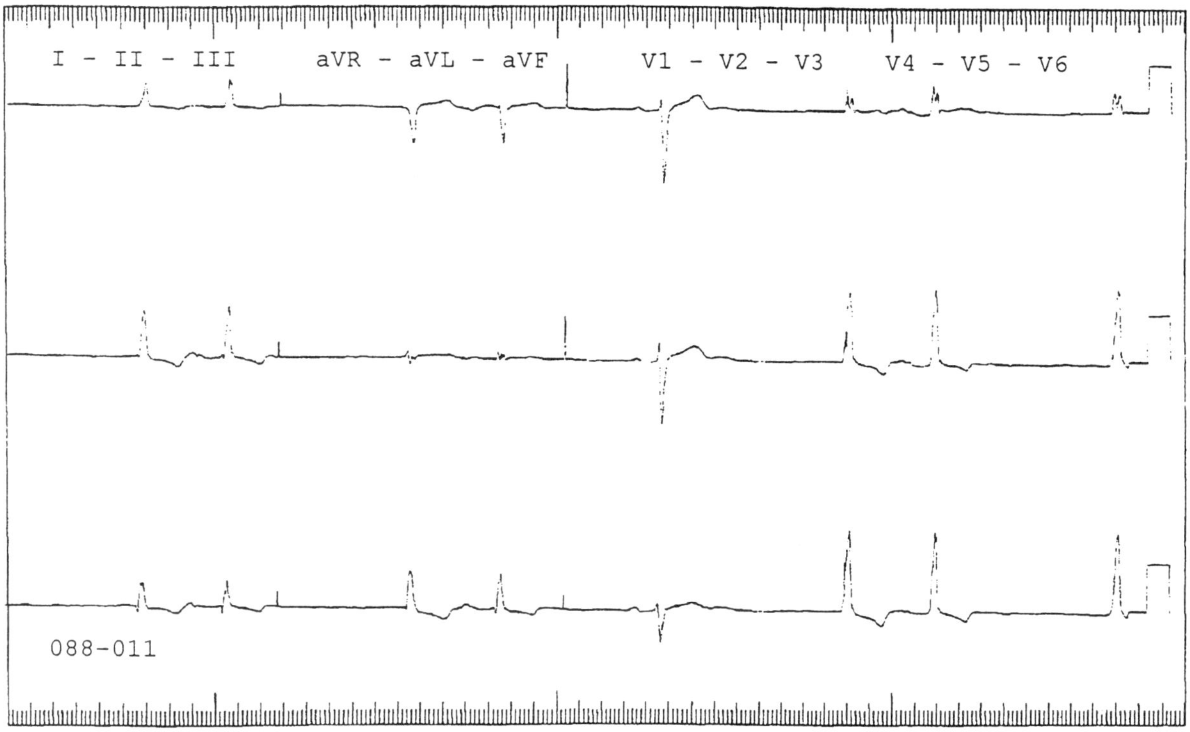

Escape-Capture Bigeminy, ST-T Abnormalities, Probably LVO

```
±50   ±50   24   10   40   see below
+60    2:15    V3½    15:0  normal
              none
          related to T
-90    pos V1-2  ±V3-4   neg V5-6

(1) Sinus arrhythmia, rate
    about 40, with borderline
    AV conduction time
(2) Junctional escape, rate ±40
(3) ST-T abnormalities,
    probably left ventricular
    overload
```

This is a good example of several principles of cardiac electrophysiology learned very early in medical school. First, the fastest functioning pacemaker available to a chamber determines the rate at which it beats; second, the normal sinus rhythm is not perfectly regular; and third, a default pacemaker is available as a backup when a faster one fails (122). These are all expressed as "sinus arrhythmia." In this case, the sinus node is functioning normally but its rate varies a bit more than usual. When an impulse from it fails to reach the junction after an interval representing its inherent rate, that focus escapes and drives the ventricles. If this occurs every other beat, there is escape/capture bigeminy (146).

Whether to call a PR of 0.24 s at a rate of 50 first degree AV block, is a an arbitrary decision, and not very important.

The ST-T pattern is abnormal, nonspecific, but suggestive of left ventricular overload.

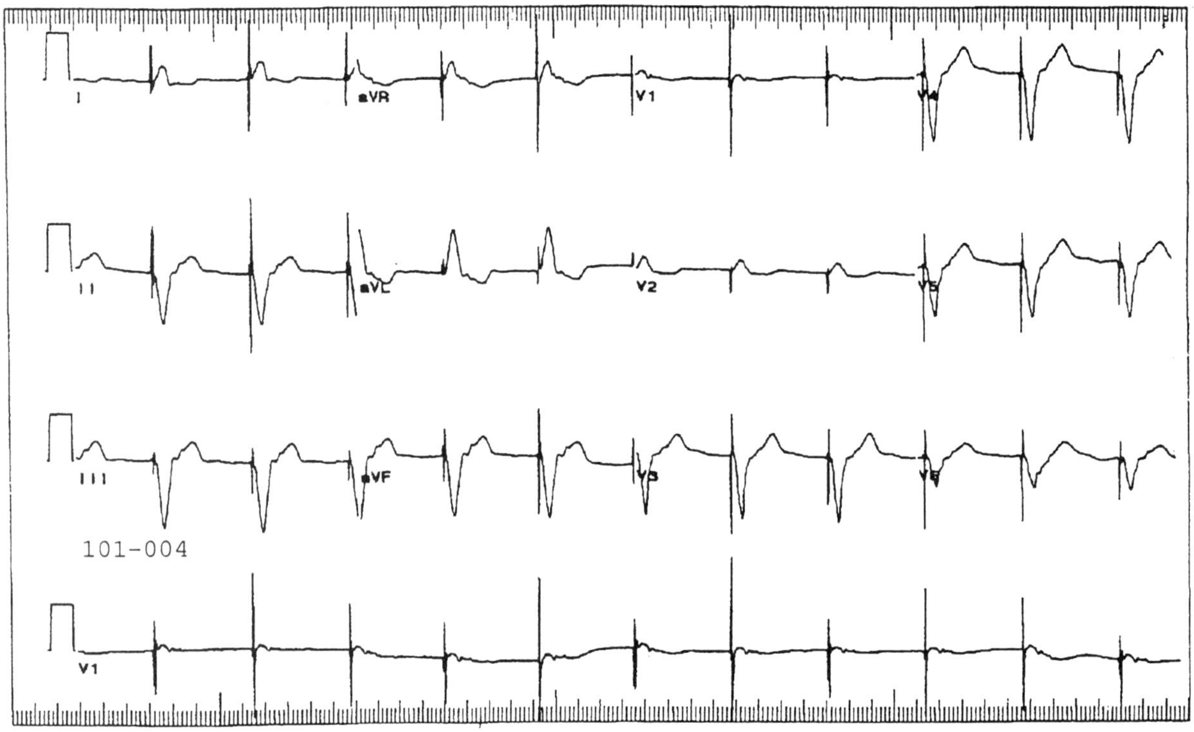

Artificial Ventricular Pacemaker with Retrograde P

QRS rhythm is perfectly regular, and each complex is introduced by a spike typical of the signal of an artificial pacemaker. They are abnormally wide, directed to the left, and of bizarre configuration approaching that of left bundle branch block. All these features identify an artificial pacemaker in the right ventricle. Note that even when driven by an electronic device there is variation in detail from beat to beat.

Description of the mechanism is not complete until the atria have been accounted for. If atrial activity is not identifiable, this must be noted. In this case, P is easily seen as a little notch early in ST. Its cephalad orientation says that the atria are depolarized retrograde, and its timing at the same interval following each QRS implies that it is transmitted from the ventricles. The artificial pacemaker is driving the atria as well as the ventricles.

```
70  70   --   16  44     see below
-75   2:0    --    0:8  diff slur
               none
          not remarkable
+90      ±V1-2     positive V3-6

(1) Artificial ventricular
    pacemaker capturing regu-
    larly, rate 70
(2) Atria depolarized from
    ventricles
```

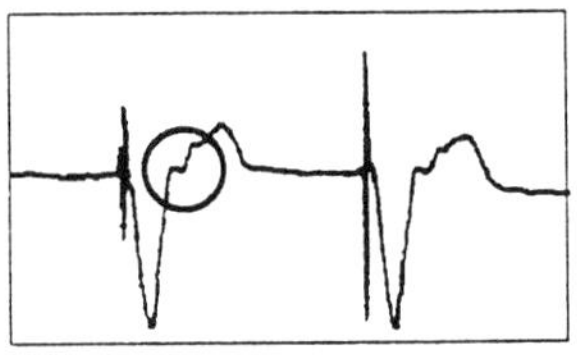

aVF from above

When ventricular depolarization is from a focus other than supraventricular, repolarization is changed proportionally, and the ST-T complex cannot be interpreted by the usual rules.

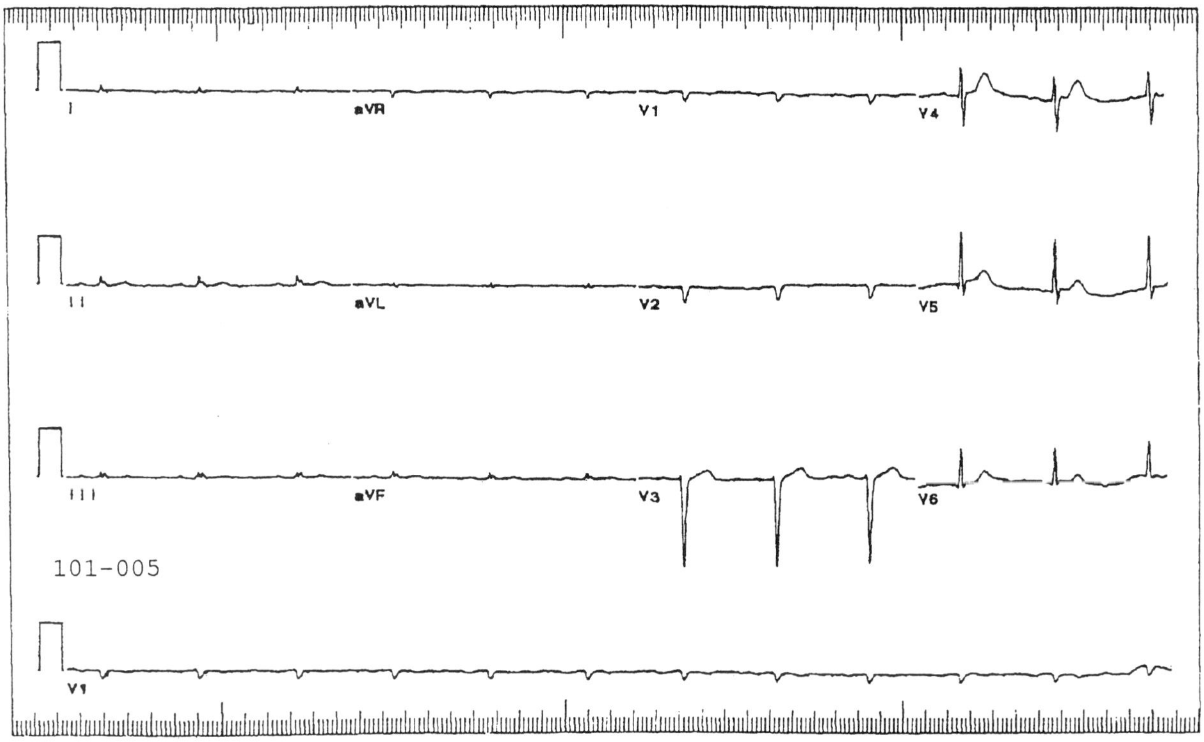

Calcium

```
70  70    20   08   36       sinus
+60 low    0:2  V4   7:0    normal
              none
             normal
?+60     ±V1-2  positive V3-6

(1) Sinus mechanism, rate 70
(2) Within normal limits
```

The potential value of the electrocardiographic picture of hypo- or hypercalcemia is as a suggestion for the direction for further study. The relation is far from linear, and with serum calcium levels so readily available now, its usefulness is small (231). This tracing is within normal limits and was chosen for illustration of these comments partly because prototypes are so hard to find, and partly to indicate the relative unimportance of the subject. The serum calcium level at the time it was recorded was 13.7 mg/dL. The traditional picture of hypercalcemia is short QT with the trace rising almost straight from J to the peak of T. The computer produced a "QTc" of 0.352 s in this case, short, but a value that is beyond the limits of credibility.

The traditional EKG picture of low calcium, a long, flat ST with low T, basically nonspecific ST-T abnormalities, is very unlikely to be the first indication of metabolic imbalance. Its significance is appreciated only after the serum calcium level is known.

This patient had none of the known explanations for low voltage (228), but low voltage is not often anything more than a finding, of little value by itself, comparable to short stature.

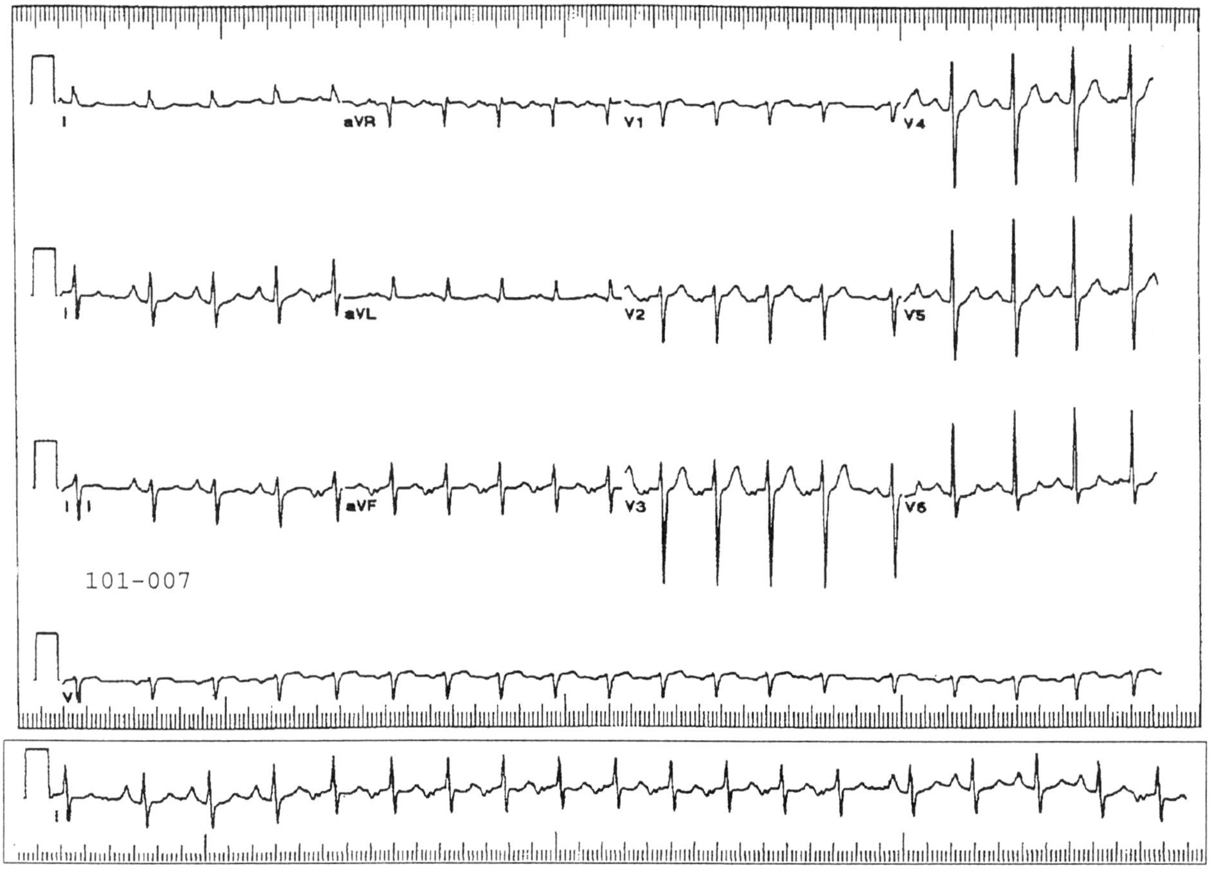

The full tracing as Lead II

Paroxysmal Atrial Tachycardia (PAT)

The rate is usually much greater than 135 when there is usurping atrial ectopy with regular rhythm and 1:1 AV conduction, but this is about as clear an example of a paroxysm that as one is likely to see.

Supraventricular tachycardia, or "SVT," seems to have usurped the title for this entity, but that is not necessarily a good thing; paroxysmal atrial tachycardia is a lot more specific. There is more information in knowing the rate and the locus of the pacemaker than just that the heart is beating rapidly; also, "SVT" could be of sinus origin, atrial flutter, atrial fibrillation, or junctional, high, middle, or low. Be as specific as possible. It may make a difference (129).

100 100 16 08 32 see below
±0 1:5 V4½ 15:3 normal
none
normal
low ±V1 positive V2-6 low V6

(1) Sinus mechanism, rate 100
(2) Paroxysmal atrial tachycardia, rate 135
(3) Otherwise WNL

Beginning of paroxysm

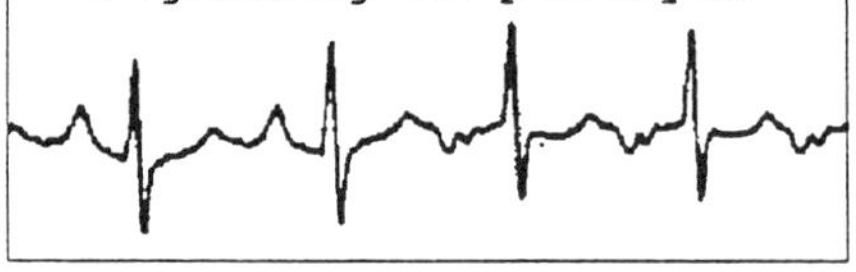

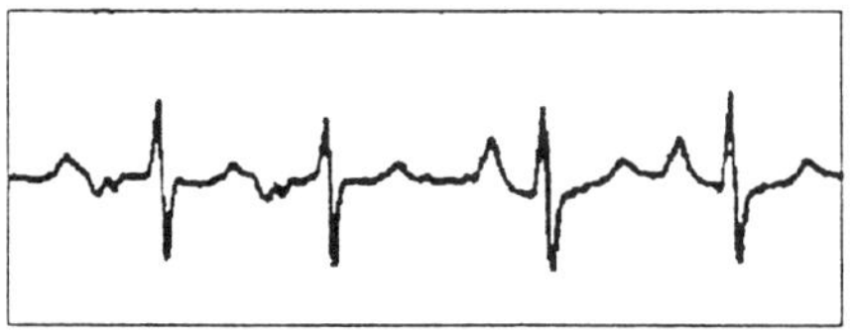

End of paroxysm

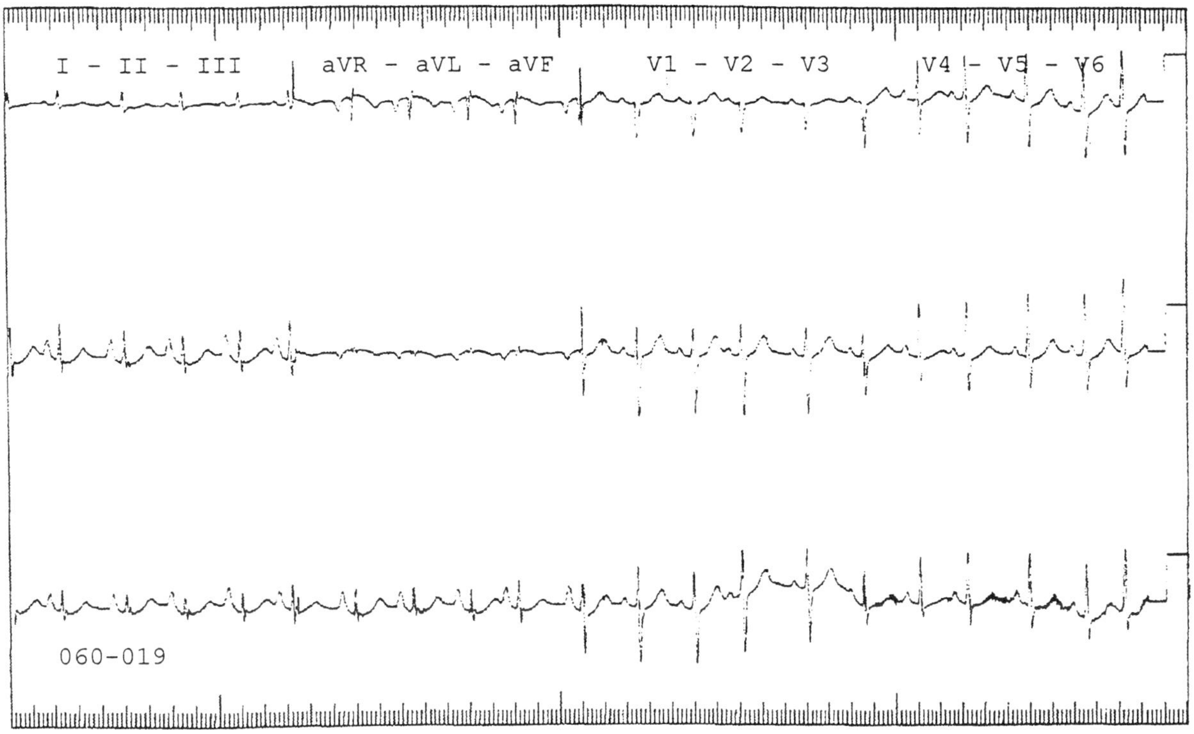

Right Atrial Enlargement, Pulmonary Emphysema

120 120 12 08 36 sinus
+60 1:6 V4 10:4 normal
none
some sagging
low +60 positive V1-6
P: tall, peaked II, III, aVF

(1) Sinus mechanism, rate 120
(2) Right atrial enlargement
(3) Otherwise probably WNL, at worst only small ST-T ab normalities

--The P-ST-T pattern suggests pulmonary emphysema

EKG reports often include words implying that the tracing reflects pulmonary disease, and this can be defended easily, but it assumes that the doctor realizes that it is not literally true; EKGs show the electrical activity of the heart, not the lungs. A better policy is to be specific, to say first what the tracing itself shows, and supplement that with whatever comment seems appropriate.

This tracing shows a pattern that correlates well with pulmonary emphysema (233), a smooth curve from the top of a large P, suggesting right atrial enlargement (188), to the top of T, which need not be large. See insets. Atrial repolarization may be a factor in this configuration, but in the final analysis the correlation is simply empirical. Evidence of right ventricular enlargement, as often seen with respiratory disease, may be present, and T voltage may be low.

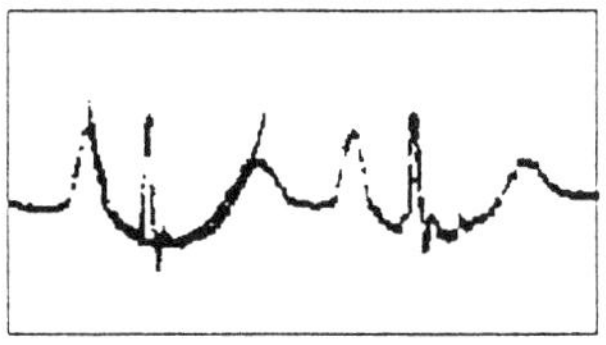
aVF from above

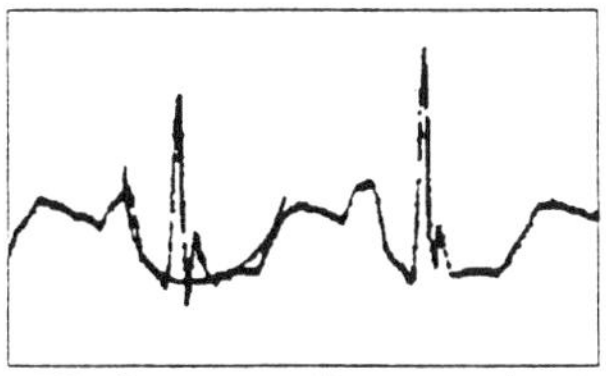
aVF from another patient

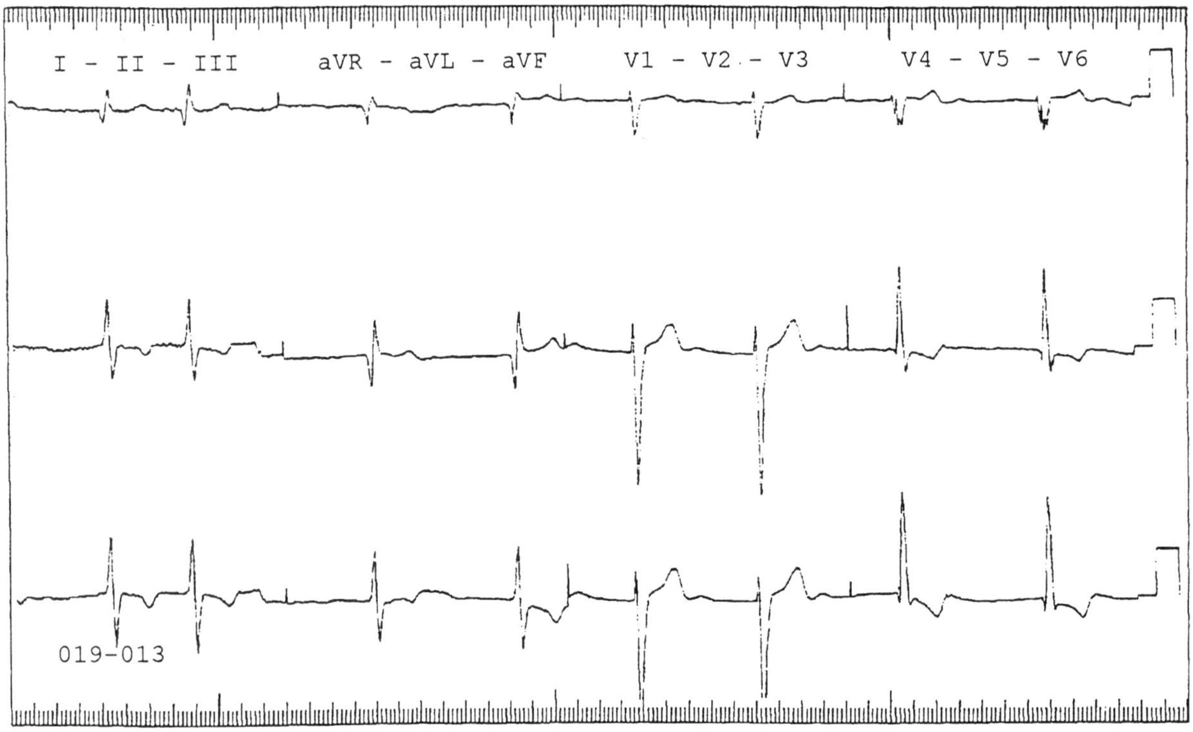

Old Lateral Myocardial Infarct

(Or crossed arm leads?)

--	50	12	48	AF
??	2:6	V4½	20:1	Q1,aVL,V5-6
		none		
		related to T		
-60	±V1	pos V2-4	±V5	neg V6

(1) AF, rate about 50
(2) ST-T abnormalities suggestive of left ventricular overload
(3) Atypical IV conduction defect, ??peri-infarction block
(4) Old lateral myocardial infarct, probable.

The mechanism is clear here, and the otherwise normal T oriented nearly opposite QRS suggests left ventricular overload, but the QRS pattern offers several options for explanation. The grossly broad, slurred Q in views from the left, I, aVL, and, less obviously, V6, is probably evidence of a scar deep in the myocardium. The machine called it a lateral infarct, and, knowing only that the patient is a 71-one-year-old man, that is probably an appropriate interpretation. An alternative is crossed arm leads. Correcting for that would get rid of the QI, but still leave a prominent Q in aVL and V5-6. Prolongation of IV conduction time may mean periinfarction block (184), diffuse patchy fibrosis, or the effects of quinidine or some other drug. QT is long, but that adds nothing.

"Lateral" is one of those words whose meaning is obvious, but is not used consistently in reporting EKG's. Sometimes it refers to views from the left, as here, sometimes to views from the left side of the front, V4-6. The latter usage seems to differentiate between lateral, a view, and septal, a structure, is hard to understand, and adds little (177).

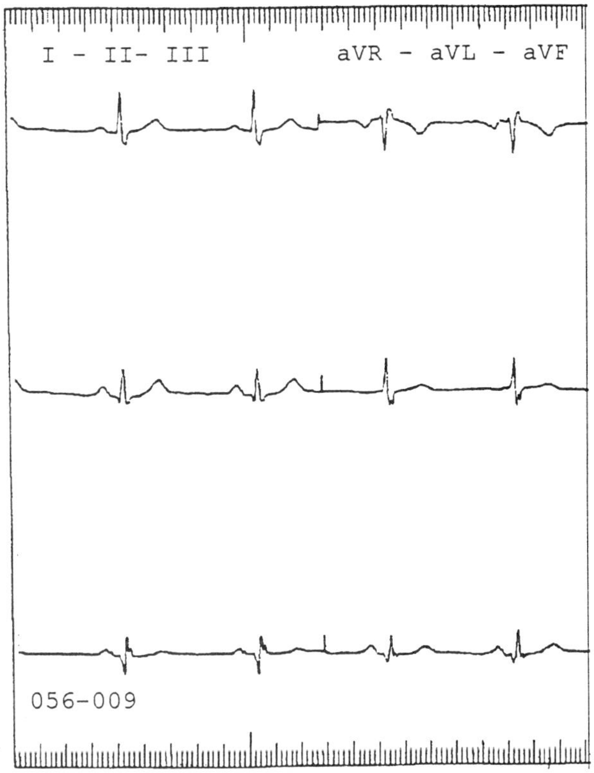

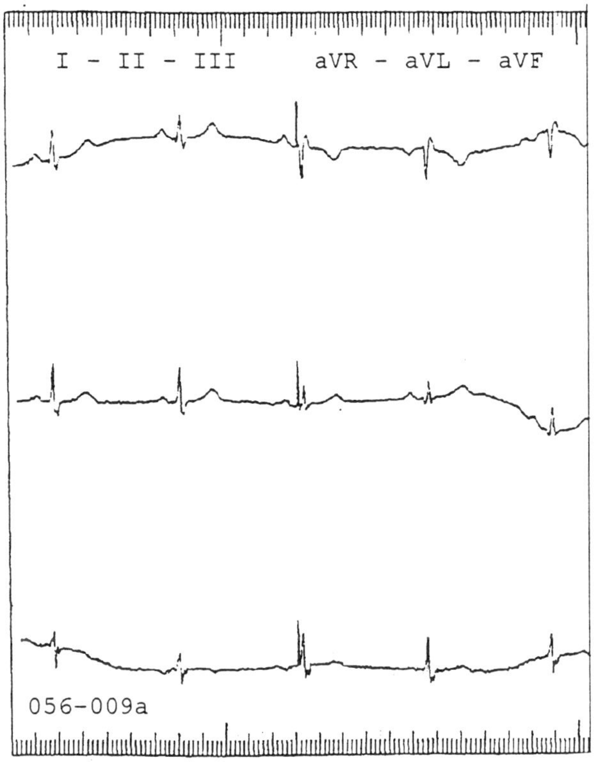

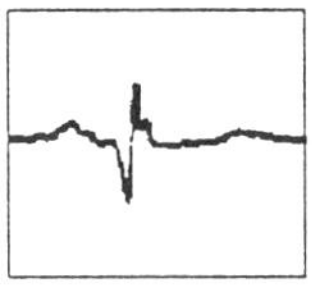
Lead III

60 60 16 08 40 sinus
+30 ----------------- Q2,3,F
none
normal
+45 ----------------------

(1) Sinus mechanism, rate 60
(2) Old inf mci, prob
(3) Otherwise WNL, but incomplete, frontal leads only

--Nothing looks new.

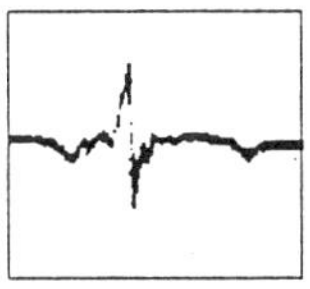
Lead III

55 55 16 08 40 sinus
+30 --------------------normal
none
normal
+15 --------------------

(1) Sinus mechanism, rate 55
(2) Old inf mci, prob
(3) Otherwise WNL, but incomplete, frontal leads only

--Nothing looks new.
--Interpretation corrects for transposition of left arm and leg leads.

Old Inferior Myocardial Infarct

Evidence obliterated by transposition of left arm and leg leads

The properly recorded tracing, at left, shows a prominent Q3. Crossing of the left arm and leg leads in the tracing on the right reverses the polarity, changing the complex from a QR to an RS, and swaps Leads I and II, and aVL and aVF. aVR and the precordial leads are not affected. The problem is likely to be greater when it is the artifact that simulates an infarct than when it obliterates evidence of one. With only one tracing, the error can only be suspected. The negative P and T in Lead III are the key, but neither is abnormal in itself. Another suggestion of the artifact is EKG evidence for an inferior infarct in a patient not thought to have had one. The tracing is complete and correction is easy (104).

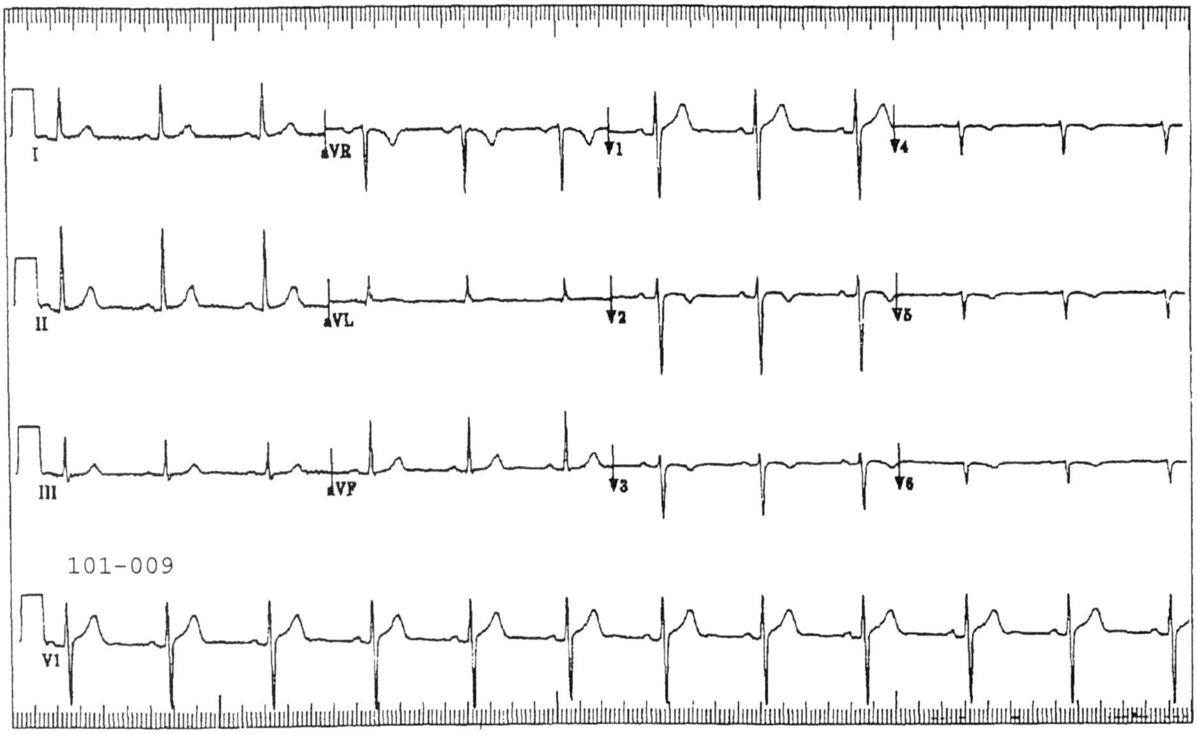

Precordial Leads on the Right

Within normal limits, but incomplete

```
70    70    16    06    36     sinus
+45    5:16    --    --      normal
              none
             normal
(1) Sinus mechanism, rate 70
(2) Within normal limits, but
    incomplete

--V1 and V2 are transposed,
  and V3-6 are really V3R-6R
```

The program, having been instructed that the chest leads were positioned properly, called this a "possible lateral infarct," becoming part of the problem instead of part of the solution. Of course, an infarct is possible, the alternative is impossible, "ruled out," and the EKG cannot show this. "Lateral" is used in the sense of the left side of the front. If the leads were positioned as labeled, this would be an appropriate interpretation, but they are not. The tracing contains useful information, but is not complete, and the error cannot be corrected.

The giveaway is that QRS points to both the left (Lead I) and the right (V6). The progression of precordial P and QRS is backward for V1-6, but proper for V2-V6R. The differential includes dextrocardia and right ventricular enlargement, as well as an old anterior infarct (108).

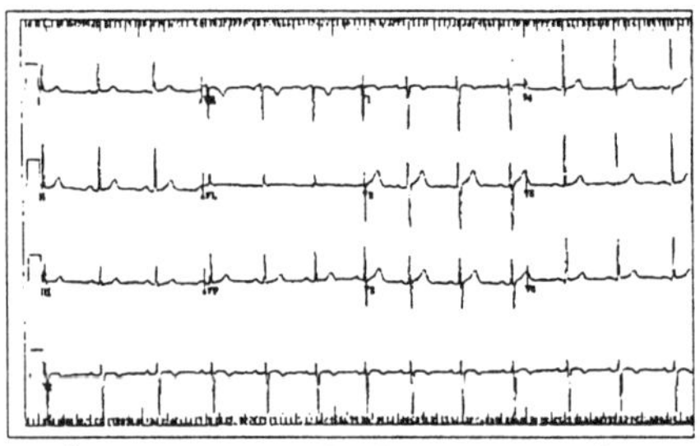

#173 recorded correctly

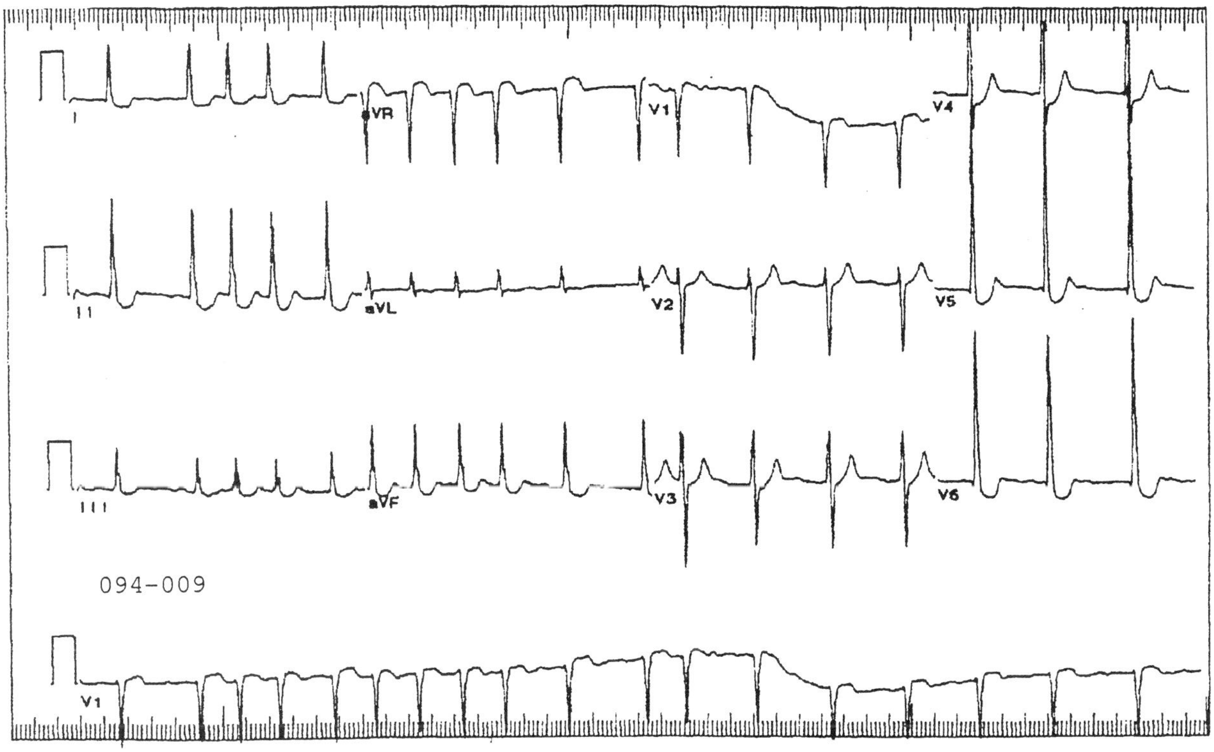

Atrial Fibrillation, Digitalis Effect, Coronary Insufficiency, Left Ventricular Hypertrophy

```
--   110   --   08  32   see below
+45   1:12    V3   (V5)40:0   nl
  down I,II,aVF,V4-6,  up aVR
    sagging/flattened/arched
low   ±V1   pos V2-5,   flat V6

(1) Atrial fibrillation, rato
    about 110
(2) ST-T abnormalities with el-
    ements to suggest digitalis
    effect, left ventricular
    overload, and coronary in-
    sufficiency
(3) Left ventricular hyper-
    trophy, probable
```

This is almost a classic portrait of an old person with angina, hypertension, and congestive heart failure. The tracing shows none of these, of course, only what is reported in the box at right. Discordant ST displacement, flattened in some leads, is typical of coronary insufficiency (207), short QT with sagging/arched ST in some leads suggests digitalis effect (229), and high QRS voltage suggests left ventricular hypertrophy (192). The evidence for left ventricular overload is not so clear, but that would be in ST-T, and the pattern there looks more like digitalis effect and coronary insufficiency. If there is left ventricular hypertrophy, the left ventricle must be, or have been, overloaded.

Applying the law of parsimony, or Occam's razor, as we always do in making a diagnosis, one tries to explain everything with the simplest possible answer. The single pathologic process that could explain everything here is atherosclerosis, found in old people, and the lesions suggested imply the manifestations noted above.

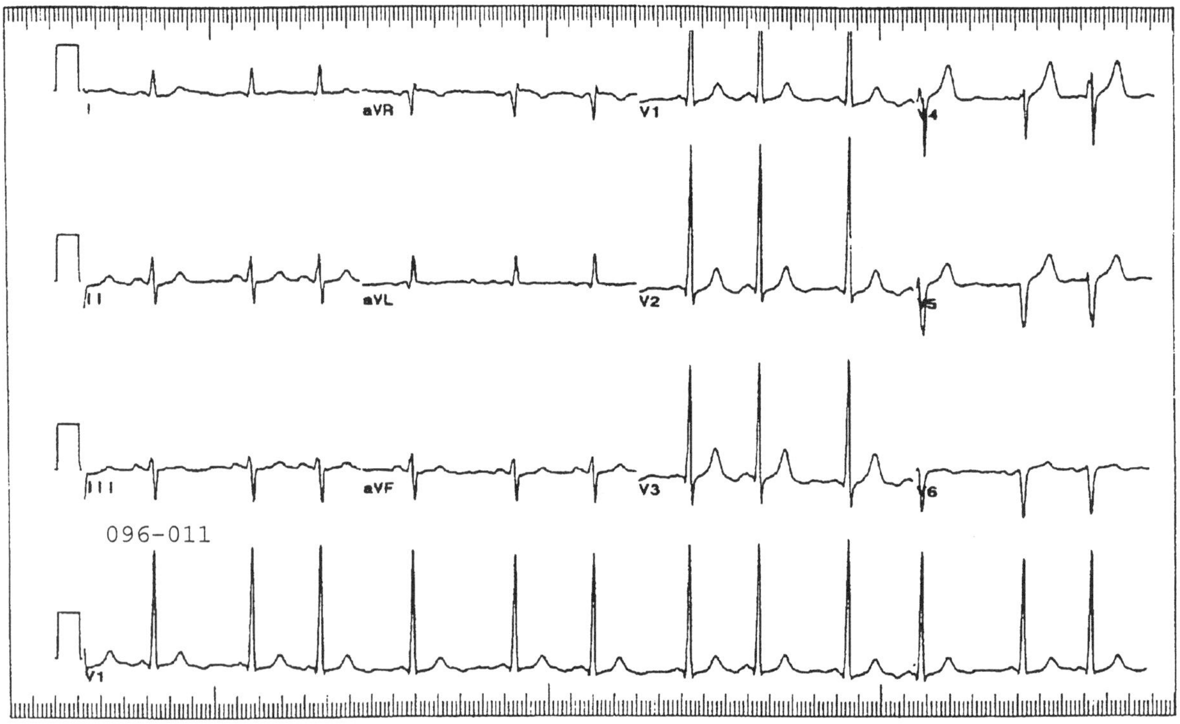

Artifact Called Infarct, Precordial Leads in Reverse Order

This represents an all-too-human lapse of attention by the technician recording the tracing. The problem is usually in electrode positions on the chest, but another possibility is that the lead wires are plugged in to the wrong holes in the data acquisition unit. The effect on the patient depends on the doctor who interprets the tracing (or the computer readout, or an interpretation supplied by another doctor). If the error is recognized, there is no problem, compensation being easy; if it is not, the findings can be seen as evidence of an anterior infarct, as the readout reported in this case, with unpleasant consequences. Suspecting the problem depends on awareness of the possibility; proof of it, on the conflict between QRS pointing to the left (Lead I), and the right (V6). Terminal P negativity in "V6" (not very clear here) with positive P in "V1" is even more telling (85, 109).

75 75 16 08 40 sinus
-15 1:10 V3½ 30:0 normal
none
normal
+60 positive V1-6, low V1

(1) Sinus mechanism, rate 75, with PAC's
(2) Within normal limits

--Interpretation corrects for V1-6 in reverse order.

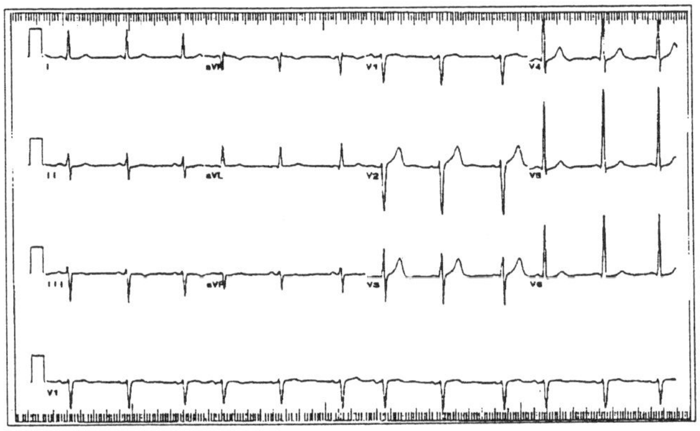

EKG #175 recorded properly

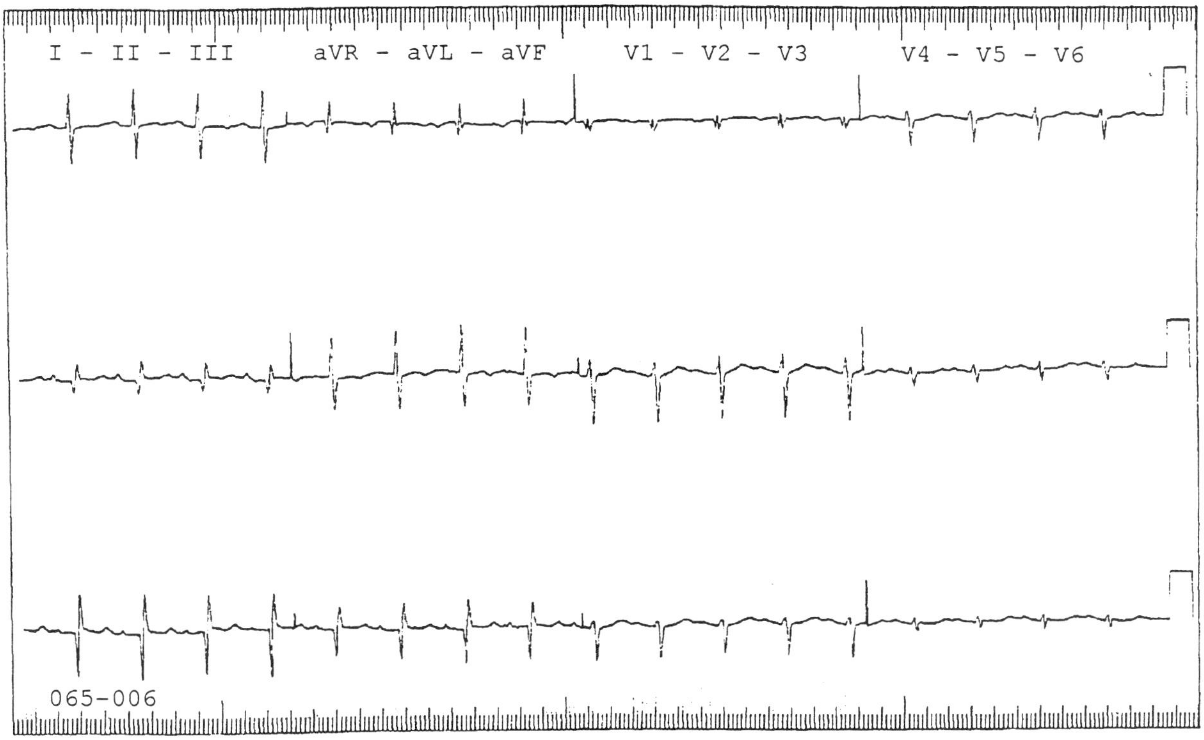

Inferior Myocardial Infarct can be Masked by Crossed Left Arm and Leg Leads

```
105   105   20   08   ?36        sinus
??    QRS1:1:2     V5-6        Q2,3,F
                none
           related to T
?+75 low    ±V1+V2-4 low      ±V5-8

(1) Sinus mechanism, rate 105
(2) Old inferior myo infarct

--Nothing looks new.
```

As always, interpretation is called for. Prominence of the inferior Q here is more a function of amplitude than either duration or contour, but it is at least probable that it is abnormal and represents an old infarct (174). An alternative interpretation is that there are only nonspecific ST-T abnormalities, and the evidence for an infarct is only suggestive. Given that there is an infarct, an additional diagnosis of nonspecific ST-T abnormality is hard to defend. The inset shows what happens if left arm and leg leads are transposed, a common problem (104). The tracing is complete, and correction requires only application of Einthoven's premises (see "Summary of Rules, Assumptions..." No. 3, in Chapter 2), but if there is only one tracing it may be hard to tell whether the Q3 is valid or an artifact (EKG 179), especially if P is small. In that case, at least one other tracing is needed.

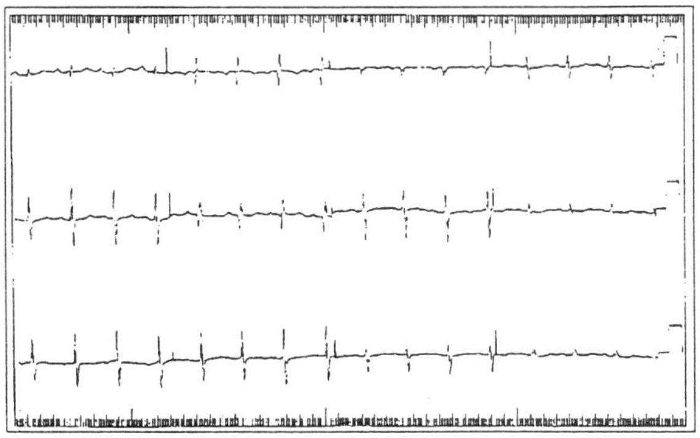

#176 recorded with left arm and leg leads transposed

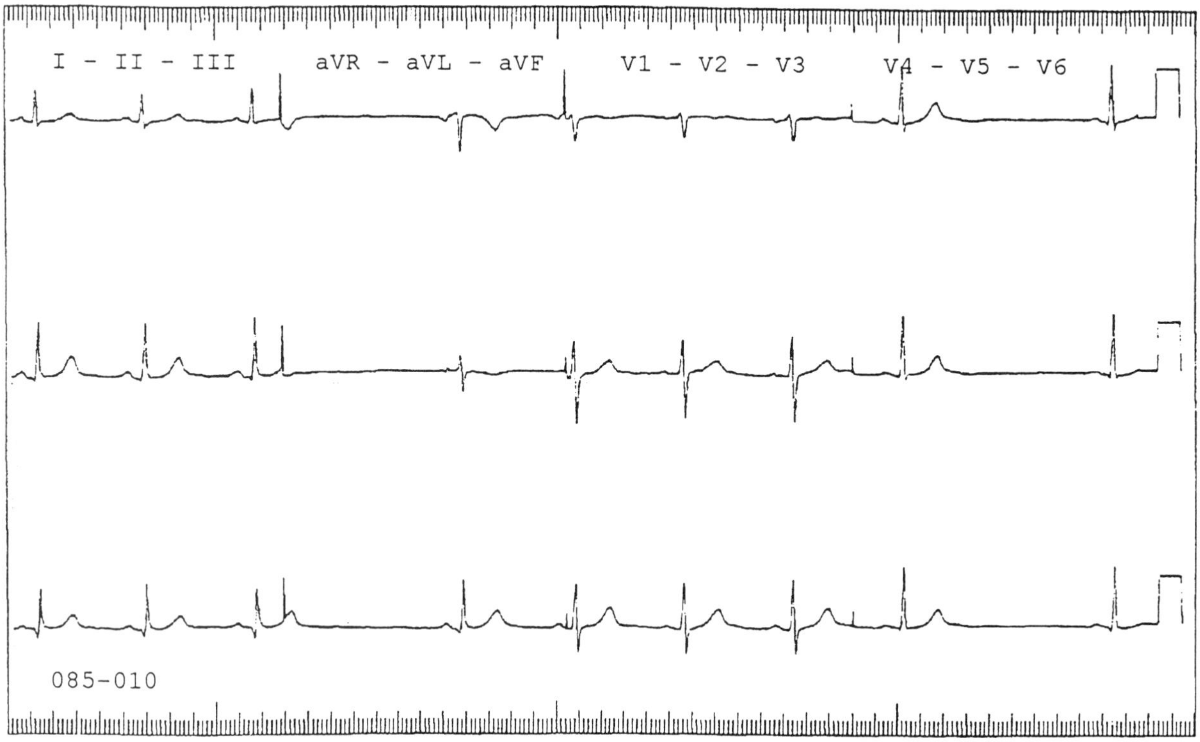

Sinus Pauses, Bigeminy

50	50	16	08	40	see below
+60	1:4	V2	12:0		normal
		none			
		normal			
+75	isoelectric V1				pos V2-6

(1) Sinus mechanism, rate 50
(2) Sinus pauses
(3) Otherwise WNL

This is a fairly common finding in normals, with little if any clinical significance by itself. The most common alternative is simply marked sinus arrhythmia, but blocked PACs, and second degree AV block, are in the differential. The answer may depend on more than the 10 s documented in a routine 12-lead tracing. Especially when P is not clear, a longer strip may be needed (123).

The explanation for sinus pauses involves the concept of sinoatrial (SA) block. There is a lot of support for this hypothesis, even leading some to distinguish between Type I and Type II SA block, but proof requires more information than can be had from the surface tracing. A related subject defines SA nodal reentry as an explanation for sinus tachycardia in some instances.

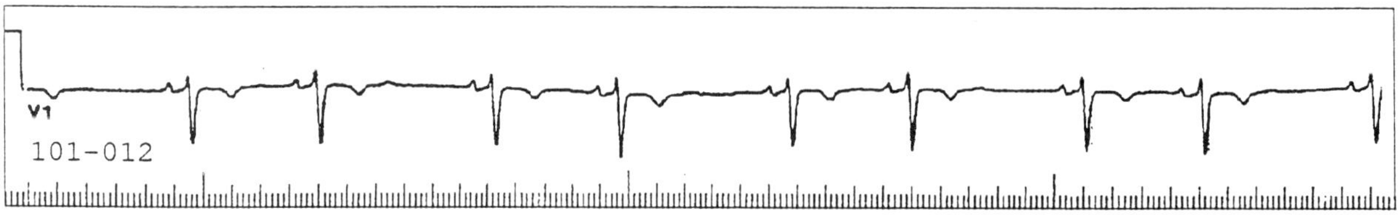

Bigeminy due to sinus pauses (not the same patient as above)

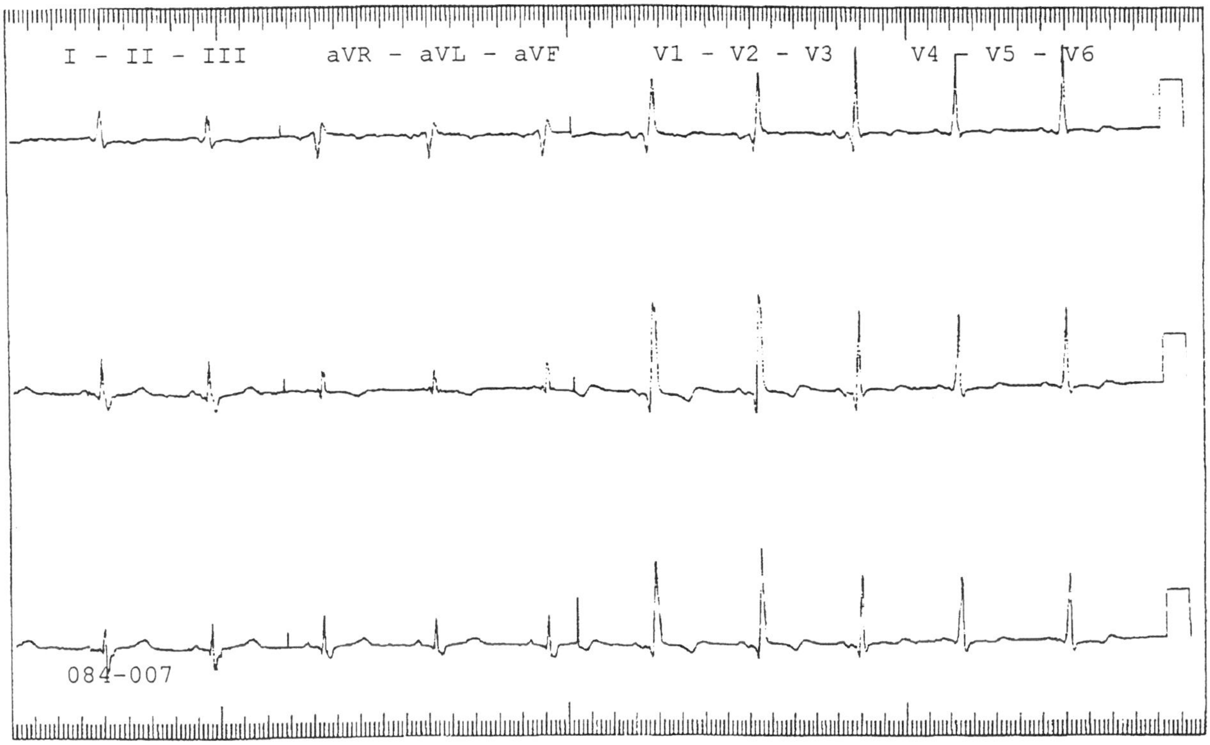

Atypical IV Conduction Defect, Old Anterior Myocardial Infarct, Peri-Infarction Block? Etc.?

```
65   65    16    12?    44?    sinus
?+15  QR,4:10   --   15:1   QV1-3
                     terminal slur
                none
           related to T
+90   ±V1    neg V2-3       +V4-6
U: prominent

(1) Sinus mechanism, rate 65
(2) Old anterior myo infarct
(3) Atypical prolongation of IV
    conduction time, ?peri-in-
    farction block
```

Few would doubt the evidence for an old anterior scar in this tracing, or see fit to make anything of the prominent U, or the arbitrarily long QT (which the computer called 0.510). The computer measured QRS duration as 0.110 s. This figure need not be taken as absolute, but QRS does look wide, an abnormality that must be accounted for (as specifically as possible). The fact that the abnormality affects the terminal forces, directing them anteriorly, suggests right bundle branch block (q.v.), and that may be the explanation, but the contour is not broad and irregular enough to be typical. Right ventricular hypertrophy is in the differential, but would not explain prolongation of QRS. Abnormal widening of QRS without the other features of the usual explanations has been attributed to "arborization block", "parietal block," "peripheral block," and, when there is also evidence of an infarct, "periinfarction" block. In this case, the latter seems most likely. The term was proposed early for what has come to be known as left anterior hemi (or fascicular) block (168). It implies that the infarct somehow slows depolarization, but lacks much usefulness.

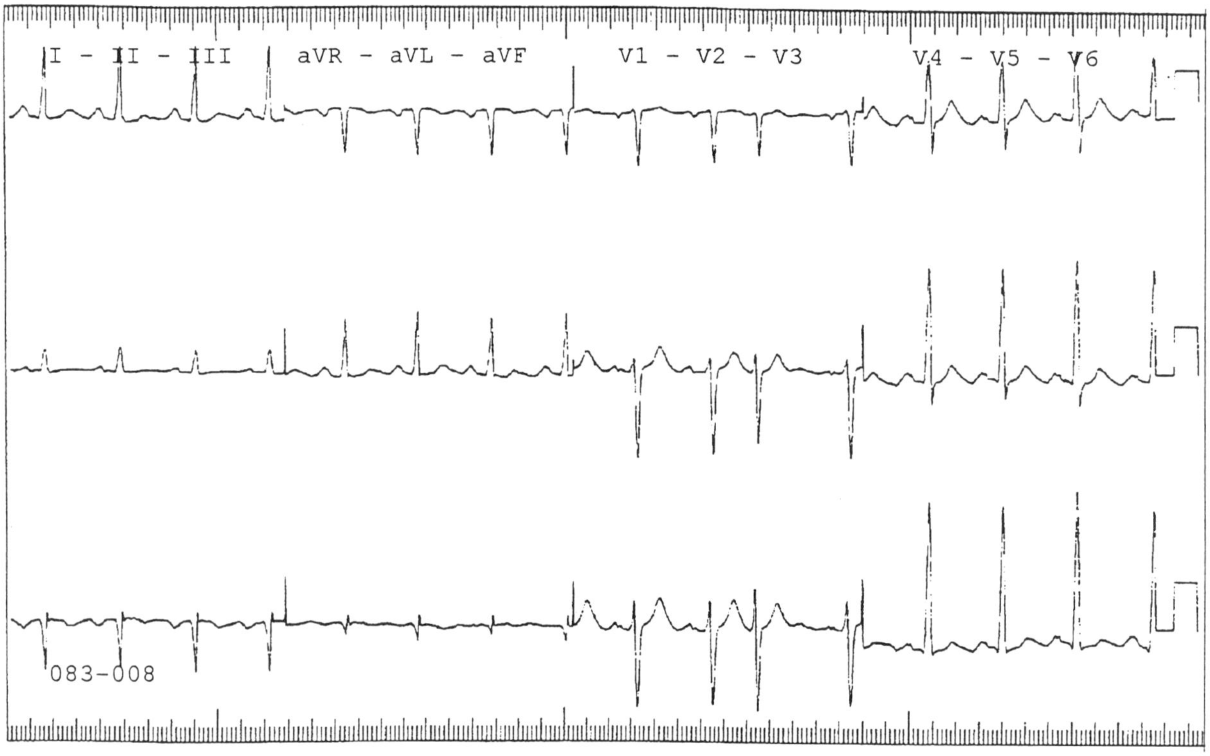

Crossed Left Arm and Leg Leads Simulate Inferior Myocardial Infarct

Crossed left leads is one of the commonest technical artifacts. It is harder to recognize than one that produces a flat line in a lead. All three corners of the triangle are represented, and the tracing is complete. V leads are not affected. Correction is easy once the problem is suspected (104), and the key to that is the negative P3. With experience, especially if the patient is not thought to have had an infarct, the P-QRS-T pattern in III looks upside down. If there is no P, or P is too small to evaluate, the problem will be missed. Proof depends on a control tracing. The one in the inset here was made several months after the one above, and is not exactly like that one; EKG findings are not always fixed. Note variation in QRS voltage, irrelevant here, but sometimes a problem.

```
95    95    20    08    36     sinus
+60    1:10    V3½  25:0    normal
             none
            normal
+90    ±V1    positive V2-6

(1) Sinus mechanism, rate 95,
    with PAC's
(2) Within normal limits

--Interpretation corrects for
  recording with left arm and
  leg leads transposed.
```

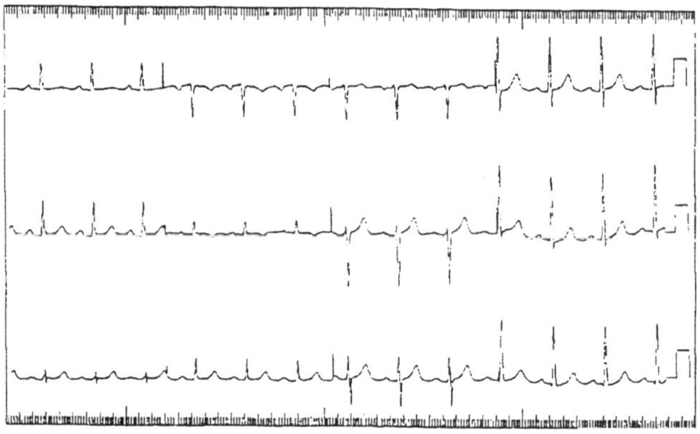

EKG #179 recorded correctly

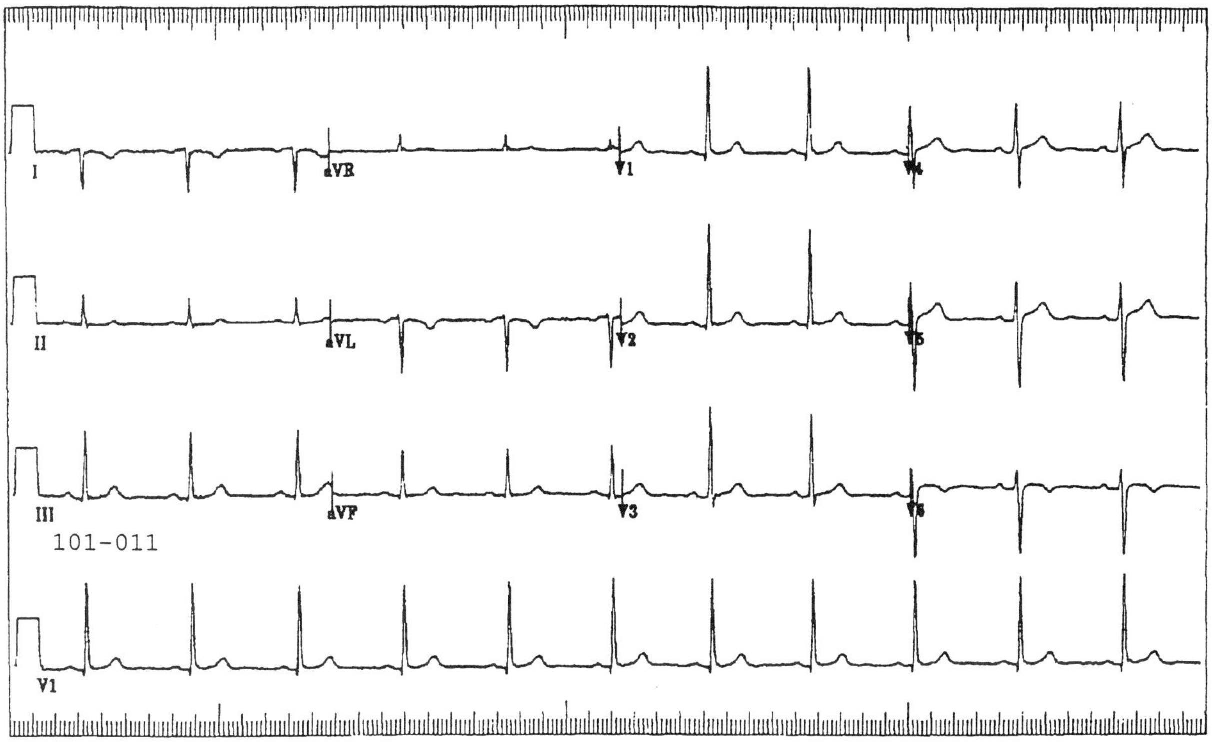

Crossed Arm Leads, Precordial Leads in Reverse Order

```
65    65    16    08    40      sinus
+45    5:15    V3    18:0...normal
              none
             normal
+45   negative V1, positive V2-6

(1) Sinus mechanism, rate 65
(20 Within normal limits

--Description and interpreta-
  tion correct for crossed arm
  leads and precordial leads in
  reverse order.
```

Once suspected, this double artifact is easy to understand. It represents only momentary inattention on the part of the technician, and correction for it is simple (104). If there is terminal P negativity in V1, as there frequently is, the nature of the problem may be even clearer than here. Real abnormality in the tracing may complicate matters.

Interpretations with which this picture may be confused include crossed arm leads, right ventricular hypertrophy (as the computer called it in this tracing), and dextrocardia. See the Index for examples of these.

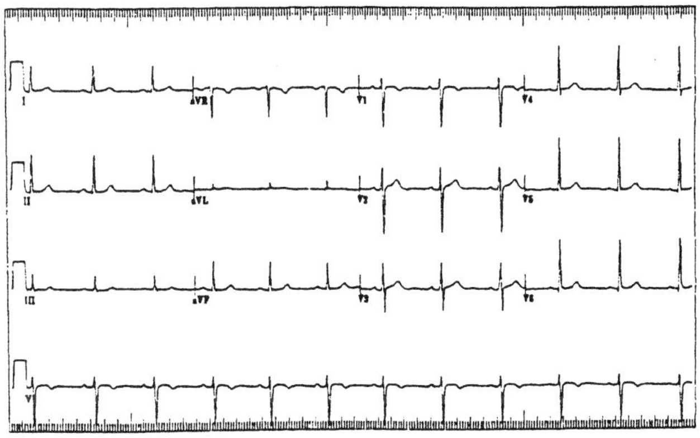

EKG #180 recorded properly

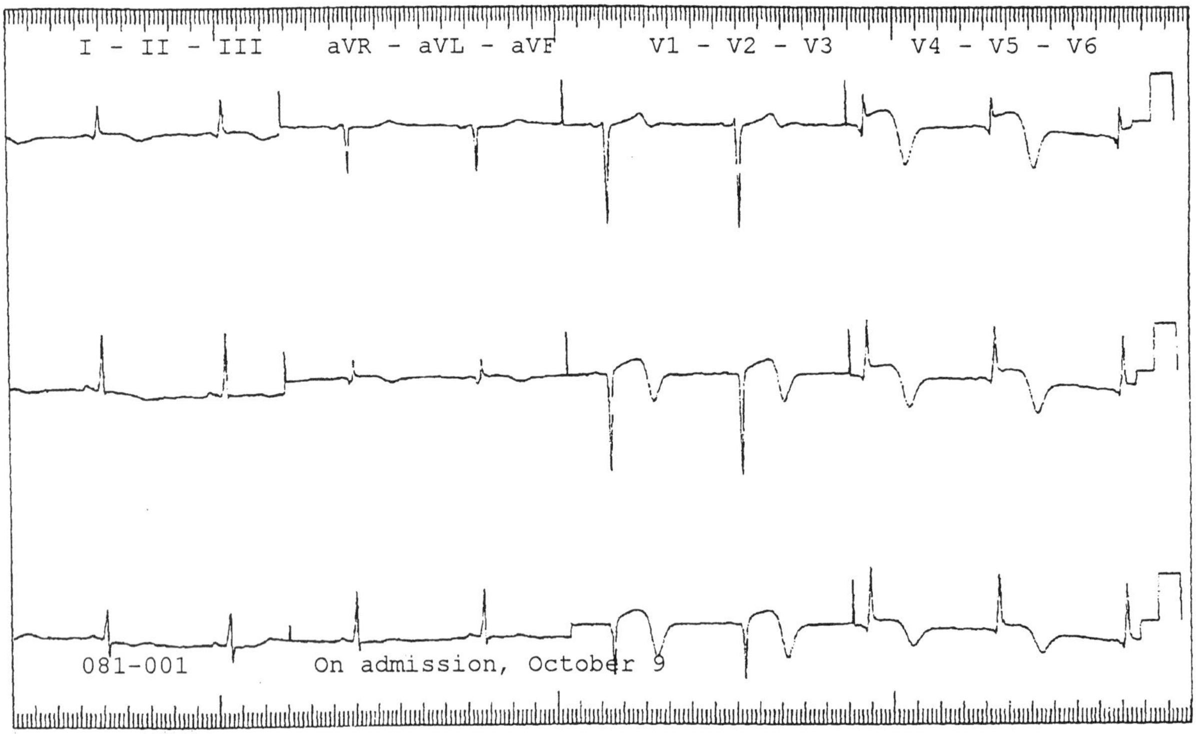

Acute Anterior Myocardial Infarct, Evolutionary Change

The admission tracing above shows all the classic findings of an acute anterior infarct, abnormality of the initial part of QRS accompanied by elevation and arching of ST in precordial leads (173). A small lateral component is visible as a prominent QaVL, but most of the abnormal forces are perpendicular to the frontal plane. As the lesion evolves, ST displacement diminishes and its contour segues into a negative T that is continuous with a prominent U. Later, T becomes positive, with an almost normal ST contour. This course is typical, but the range to be expected is very, very wide, all the way from near stability of the STT pattern of injury to its resolution within hours. U is prominent and can be separated from T only in V1 in this tracing.

```
55    55    12    08    40.. .sinus
+45   1:20  V4   12:0   QSV2-3,QV4
         up V2-6
      arched into T
low ±180  pos V2, negative V3-6
U: prominent, negative V2-6

(1) Sinus mechanism, rate 55
(2) Acute anterior myo infarct
```

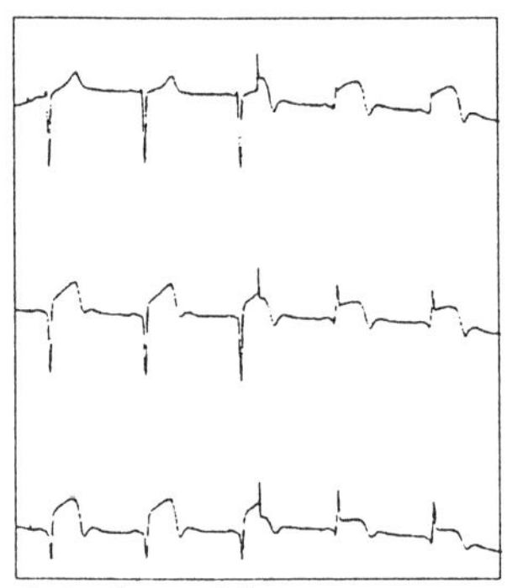

October 10

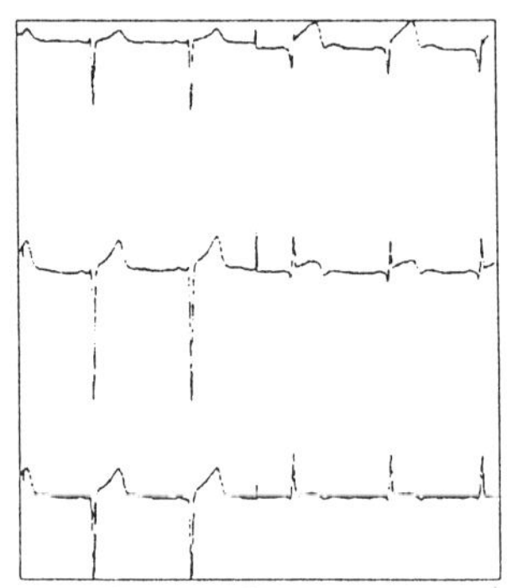

October 12

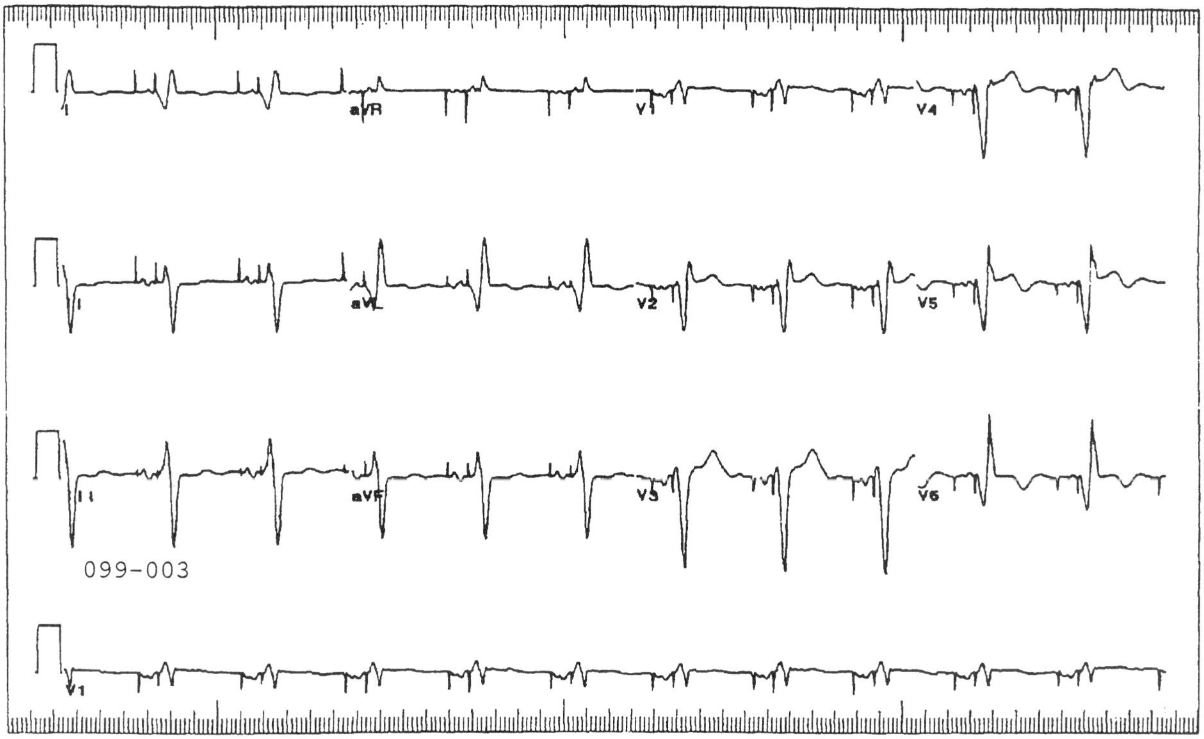

Artificial Atrial and Ventricular Pacemakers, Capturing Regularly (DDD)

```
75   75   20   16   44     see below
-60  2:3  V5½  QR6:12   diff slur
               sl up v5
              related to T
low   ±V1   pos V2-4    neg V5-6

(1) Artificial atrial and ven-
    tricular pacemakers, cap-
    turing regularly, rate 75

--When all beats are paced, no
  further interpretation is
  very helpful in a single
  tracing out of context.
```

The technology of artificial pacemakers grows increasingly elaborate as more and more options are introduced. The knowledge and skills needed to choose and install a system, and, especially, to correct its dysfunction, are recognized now as a subspecialty, but most patients with pacemakers are followed by doctors with broader interests. The function of a unit can be evaluated satisfactorily from a routine 12-lead EKG in most instances, but the language used in reports can be confusing. The basic code consists of three letters: the first indicates the chamber(s) paced (V or A); the second, those sensed; and the third, the "mode," whether inhibited (I) or triggered (T); D stands for dual, both atria and ventricles. The DDD designation is the most confusing. It implies the capacity for both sensing and pacing in either or both chambers, approaching an ideal arrangement. Beyond this simplistic summary, things get complicated. For those not secure with the jargon of the method, a report such as the one above has more meaning.

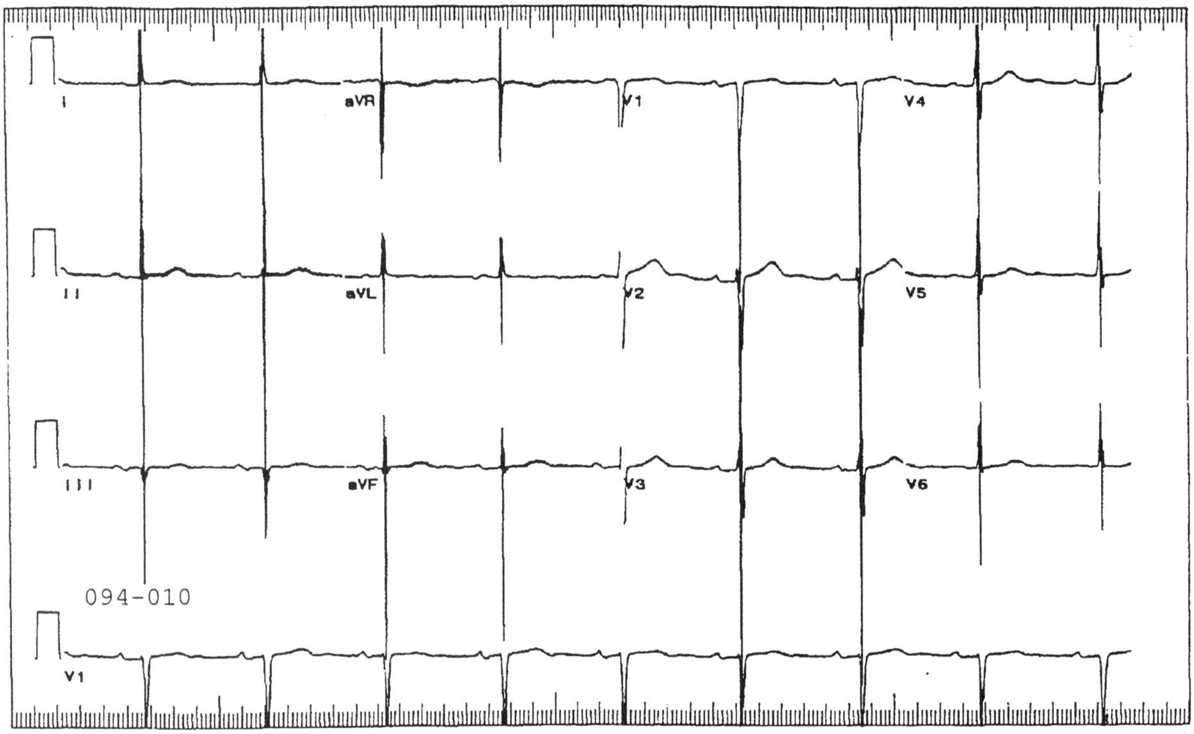

QRS-Triggered Artificial Ventricular Pacemaker, Functioning Properly (VVT)

```
55   55   20   08   44      see below
??   0:?10   V3½   ?8:1?     normal
                none
          not remarkable
low +60  positive V1-6, low V1

(1) Sinus mechanism, rate 55
(2) QRS-triggered artificial ven-
    tricular pacemaker function-
    ing properly.
```

Choice of a pacemaker, and management of its function (or dysfunction), requires familiarity with an ever increasing array of equipment and methods. The terminology of this complex field can be bewildering to the primary physician whose concern is chiefly with whether the system is working, and this can usually be assessed satisfactorily in a routine 12-lead tracing.

In this tracing, the ventricle (the first V of the three letter code) is subject to pacing. The second V indicates the chamber whose activity is sensed, in this case also the ventricles. The third letter indicates the mode of response, triggered (T) or in-hibited (I). The large amplitude of the pacemaker artifact indicates a unipolar setup; a bipolar one produces a smaller spike, and the orientation of the artifact is influenced by the position in the heart of the pacing electrode(s). The ventricles here are responding to the sinus impulse; the pacemaker spike falls within QRS. It is available, and if intrinsic activation does not occur it will come into play. It is almost obliterated by a lead change in the beat in the middle of the tracing.

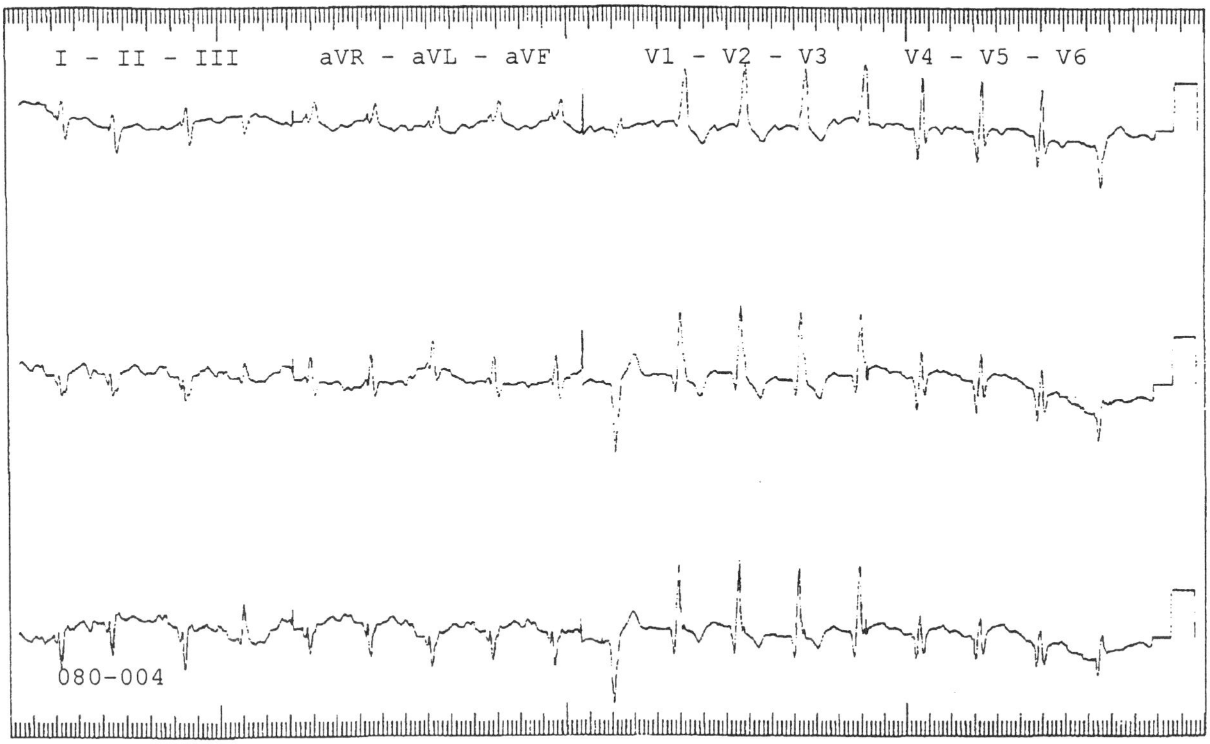

Time and Three Dimensions

```
115    115    20    12    36  sinus
?? 12:0 -- QRS/3:5:3      BSTDRA,
                   QS2,3,F, QV2-6
                 none
           related to T
+60     negative V1-3,   ±V4-6

(1) Sinus mechanism, rate 115
(2) Right bundle branch block
(3) Old anterior myo infarct
(4) Old inferior myo infarct
```

This shows the value of thinking of the EKG as a map of a point moving in both time and space. Information in the initial part of QRS can be separated from that in the terminal part, and forces in one plane have no projection on one per pendicular to it. An inferior infarct,presumably evidence of a right coronary artery lesion, is seen inthe initial components of leads II, III, and aVF; the anterior one,a left anterior descending artery lesion, in precordial leads (177).

The architecture of the heart is not limited by rectilinear coordinates, and the distribution of the coronary arteries is subject to wide variation. V6 is in both frontal and horizontal planes, and the findings here may represent a single lesion seen in two projections. Long experience, however, has shown that left anterior descending artery lesions do not show in inferior leads, and right coronary artery lesions do not show in those in the horizontal plane. The findings justify diagnosis of two infarcts.

Right bundle branch block is seen in both planes (159). It involves terminal QRS forces selectively and the presence of infarct(s) does not interfere with its recognition.

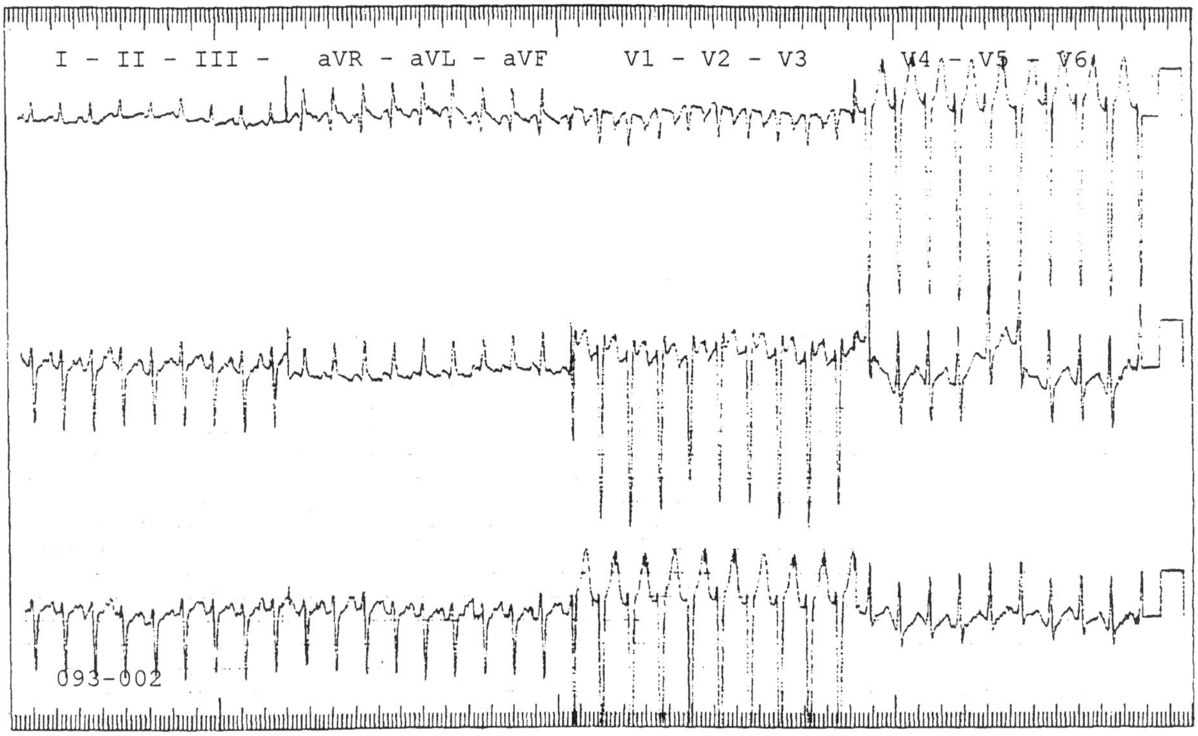

Sinus Mechanism, Rate 230

```
230   230   ±10   08   28       sinus
-75    0:5    V5   10:2       normal
              none
         related to T
low      ±V1     positive V2-6
P: prominently negative V1

(1) Sinus mechanism, rate 230
(2) Left atrial enlargement
(3) Left anterior hemiblock
(3) Otherwise WNL
```

There is no specific rate that defines fast (tachycardia) and no fixed upper limit to sinus rate. A ventricular rate above 140 with no QRS widening usually means usurping supraventricular ectopy, but not always. If a crisis such as cardiorespiratory failure. blood loss, or hyperthyroidism, exists, the rate would present no problem. (This patient was 50-years-old and the tracing was made at 2:45 A.M.) Given the tracing and readout alone though, it could become part of the problem instead part of the solution. The computer called this atrial flutter, and many doctors would have called it "SVT," or "EAT" (ectopic atrial tachycardia), a strange and redundant name but in common use, probably intended to imply repetitive firing of an atrial focus as the means by which activity is sustained). Despite the rate, though, P is clear, and directed to the left (positive in I), caudad (positive in aVF), and terminally dorsad (negative in V1), identifying a sinus origin. Flutter would require more Ps than QRSs, and, since QRS rhythm is regular, atrial rate would have to be a multiple of 230, which is so unlikely as to be negligible. Also, another P would be identifiable. The readout also said "septal" infarct, age indeterminate, but there is no identifiable evidence of one.

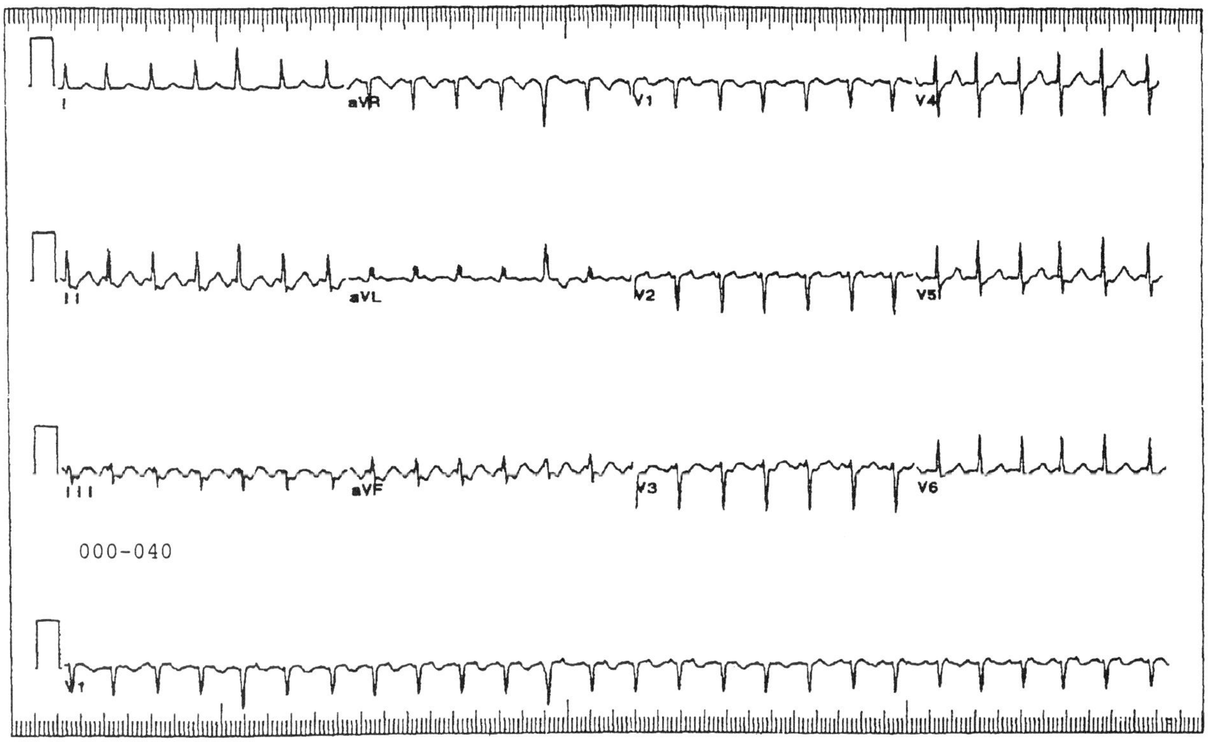

Atrial Flutter, Effect of Adenosine

```
300   150   --   06   24  see below
+15    0:5     V4   6:0     normal
              none
             normal
?+60         ±V1-2          +V3-6

1. Atrial flutter, 300/150
2. Otherwise within normal
   limits
```

Atrial flutter is present when all QRSs are derived from regularly repetitive atrial depolarization at a rate greater than the sinus rate and greater than the AV node can conduct, typically about 200/min, so that not all atrial impulses reach the ventricles. A continuous process involving both atria, "circus conduction" or "reentry," is the usual means by which the ectopic activity is sustained. When attributable to automaticity of a single focus, the mechanism is sometimes called "PAT with block."

Adenosine can obliterate nodal function selectively, leaving atrial activity unaffected.

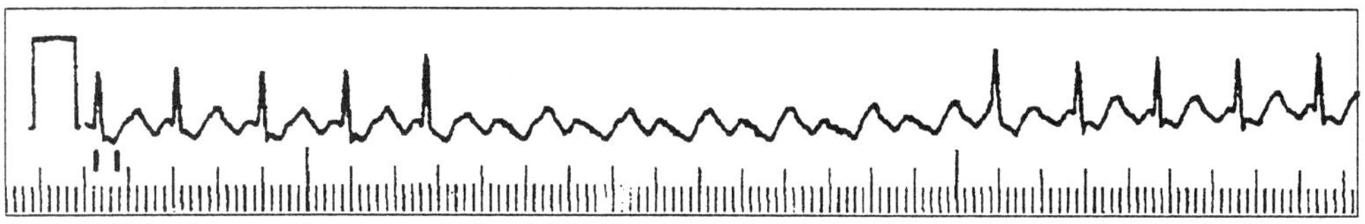

Lead II from above with QRS removed to expose atrial activity

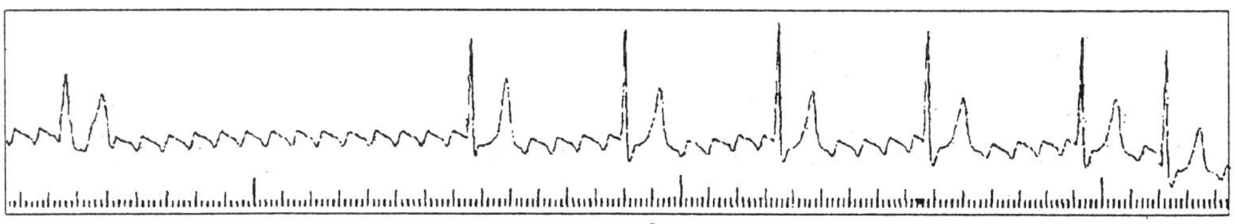

Lead II from monitor: transient 3° AV block following adenosine

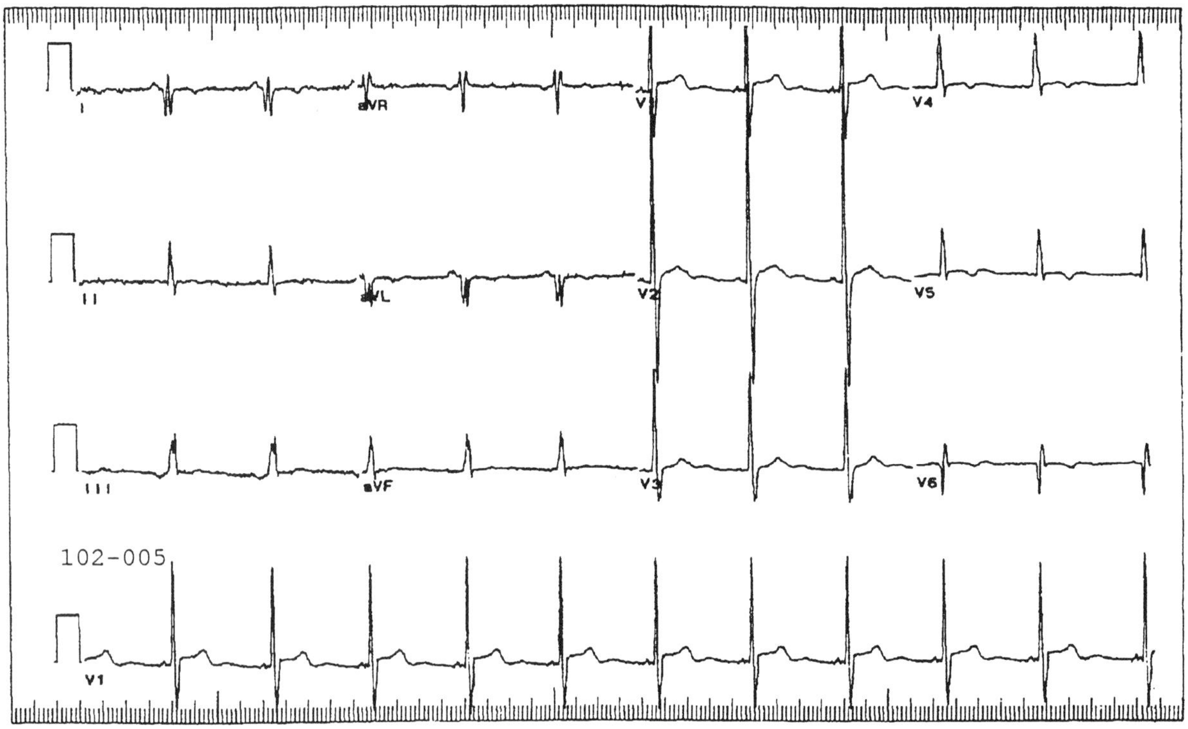

Duchenne Muscular Dystrophy

```
70    70    12    10    36          sinus
+105   20:10   V6   (QR)6:4    Q1,L,V6
                  none
              related to T
low +105      pos V1-3 .    neg V4-6

1. Sinus mechanism, rate 70
2. Old lateral myocardial scar
   typical of an infarct, but
   other explanations are pos
   sible.  The clinical setting
   and stability of the findings
   are important unknowns.
```

Recognition of myocardial infarction is perhaps the most useful application of electrocardiography. If we respect the rule to be as specific as possible, however, it is beyond the limits of the method; the tracing shows electrical inactivity deep in the myocardium, a scar, but not its cause (174). Other explanations include the limits of the method for defining abnormality of initial QRS forces, artifacts, and diseases other than those depriving the tissue of oxygen, e.g., various forms of idiopathic cardiomyopathy (182). This tracing is from a 22-year-old known to have Duchenne muscular dystrophy and severe congestive heart failure. It was reported as showing an old lateral infarct, an altogether reasonable interpretation, given that the interpreter did not know the patient's age or why the tracing was ordered, and that infarction is by far the most likely explanation for the findings.

The tall initial R in V1-5 is probably evidence of the same force expressed as a Q in Leads I, aVL, and V6.

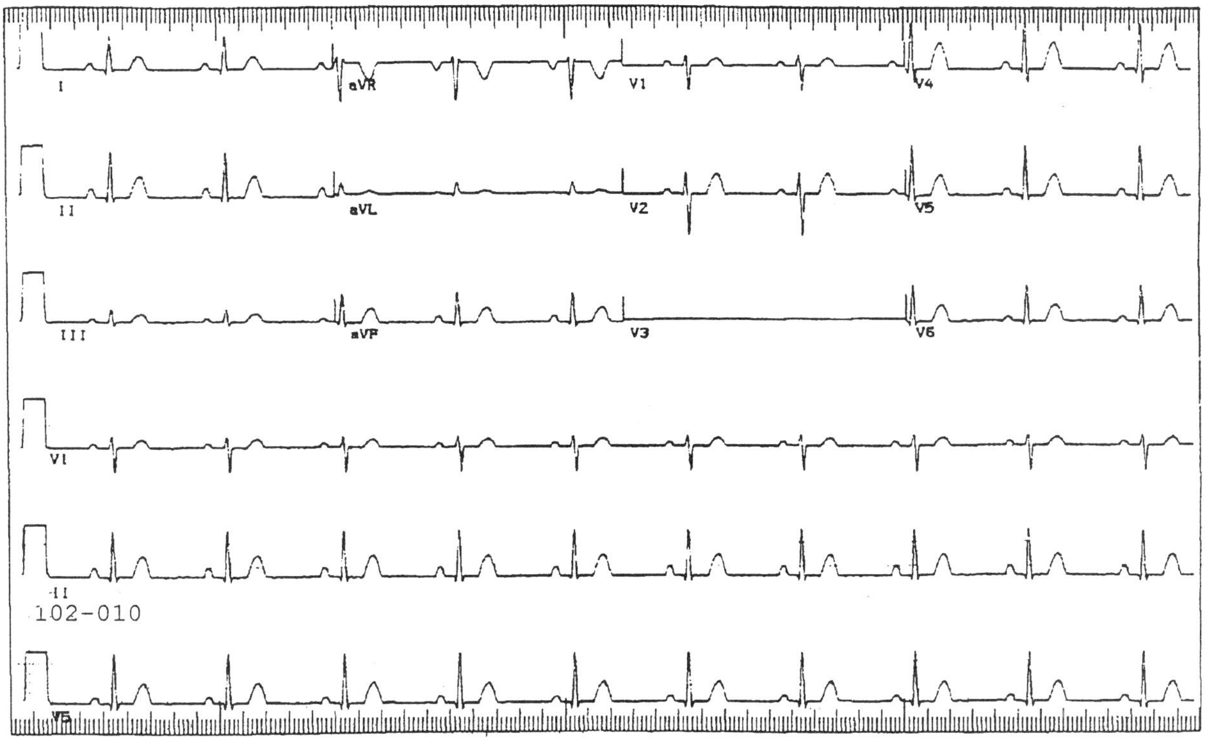

Simulator

```
60    60    16    08    36      sinus
+45    1:8    V3    8:0       normal
              normal
               flat
+45  negative V1, positive V2-6

(1) Simuulator; not a real EKG
```

Maintenance of EKG machines often requires testing such features as frequency response for conformity to established standards (94). It was once common to see repair technicians with patient cables attached to themselves, using their own hearts as input. Now, though, signals approximating those from a heart are generated electronically by a small unit known as a simulator.

It is possible for such tracings to be labeled with a patient's name and number and seen as representing a patient. It is unlikely that any real harm would result, but the error can lead to confusion and uncertainty.

In this case, the absence of V3 is not much of a problem; precordial leads often must be omitted because their positions are covered by a bandage, or inaccessible for some other reason. The things that give this away as a total artifact are a combination of the perfectly flat ST with a clear demarcation from T, and the perfectly repetitious pattern of the whole P-QRS-ST-T pattern. Absolutes such as these are not found in real tracings; awareness of the limits of the method, variations to be expected from beat to beat, are things that comes with experience.

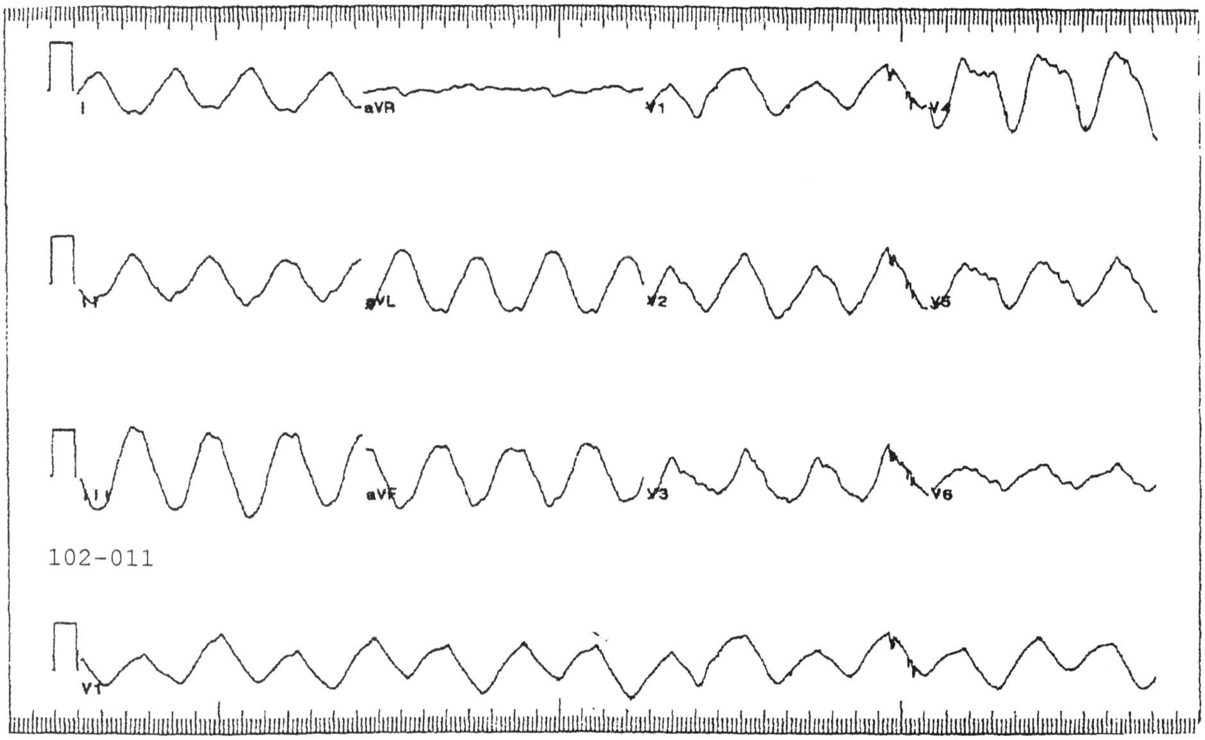

Agonal

This tracing probably would pose no problem for the one taking care of the patient, but for the one responsible for writing a complete and adequate report of it (p. 7) (56), it presents a real challenge. To say it represents a dying heart would not hurt the patient if that is not accurate, because the primary doctor would recognize it as wrong, but it also would not help. The differential includes not only a ventricular origin, but also an inseparable combination of supraventricular origin and QRS, ST, T, and U abnormalities that may represent more than one thing. A recent myocardial infarct would explain much, and ST-T evidence of injury, and/or of intoxication with potassium, tricyclic antidepressants, quinidine, or other drug or electrolyte also must be considered.

-- 90 ?? ?40 see below
?? ?:? ?±V6 ?:? indet
??
related to T
?-60 neg V1-3?, pos V4-6?

1. Atrial activity is not identifiable
2. Ventricular rate 90 with regular rhythm, probably of sinus origin with complex QRS-T-U abnormality, but almost as easily ventricular

--The clinical setting and stability of the findings are important unknowns.

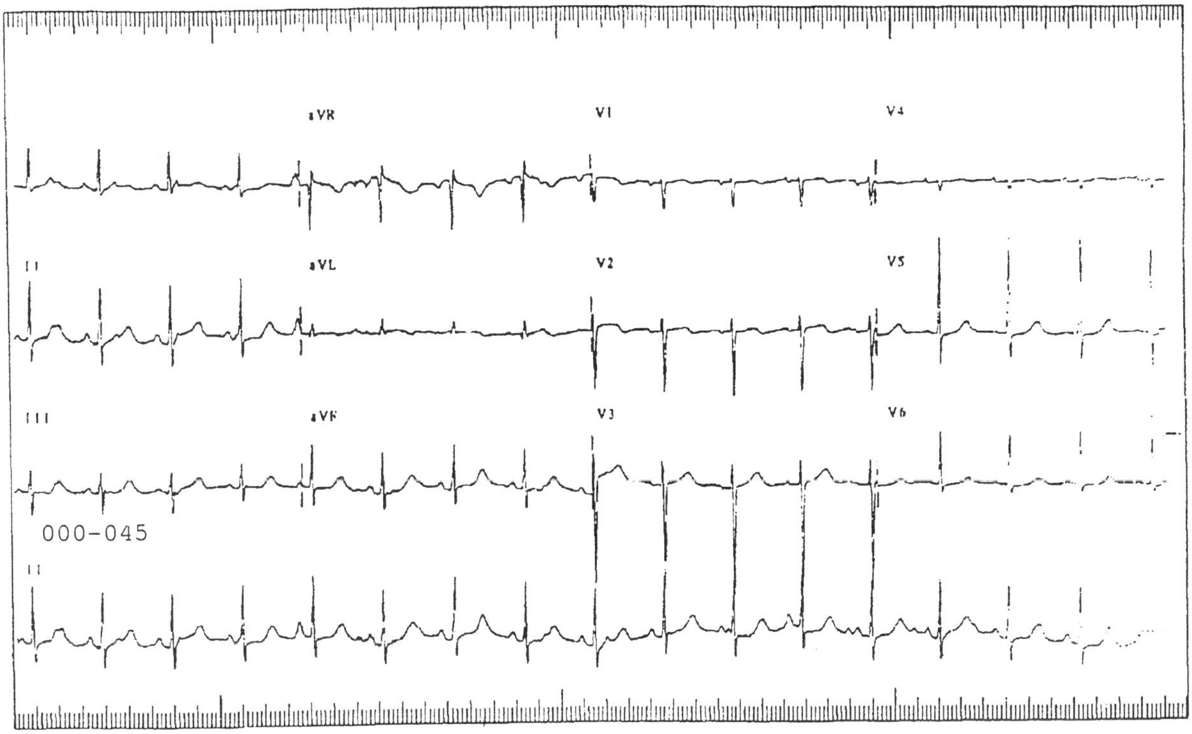

Cardiac Transplant, Two Sets of P Waves

Depending on how much of the native atria remains, two sets of P waves may be seen following cardiac transplant, native and transplanted. There are not many alternatives in the differential, but, if the clinical setting is not known to the one reporting the tracing, and the rates of the two sets are close, atrial dissociation (124) may be considered.

```
100   100   16   08   40        sinus
+30   1:5    V4    10:1         normal
                none
               normal
+75    ± V1-2          positive V3-4

1. Sinus mechanism, rate 100
2. Within normal limits
--Note two sets of P waves,
  native and transplant.
```

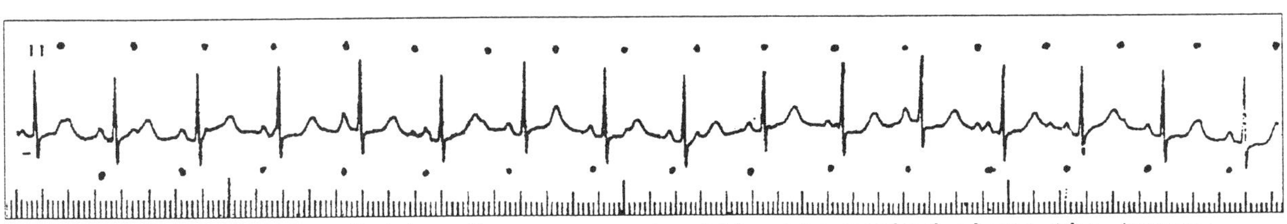

Lead II from above. Native P waves, rate 110, are marked above the trace; those from the transplanted heart, rate 100, below it.

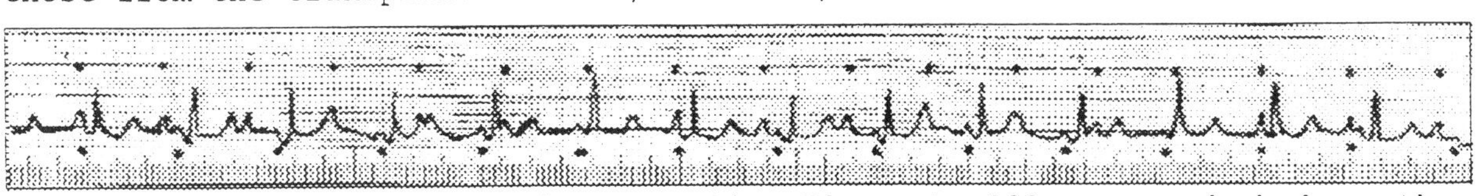

Lead II from a different patient. Native P's, rate 100, are marked above the trace; those from the transplanted heart, rate 90, below it.

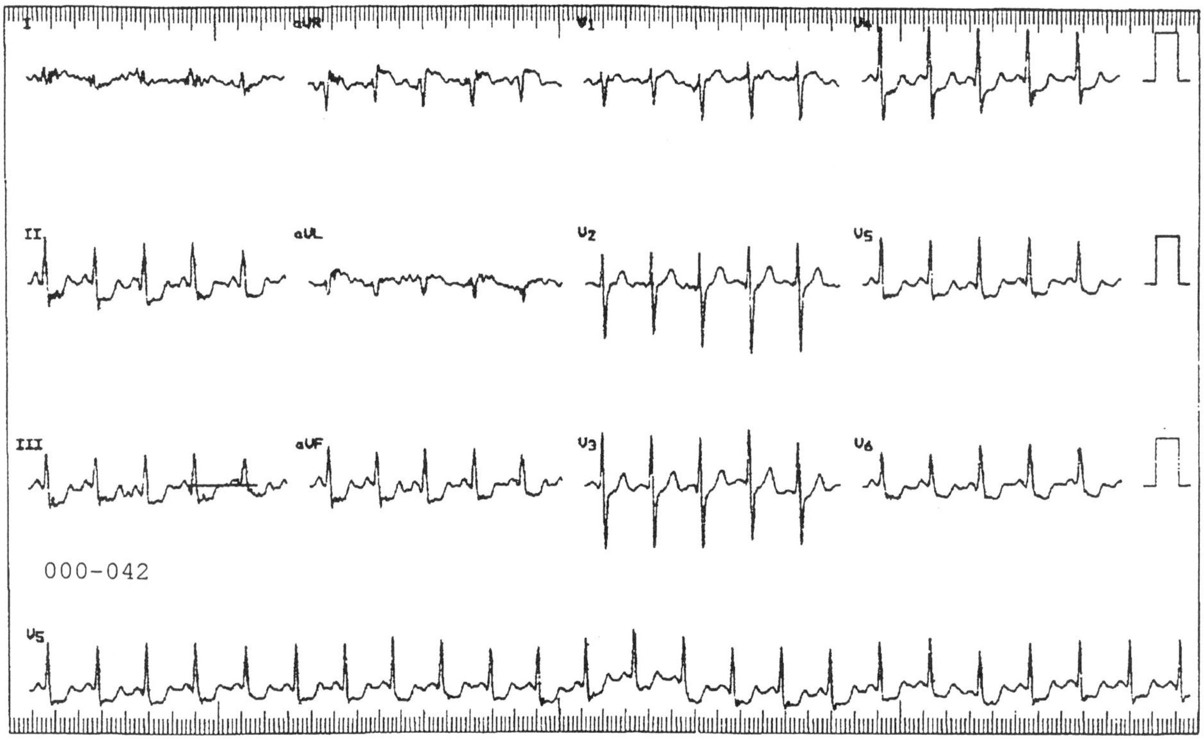

Exercise: rate 140, flattened depression ST2, 3, F, V4-6

POSITIVE EXERCISE TEST

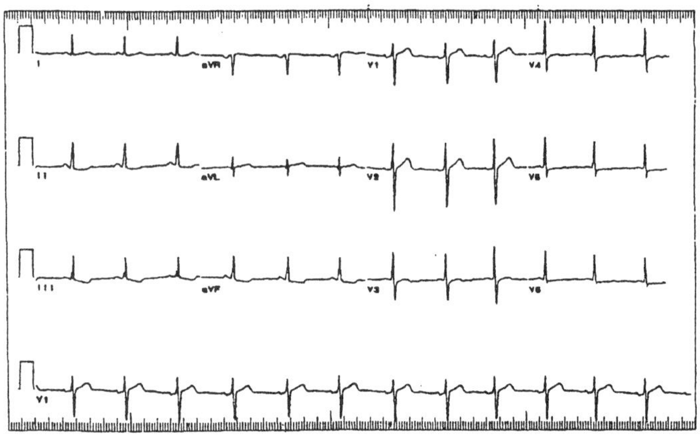

Control: rate 75, nonspecific ST-T abnormalities

```
75    75    12    08    36     sinus
+60   5:10    V3    8:1   ...normal
              none
           related to T
low -45     pos V1-2    ±V4-6

Control: rate 75, nonspecific
    ST-T abnormalities
Exercise (Bruce Stage II):
    rate 140, flattened depres-
    sion ST2,3,F,V4-6
Recovery: return to control
    (not shown)

1. Positive EKG response to
   exercise.
```

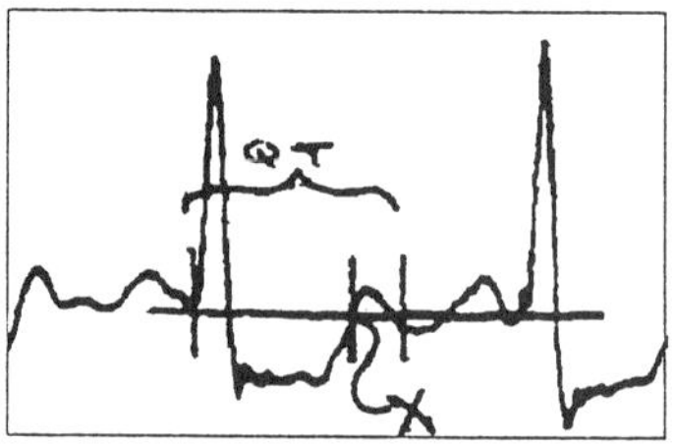

Lepeschkin's QX:QT

Positive Exercise Test

Several protocols for exercise are available (219), and EKG evidence of subendocardial injury, representing inability of the coronary circulation to compensate for a controlled increase in need for oxygen, i.e., coronary insufficiency, is the marker of a positive response. Criteria for this are not standard, but all utilize depression *and* *flattening* of ST. The cleanest definition of both is Lepeschkin's QX:QT greater than 50% (inset) (221).

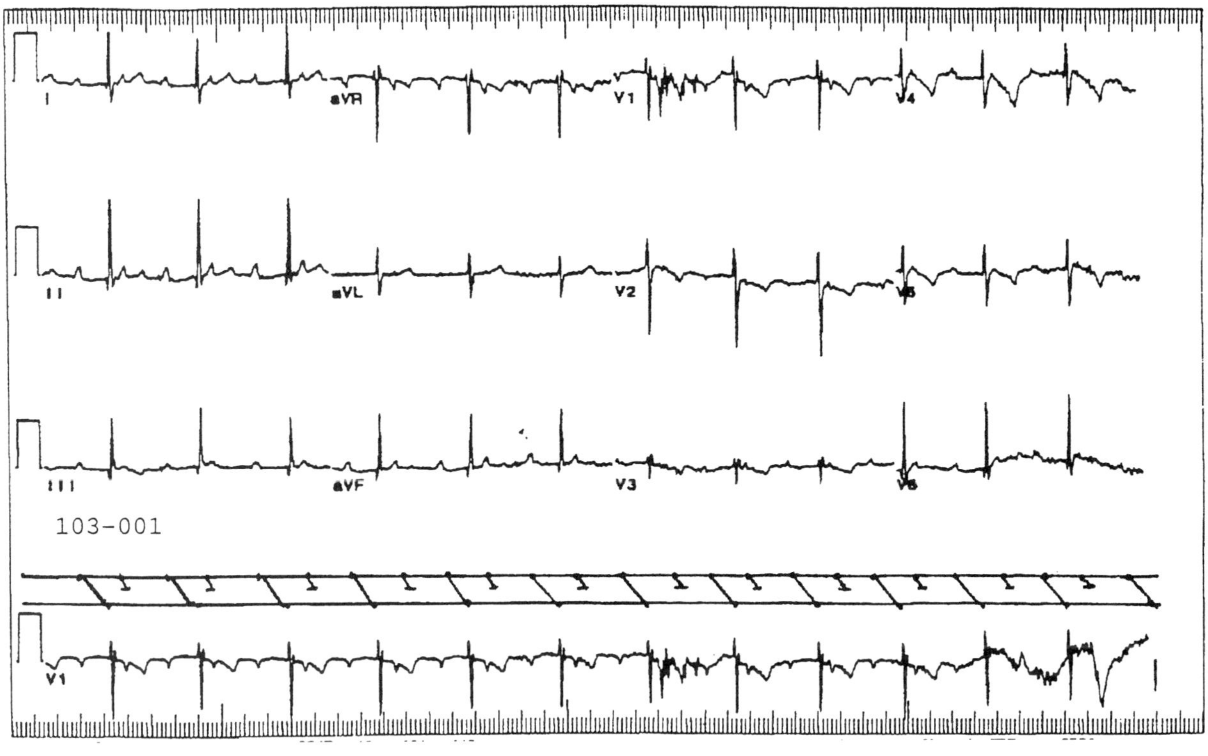

AV Block in an Infant

160   80   --   06   36   see below
+60   rSr 4:12:1,   V4-5,   15:2   nl
none
normal
+30   neg V1-2, ±V3, neg V4-5, ±V6

1. Sinus mechanism, rate 160
2. 2° AV block, 2:1, ventricular rate 80
3. Otherwise within normal limits

--Isolated precordial T negativity is not abnormal by itself in a child.

Methods for analysis of an EKG, rates and intervals, and orientation, duration, amplitude, and contour of P, QRS, ST and T, are the same no matter what the patient's age. Names for the findings may not be consistent from infancy to old age, though, and the pathologic anatomy and physiology that explain them do change. Ischemia, the penultimate etiology for most abnormalities in tracings of adults, is rare in infants, and the opposite is true of congenital malformations. In any case, the EKG shows only what is present, not its etiology. This patient was ten months old.

In this tracing, all QRSs are of supraventricular origin (not wide), but not all atrial beats are followed by QRSs, i.e., there is second degree AV block, neither Type I (Wenckebach) nor Type II (Mobitz), just 2:1 (121, 152). The basis for this unusual finding in an infant depends on the clinical setting. Reasonable possibilities include a congenital lesion such as an endocardial cushion defect (234), surgery, inflammatory disease, and drugs.

Isolated precordial T negativity may be seen in normal children (212).

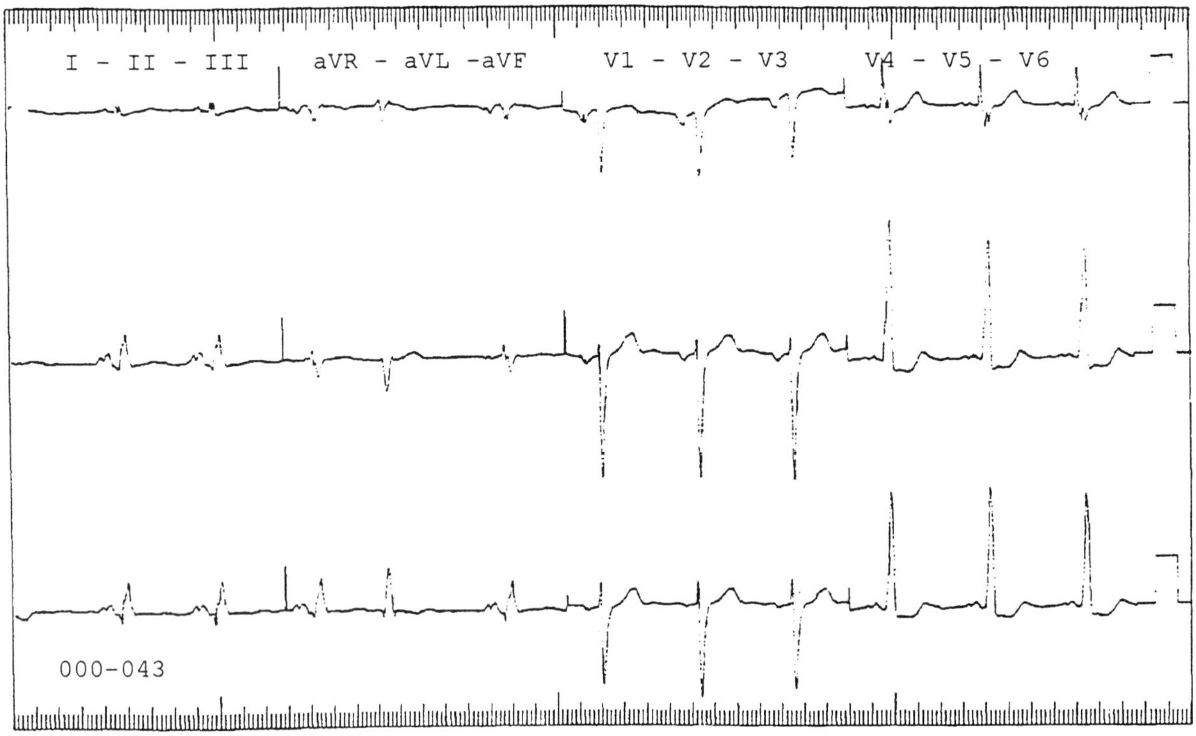

P "Mitrale"

Left atrial enlargement (188) is a useful EKG interpretation that identifies a specific chamber of the heart as having responded to either increase in resistance to outflow and/or increase in flow. To the extent that it is valid, it can suggest specific lesions. Its expression as a wide, notched P in Leads II and III, P "mitrale" (inset), was considered almost diagnostic of mitral stenosis by Sir Thomas Lewis as early as 1912 (67). With the advent of precordial leads, it became possible to assess forces perpendicular to the frontal plane, such as those generated by dorsad activation of the left atrium, and responsible for the last part of P. Since about 1964, prominence of P terminal negativity in V1 has been the usual criterion. Left atrial enlargement is badly overinterpreted by most computer programs, but this is because it is so hard to define quantitative criteria for such a small and inconstant finding.

```
70    70    16    10    40      sinus
+75   0:15  V3½  25:0        normal
            down V5-6
   flattened and related to T
low    ±V1    pos V2-6, low V5-8

P: Prominent II,III,aVF and V1,
   notched II

1. Sinus mechanism, rate 70
2. Left atrial enlargement
3. ST-T abnormalities typical
   of coronary insufficiency
4. Suggests old inferior myo-
   cardial infarct.
```

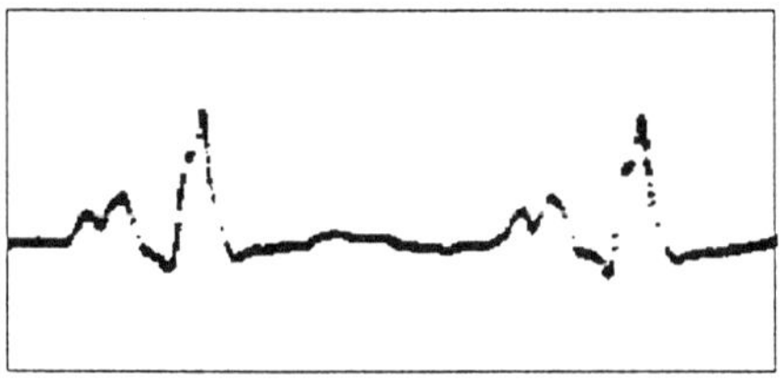

Lead II from above
P "mitrale"

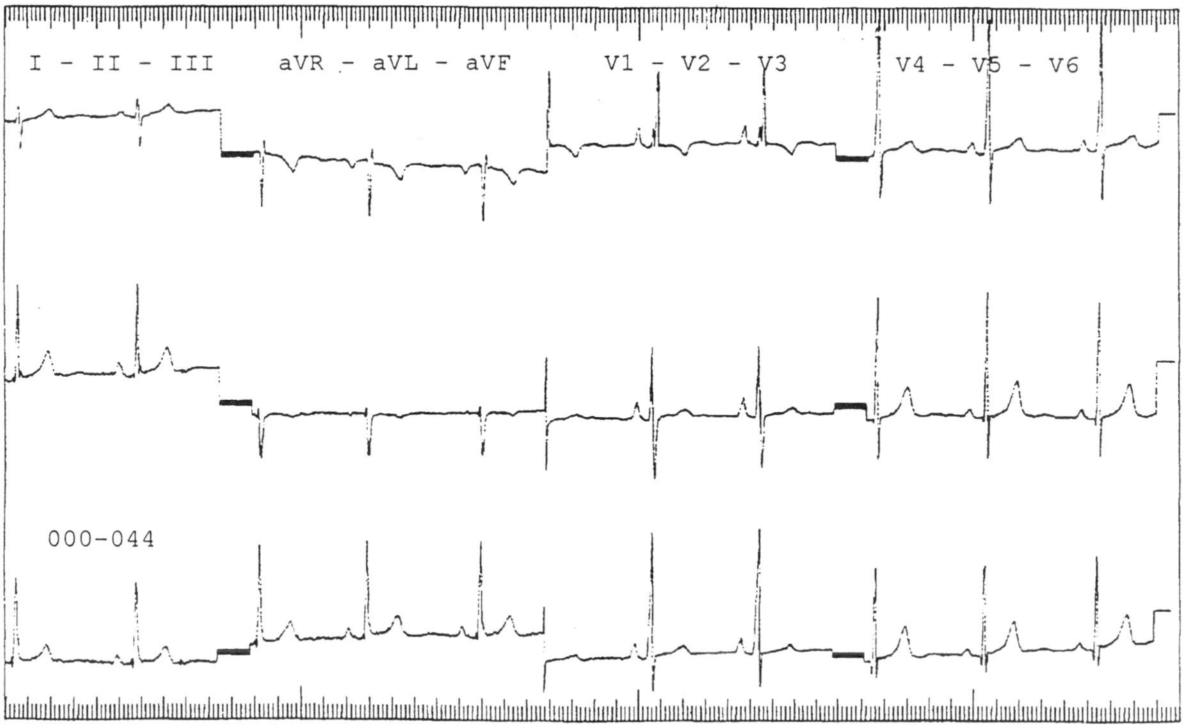

P "Congenitale"

P "congenitale" (188) is invoked only rarely as an interpretation, and is not likely to be of much importance. It is included in this collection mostly for the sake of completeness. The classic patterns known as P "pulmonale" and P "mitrale" not only identify one atrium or the other as enlarged, but also suggest an explanation for the enlargement. This one suggests an explanation without saying which atrium is involved.

In effect, the pattern is evidence of enlargement of the right atrium. More typically, this is recognized by its projection on the frontal plane, and the prominence and symmetry of P in Leads II, III, and aVF, reflecting leftward and caudad depolarization. There is also a ventrad component of these forces that produces the positive initial part of P in V1. This is usually small, but in P "congenitale" it is exaggerated, sometimes very markedly. The objective base for these observations is ill-defined.

```
60    60   16   08   40        sinus
+90   15:0   V2   20:2         normal
               none
              normal
+75    neg V1   ±V2. .pos V3-6

P: peaked II III, aVF, tall V1

1. Sinus mechanism, rate 60
2. Right atrial enlargement, prob-
   able, in an unusual pattern
   often associated with congeni-
   tal heart disease.
3. Right ventricular hypertrophy
4. Otherwise within normal limits
```

Note half-gain in the top and bottom channels.

This patient was identified only as 19 years old.

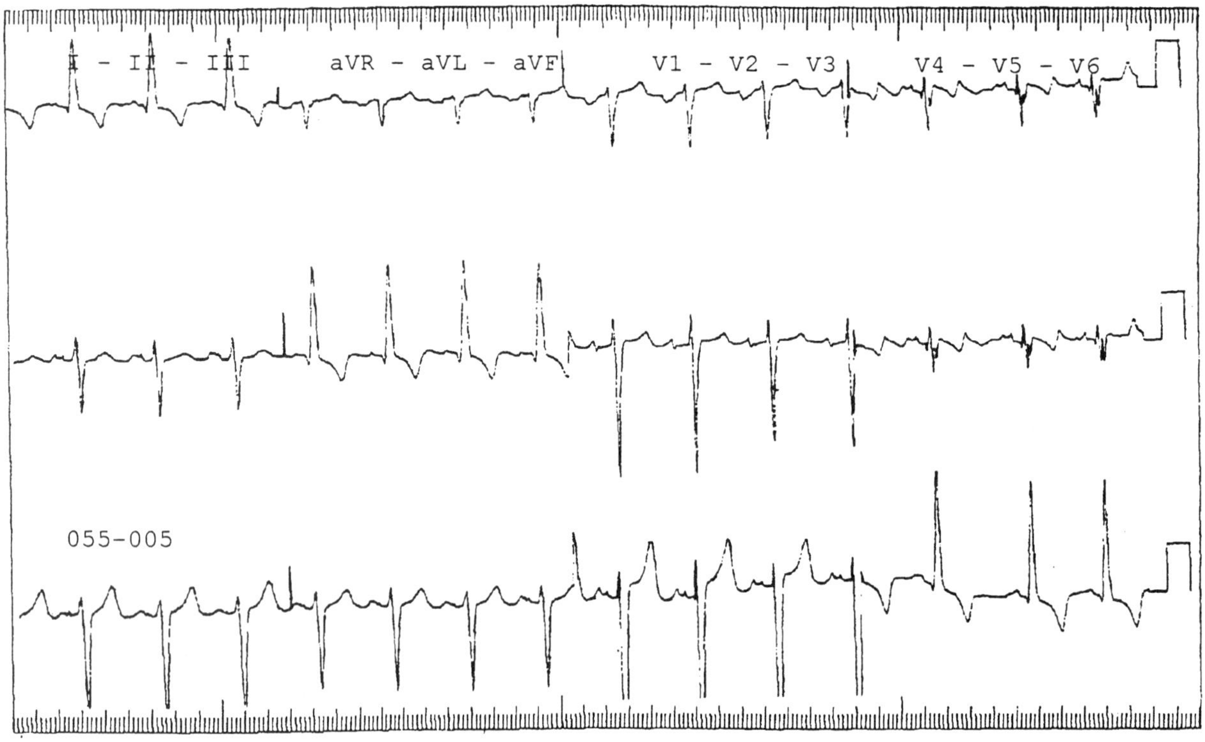

Left Atrial Enlargement, Left Ventricular Overload

```
90    90    20    10    40     sinus
-45   1:12   V4   25:0    normal
            none
         related to T
+135  pos V1-3  ± V4-5   neg V6

1 Sinus mechanism, rate 90
2 Left atrial enlargement
3 ST-T abnormalities, probab-
  ly left ventricular overload
```

The findings in this tracing suggest a train of events that would result from overload, or strain, of the left ventricle: i.e., increase in resistance against which blood must be ejected in order to maintain adequate flow, and/or increase in the volume of blood that must be pumped (189). If this produces enough electrophysiologic change to show in the EKG, it should appear first in the most sensitive part of the tracing, the T wave, and experience has shown that this is true; T is reoriented nearly opposite QRS without change in its amplitude, duration, or contour. Enough strain of a muscle produces hypertrophy, a structural change that would be expected to show in QRS, and many sets of numbers have been proposed to identify this (192). All involve QRS amplitude, but this is subject to many determinants (228), and is inconstant, and criteria for the anatomic definition of hypertrophy, by which they must be validated, are not standard. None of these is fulfilled here, but absence of evidence is not evidence of absence. Loss of compliance may precede hypertrophy, increasing the resistance to flow from the left atrium, and left atrial enlargement is suggested here by the prominent P terminal negativity in V1 (188). Together, the findings should direct attention to overload of the left ventricle selectively.

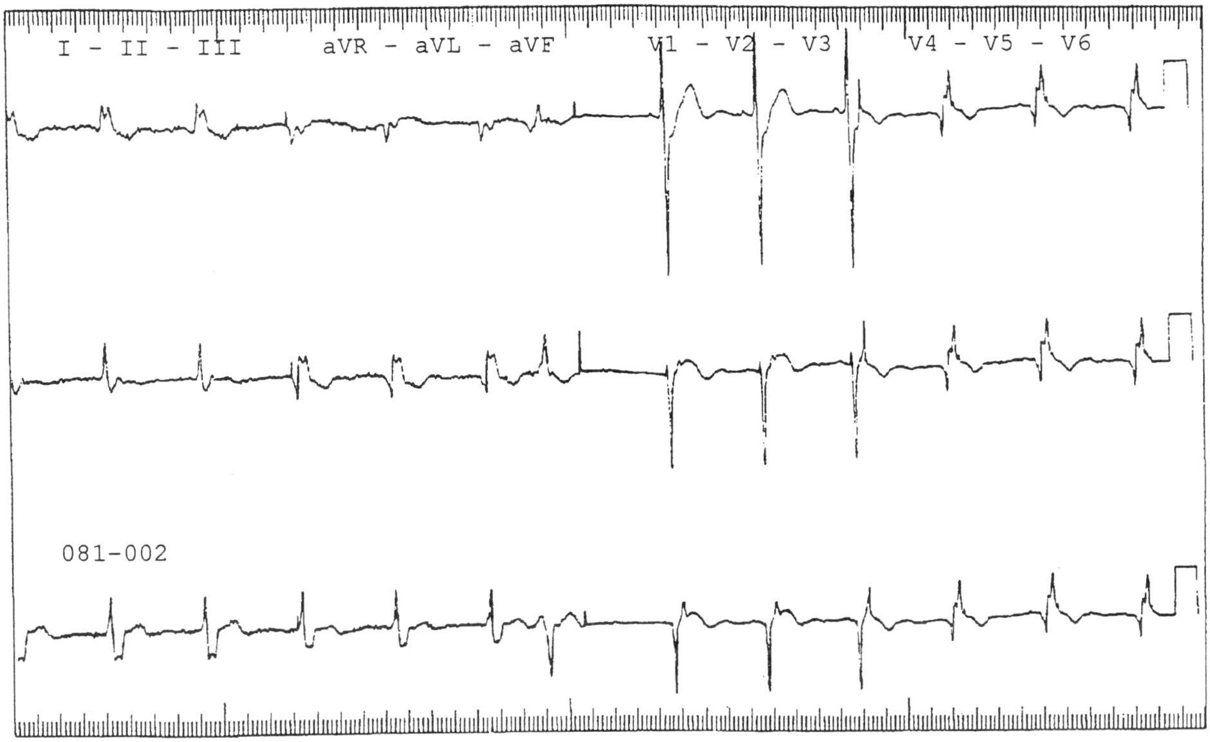

Left Bundle Branch Block, Anterior Myocardial Infarct

```
75    75    16    16    40       sinus
-45    15:30    V4-6...(QR)5:8 diff
                        slur, QV3-6
                 none
              related to T
low +185  pos V1   ±V2-3..neg V4-6

1. Sinus mechanism, rate 75
2. Left bundle branch block
3. Anterior myocardial infarct,
   probably old
```

Not many of us have dissected the left branch of the bundle of His, and proof of impairment of its ability to conduct electricity is difficult, but left bundle branch block is one of the most uncontroversial of all EKG diagnoses (160). It says what is present, but does not speculate about what caused it, whether new or old, or how long it will last. It was once called complete or incomplete, and typical or atypical, but those terms have given way to identification of its anterior and posterior subdivisions.

There is a tradition that the presence of LBBB precludes recognition of an infarct, and this has a reasonable basis. Infarction is recognized in the initial part of QRS, and LBBB, if proximal enough, affects the same area, invalidating the logic behind the diagnosis of an infarct (177). Nevertheless, there are instances, such as this one, when evidence of both is compelling (170). It is easy to assume that the bundle branch is included in the infarcted area, explaining the block. Change in the route of repolarization must follow change in that of depolarization, and if electrophysiologic function is not affected, T is directed opposite the blocked part of QRS (in both left and right bundle branch block).

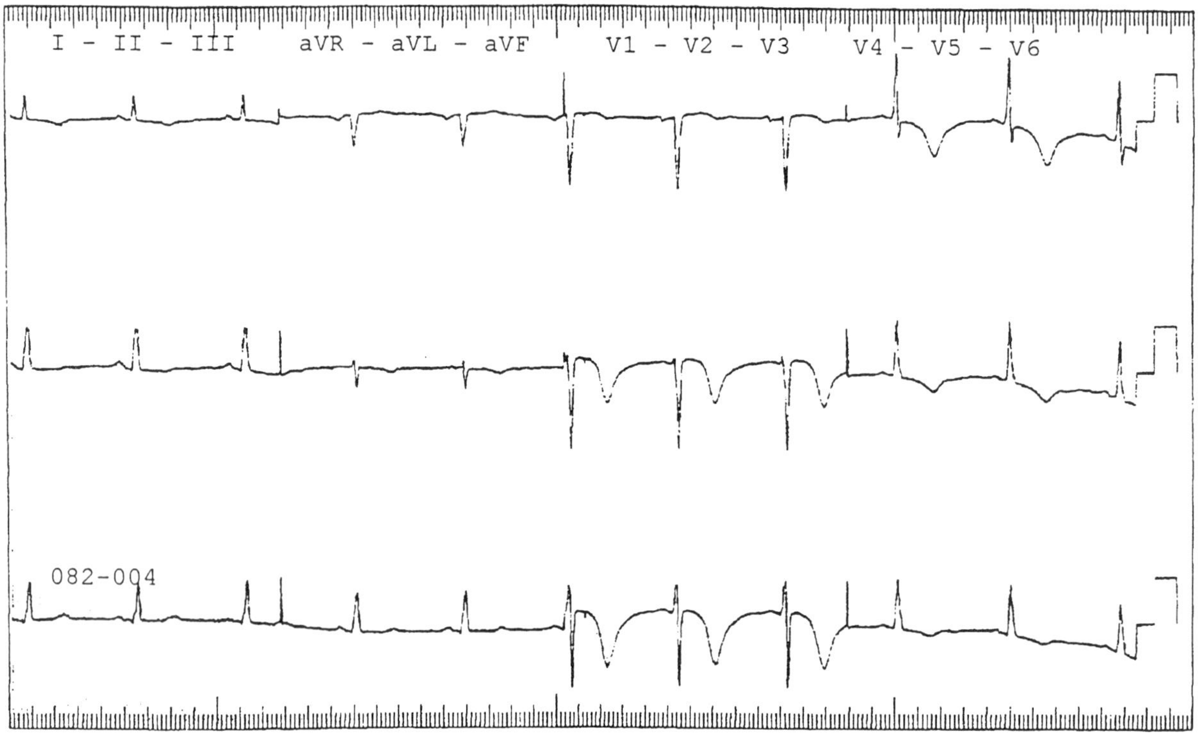

Mid-Precordial ST-T-U Pattern as with Coronary Insufficiency

Like the electrocardiogram itself, and most visits to the doctor for that matter, the U wave is not very important...except when it is (217). It is a part of the normal tracing, following T by a very short interval, and often identifiable with the most confidence in V1 or V2. It may be merged with T and read as a long QT (a factor in minimizing the value of the "QTc") (24). The finding in the "long QT syndromes" (234) sometimes associated with seizures, is probably really a long QU. When QT is read as greater than 0.44 s, there is a good chance that it is really QU. When U is prominent, a suggestion of "electrolyte imbalance" may be in order because it is seen sometimes with hypokalemia and hypocalcemia, but neither of these produces a really typical pattern very often.

```
60   60  16   08   ?50     sinus
+60  0:15  V3 ½  10:0    normal
            nine
        related to T
low +120  ±V1  neg V2-6,  deep
           and symmetrical V2-4
U: prominent, negative V2-5,
   continuous with T

1. Sinus mechanism, rate 60
2. ST-T-U abnormalities, sug-
   gestive of coronary insuf-
   ficiency
```

A negative U in any lead is abnormal. Perhaps the greatest value of the U wave is in the pattern shown here, a prominent negative U, continuous with a prominent negative T, producing a symmetrical curve deeper between V1 and V6 than in either V1 or V6 (217).

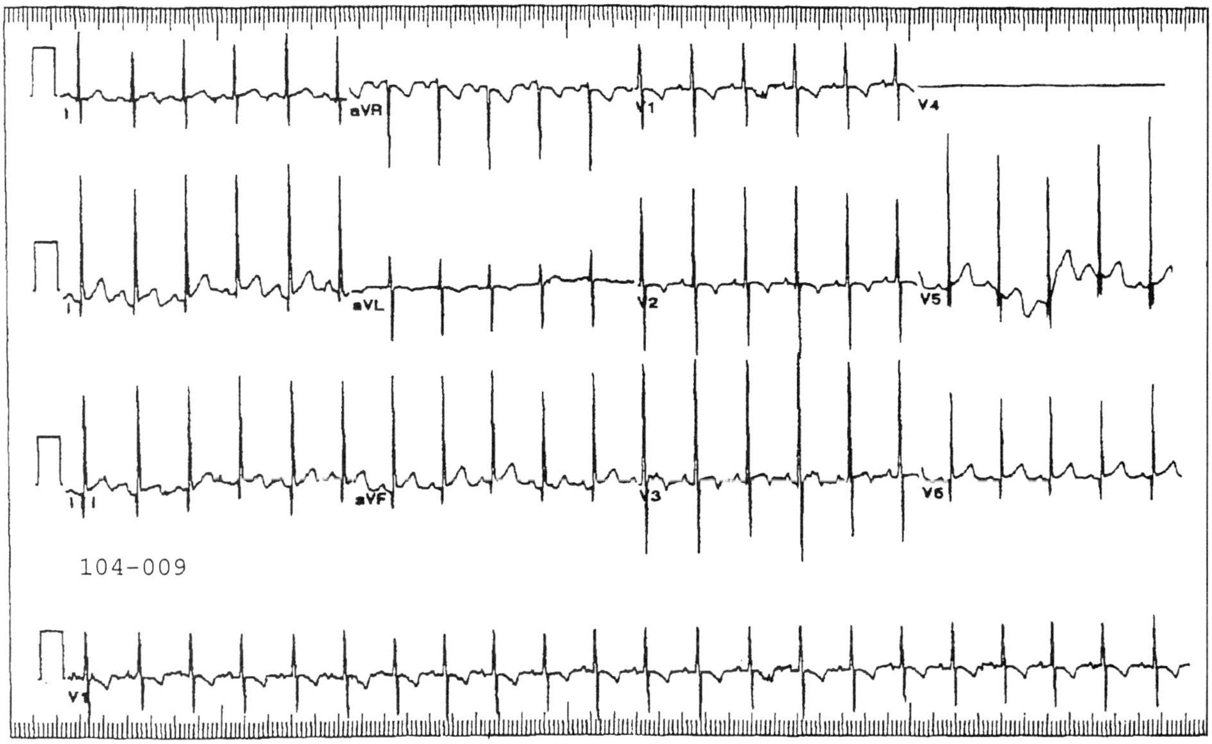

Computer Called Infarct in an Infant

```
135  135   08   04   28     sinus
+75  10:10 V1  15:0  Q2,3,F,V5-6
            sl up 2,3,F
              normal
+60      neg V1-3    pos V5-6

1. Sinus mechanism, rate 135
2. Within normal limits
```

One of the results of thinking of EKG interpretation as a technical skill, with very little regard for definitions of the universal vocabulary, is that doctors can equate Q waves with myocardial infarction (174). Loss of electrical activity in a localized area deep in the myocardium can produce abnormality of the initial QRS pattern, and this takes the form of an *abnormal* Q in most instances, but there are usually other abnormalities in the trace as well, and other explanations than infarction.

Another problem results when a doctor assumes that a computer readout is not only "right" but also that what it names is somehow a consequence of, or explanation for, the patient's complaint.

This patient was six months old, had mild pulmonary stenosis, and was asymptomatic. The clean, narrow Qs are within normal limits.

They indicate only that the motion of the theoretical point they represent is away from the positive pole of the leads in which they appear. The readout was "right" by the standards it was programmed to express, but not as a diagnosis in clinical context. In an older patient, especially one with vague chest pain, it could have had unpleasant consequences.

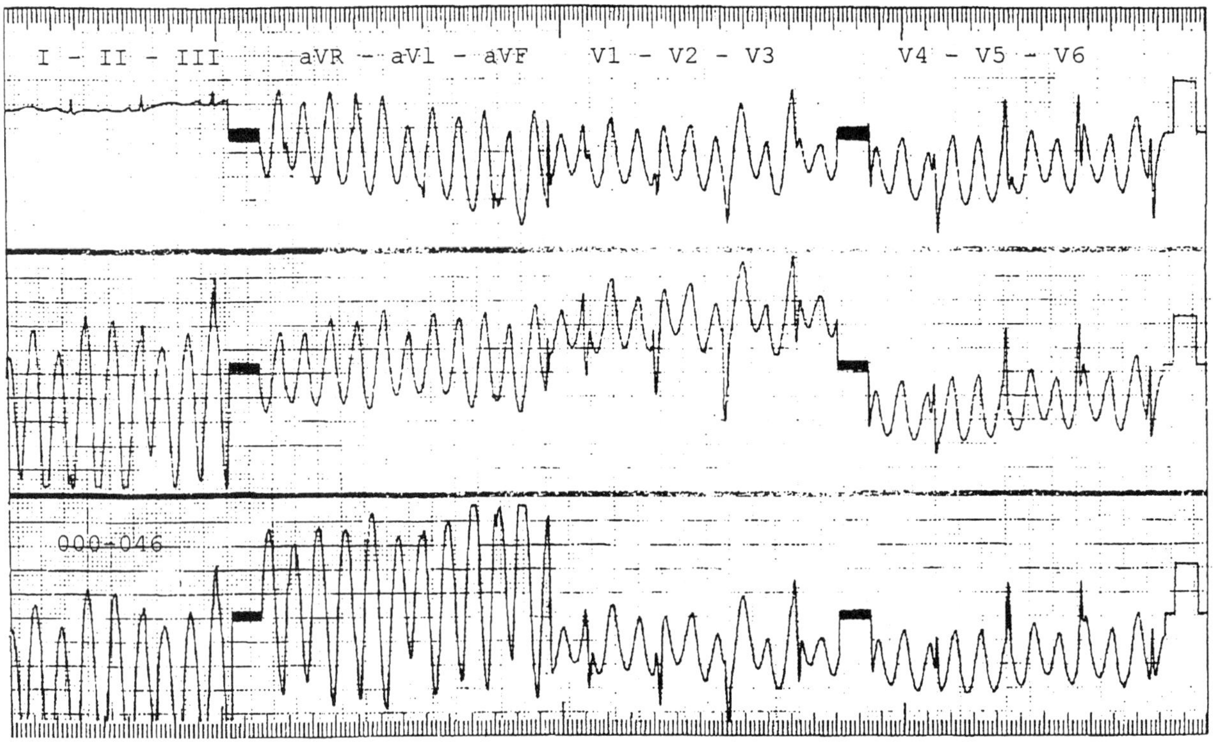

Artifact Mimics Ventricular Tachycardia

```
100     100    12    06     --     sinus
??      ??    V4?   ?15:0          normal
                 none?
                normal?
??    ??V1-6

1. Sinus mechanism, rate 100
2. Probably within normal limits
   or at worst only small ST-T
   abnormalities

--Detail is obscured by artifact
  due to muscle tremor and loose
  connection to the left leg.
```

The readout called this "undetermined rhythm," an accurate statement as far as it goes but not very helpful. The interpreter had no clinical information other than that the patient was a man about fifty years old. The potential risk to the patient is that the large oscillations with an almost regular rhythm, rate 250/min, could be seen as ventricular in origin, i.e., ventricular tachycardia or fibrillation. The key to the proper interpretation is the clean, narrow QRSs in Lead I with regular rhythm at 100/min, each preceded by a P, identifying the mechanism as sinus. Once this has been recognized, it is easy to see the normal QRSs embedded in the muscle tremor artifact (102) in other leads (inset). Muscle tremor usually produces a more "noisy" picture. Paralysis agitans may present a pattern like this, but also may not be noticeable in the tracing at all. Understanding why the artifact is visible in some leads and not others depends on knowledge of how the components of the several leads are interrelated (83). In this case, at least part of the problem lies in imperfect connection to the left leg.

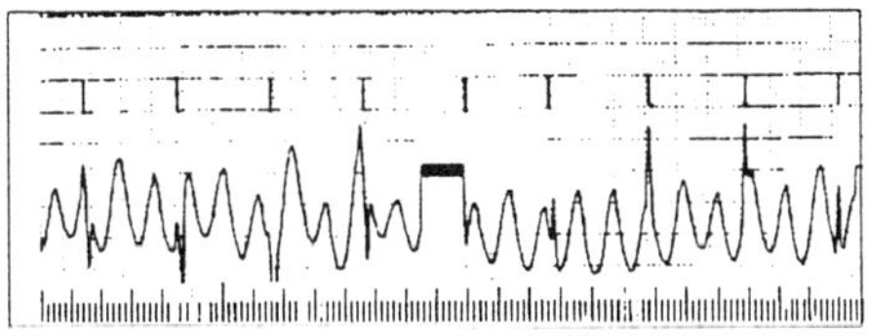
V3 and V6 with QRS's marked

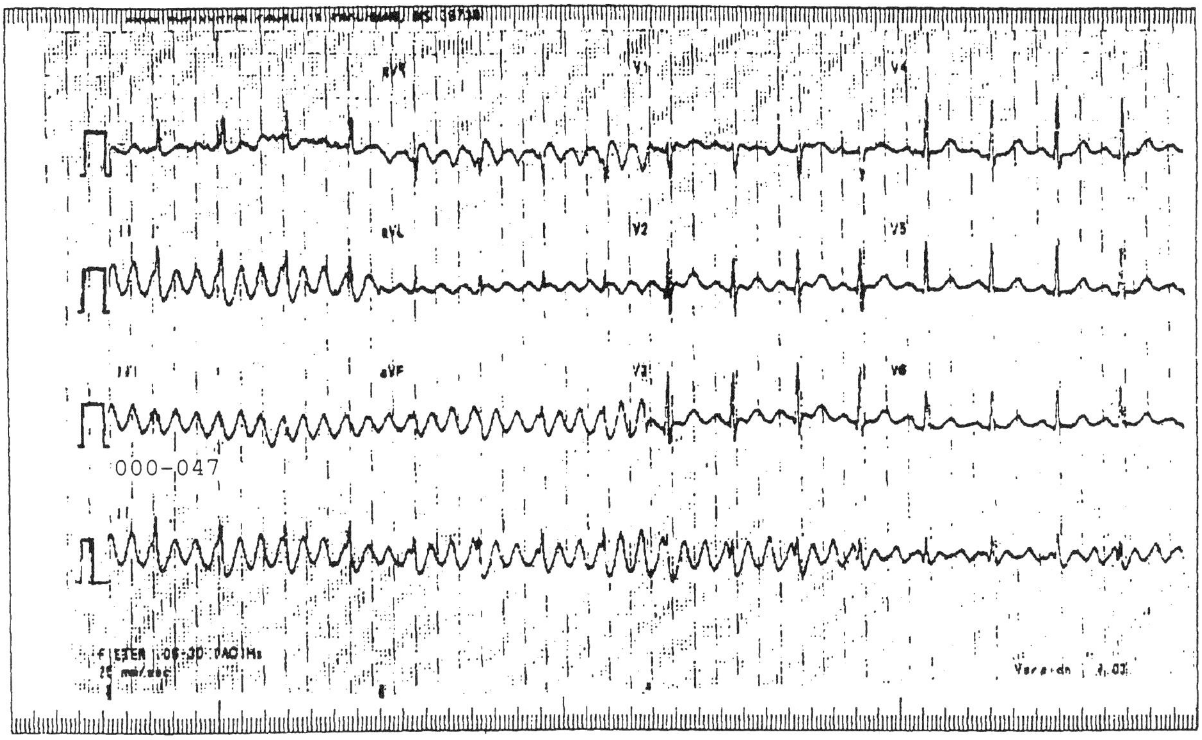

Muscle Tremor Simulates VT/VF

100 100 16 06 36 sinus
?+45 1:5 V1½ 8:0 normal
none
normal
?? isoelectric V1, pos V2-6

1. Sinus mechanism, rate 100
2. Within normal lifts

--Muscle tremor simulates ventricular ectopy and obscures some detail.

Evidence of striated muscle activity is typically of less amplitude than here, and higher frequency, "noise" instead of smooth oscillations, but can vary widely. It may not only mask potentially important information, but also simulate it. The doctor treating this patient, a 66-year-old man with chest pain in the ER at 9:45 P.M., knew his pulse was regular at 100/min, and probably would not have been disturbed by the computer readout of "atrial rhythm with occasional ectopic ventricular beat." The unequivocal statement that the tracing shows an "old inferior infarct," however, and the admonition to "consider acute process," could easily have become part of the problem instead of part of the answer. The one reporting the findings, not knowing the whole clinical picture, might mistake the muscle tremor for ventricular ectopy (144), rate about 300, the distinction between "tachycardia" and fibrillation not always being clear. The view in Leads III and aVF even comes close to the picture of "torsades des pointes" (146). P waves are usually seen best in II, III, aVF, or V1, but in this case they are clearest in V5-6. There is no identifiable evidence of an infarct.

Appendix I

Definitions

CONTENTS

Within the small discipline of electrocardiography there should be only one meaning for each word and symbol, and this meaning should be unambiguous. Failure of doctors to communicate confidently can have unfortunate consequences for the patient. The use of words from the everyday vocabulary of both doctors and patients, e.g., rhythm, to mean something different in electrocardiography, and of technical jargon with only vague relevance, introduces unnecessary problems and is to be avoided whenever possible. The definitions that follow are not controversial, at least for the most part, but they do not have the weight of law, either, or even tradition in some cases. Their usefulness depends upon their being accepted because they make sense. Read them and think about them, but don't memorize anything. They are used consistently in this book. If in your judgment one is not valid, note this, record your alternative, and observe the effects of the change on your decision-making process. The intent is to work from the inside out, internal electrocardiography in the same sense that we speak of internal medicine (8). The information in the tracing itself must be identified before it can be integrated with that from the history, physical examination, and other laboratory studies to produce a diagnosis. Patterns count, but they are more useful if their derivation is understood.

The Tracing and its Components

1. **Electrocardiogram (EKG or ECG):** A graphic representation of the electrical activity of the heart in a series of beats; specifically, a record of the course through time and space of the net result of this process, a single point, A, as it departs from a fixed point, B, and returns to it. The record of a single cardiac cycle, consists of a family of curves, or waves, known as P, Q, R, S, T, and U. (*see* Fig. 3-1, p. 10).
2. **B point:** The central reference point. Zero, neutral, no electrical activity. This is represented in the tracing by the point of junction of PR (or PQ) and QRS, the beginning of the QRS complex. Atrial repolarization is in progress here, and the level of the U-P segment is nearer to theoretical zero, but it is hard to define. Atrial repolarization is a negligible factor in curves recorded from the surface, and the UP segment is not often flat enough long enough to justify extrapolation from one beat to the next as a baseline. The B point is the most reproducible point on the tracing, and the one that best represents the graphic equivalent of the absence of potential, the coincidence of the components of Einthoven's single dipole. It can be equated with Wilson's central terminal of zero potential, the center of the heart, neutral. Like the middle of the fifty yard line, everything in the tracing is measured to it, from it, or, when two B points are connected to define the baseline, above it or below it (*see* **Baseline**). Definition of the B point is the starting place, a fundamental assumption.
3. **Baseline:** A line connecting the B points of two contiguous beats in as nearly flat a section of the lead as possible. When the trace is stable and flat, the UP and PQ segments, J, and the brief segment between T and U are all at the same level, This is not true, however, when there is muscle tremor,

atrial fibrillation, or flutter, or when P is too small to define clearly; or when the level of the trace varies. A clear definition is especially important in records made during or immediately after exercise when the trace is unstable and the level of ST is critical. Pragmatically, the B point is the most stable point in the tracing, and it takes two points to define a line; a horizontal line through a single B point is not enough.

There is a usage problem with the word "baseline." Defined as the reference level, an expression of zero, it cannot change. To refer to baseline instability (wandering, sway) is oxymoronic, but when the level of the trace on the chart varies, this is the way it is described.

4. **J point:** The junction of QRS and ST, really a small area, a shoulder, rather than a literal point. Its position with relation to the baseline (in a specified lead) defines orientation and amplitude of ST, e.g., elevated in Lead I, and depressed in aVF and Vl, means orientation to the left, cephalad, and dorsad.
5. **Deflection/wave:** Excursion of the trace above or below the baseline is a deflection; return to the baseline completes a wave. In practice, the two words are used almost synonymously. There may be notches (*see* **Notch**) in a wave but it is not complete until it returns to the baseline.
6. **Notch:** A sharp, transient change in direction of the trace within a wave.
7. **P:** A small wave (compared to QRS), the first one generated in a normal heartbeat. It is discrete, predictably recurrent (except in the case of premature beats of atrial origin, "PACs") , and represents excitation of the atria in a coordinated fashion. In the normal heart, it follows discharge of the sinus node and is directed leftward, downward, and initially ventrad and terminally dorsad. Of these directions, the downward (caudad) one is most important. If it arises outside the sinus node, its orientation and contour are modified accordingly, and it is said to be of ectopic origin. To identify a wave as a P is to say that the atria are being depolarized in an organized fashion, but does not imply sinus origin.
8. **P':** Sometimes a P wave thought to have originated outside the sinus node is identified as P'. This is in conflict with the standards for specificity listed above in that it substitutes interpretation for description, and uses the prime mark for a purpose other than the more traditional one of designating repeated waves; e.g., RSR'. But it is not an important problem.
9. **PR interval:** The time from the beginning of P to the beginning of QRS, whether the initial QRS deflection is positive or negative; it may really be a PQ interval.
10. **PQ segment:** The section of the trace between the end of P and the beginning of QRS.
11. ***f* waves:** Completely irregular undulation of the trace, typical of random electrical activity of muscle fibers or fascicles, chaos as distinguished from organized activity, but of lower frequency than the "noise" of skeletal muscle activity with which they may be confused. *f* waves define atrial fibrillation and are recognized best between the T of one beat and the QRS of the next (*see* **P wave**).
12. **ORS:** The complex of waves written by depolarization of the ventricles, typically three but there may be any number. It is the largest component of the tracing in most cases, consisting, when normal, of sharp angles and straight lines. The complex as a whole is known as a QRS no matter what its specific components.
13. **Q wave:** A negative wave that initiates the QRS and is followed by an R wave.
14. **R wave:** Any positive wave in the QRS; more than one, R', R'', etc.
15. **S wave:** Any negative wave in the QRS following an R wave; more than one, S', S'', etc.
16. **QS:** A completely negative QRS complex.
17. **QT interval:** The time from the beginning of QRS to the end of T. QT is a measure of the duration of ventricular repolarization, "electrical systole"; QRS coincides with the first heart sound, the return stroke of T with the second. Repolarization is assumed to begin at the same time as depolarization; QRS is inscribed during QT.
18. **Slur:** The slowing of the rate of inscription of the trace.
19. **ST segment:** The proximal, chiefly horizontal, part of the curve written by ventricular repolarization. It is continuous with T, the distal, chiefly vertical, part of the same curve.
20. **ST-T:** A term that emphasizes reference to the whole curve of ventricular repolarization, both ST and T, the ST-T complex.

21. **T wave:** The terminal, principally vertical, part of the repolarization curve. (Sometimes the whole repolarization curve is called T.)
22. **U wave:** A small, slow wave that follows T, usually seen best in a right precordial lead. It is probably related to ventricular repolarization, but delayed potentials from depolarization may be a factor. It is not identifiable in every tracing.
23. **Wave:** A round trip of the trace from baseline to baseline (*see* Deflection).

Technical Features of the Tracing

24. **Format:** The order in which the leads are presented. There is no single right or wrong format. The most common one in current use displays twelve leads in three simultaneously recorded channels, four groups of 2.5 s each; the first group is leads I, II, and III (from top to bottom) followed by aVR-aVL-aVF, Vl-V2-V3, and V4-V5-V6. (Most tracings in this collection are in this format.) In most, but not all, formats, time is continuous across lead changes, and leads are labeled or coded, An unbroken strip of Lead II, or some other lead, is often added as a fourth channel, and usually, but not always, represents the same beats as the simultaneously recorded ones in the top three channels.
25. **Calibration:** A record of the amplitude of the deflection produced by one millivolt (mV). It also documents the frequency response of the recording system. (Both upstroke and downstroke should be vertical, and the top horizontal, with square corners.) All vertical measurements in the tracing are referred to a standard: 1 mV = 10 mm. In most automatically calibrated equipment, the millivolt signal lasts 0.20 s , and its width documents the paper speed: 5 mm, 25 mm/s; 10 mm, 50 mm/s, Also, most current equipment permits recording frontal and precordial leads at different gain (qv).
26. **Paper speed:** The EKG chart consists of horizontal and vertical lines at one millimeter intervals with each fifth one accentuated. For a millimeter to represent 0.04 s, the paper must move at exactly 25 mm/s, and this is standard. The only problem likely to occur results from a paper speed of 50 mm/s, which makes the interval 0.02 s. One way to check this on modern machines is the duration of the calibration mark (qv).

Vocabulary

1. **Analysis:** Separation of the whole into constituent parts for individual study.
2. **Block:** Hindrance, stoppage, obstruction, or impairment of passage. For an impulse to be blocked is the opposite of its being conducted, or transmitted. In EKG reports, block is either, between atria and ventricles (AV), or within a ventricle (IV). It is evidence of discrepancy between input and output of information and may result from either diminution of the ability to conduct, demand that exceeds normal ability to conduct, or both. It is an objective finding. Some authors differentiate between "block" to imply impairment of AV conduction, and "nonconducted" as evidence of the normal refractory period, a judgment that takes the atrial rate into account, not intrinsic in the tracing.
3. **Conduct/conduction/conducted:** To permit passage, to lead or guide from one place to another. The intracardiac conduction system is the network of specialized tissues over which impulses are distributed. To be conducted is the opposite of being blocked.
4. **Default:** The option selected automatically. When the (normal) sinus pacemaker fails, for instance, a junctional focus drives the ventricles by default. Default, or passive, mechanisms are normal backups.
5. **Ectopy/ectopic:** Outside the normal place.
6. **Einthoven's premises:** The assumptions about anatomy and physiology that are the base for interpreting electrocardiograms (*see* p. 7).
7. **Energy:** "Power" can be considered a synonym, and "force" is used almost interchangeably. Energy exists in two states, potential (stored) and kinetic (active); "force" implies the latter, energy brought to bear to produce change. Whatever names are used, energy is not visible and must be represented symbolically. An electrocardiogram is a symbol of energy.
8. **Function:** Physiology, as distinguished from structure, anatomy, form.
9. **Galvanometer:** A device for measuring difference in potential between two points, a voltmeter. The gasoline gauge in an automobile,

registering the difference between zero and a value greater than zero, is an example of a galvanometer. Simplistically, an EKG machine is a recording galvanometer. It measures the difference in potential between point A and point B as A moves in time and space and B remains fixed, and plots the course of A against time. All information in the tracing is presented as vectors emanating from the B point and directed toward the positive pole of the named lead.

10. **Ground:** A reference point, an arbitrary zero, or neutral, for definition of potential between it and another point. The electrical system inside the heart is not accessible to true ground (the earth), but Einthoven's premises define a point at the center of the chest, a "system ground," from which potentials are measured, Wilson's central terminal of zero potential for the V leads. (*see* **B Point**, **Baseline**, and **V leads**.)
11. **Interpretation:** Explanation, translation, presentation in understandable terms. An EKG interpretation, or report, identifies mechanism, structure, and function as precisely as possible, with speculation beyond that to the degree appropriate.
12. **Inverted:** Upside down, reversed in order or direction, a judgment implying abnormality, not a description. T waves are often said to be inverted when what is meant is that they are negative in specified leads, an indication of their orientation.
13. **Ischemia:** A local area of inadequacy of blood (really oxygen). Etymologically, the word implies restriction of blood flow, but adequacy is a function of both supply and demand. Inadequacy may result from restriction of flow, increase in demand, or both. To equate "ischemia" with negative T waves is inappropriate.
14. **Junction (AV Junction):** A region of the heart, not a structure but a loosely defined area including the AV node and its vicinity. Upper junctional is synonymous with low atrial, and with upper nodal; lower junctional is synonymous with the His bundle.
15. **Lead:** The word has several meanings. First, the concept of a dipole, the difference in potential between two points, the unknown that the tracing documents, e.g., Lead II; second, the graphic expression of this, a line on a chart; and third, a component of the patient cable, a wire. Failure to respect the difference among these may result in interpretation of technical error as evidence of cardiac abnormality.
16. **Linear conductor:** The term means what it says, a conductor of electricity along a linear path; an example is a wire. The arms and legs act as linear conductors attached to a volume conductor (qv), the thorax and abdomen, at the shoulders and symphysis pubis.
17. **Meaning/meaningful/useful:** In the context of electrocardiography, applicable to the patient.
18. **Mechanism:** A statement of the focus from which atrial excitation proceeds, that for the ventricles, the rate and rhythm of each, and their causal relation in a series of beats, commonly called the "rhythm." The common practice of calling all this the "rhythm," requires thinking of the "rhythm of the rhythm."
19. **Orthogonal: Perpendicular:** "Ortho" means straight and "gonos" means angle. A straight angle can be defined as 180°, or as 90°, and also is called a right angle, typical examples of the multiple meanings of words, in this case words on the fringes of the common language.
20. **Potential:** The possibility of force. Potential can be measured as the difference between an energy value at one level and that at another. The potential of a volume of water, for instance, is defined in feet above sea level; that of electricity, as volts above ground (or zero or neutral).
21. **Rhythm:** The temporal relation of events in a series, a word from everyone's everyday language. In practice, the rhythm of the "heart" means that of the ventricles. It is regular or irregular. (*see* **Mechanism**.)
22. **Structure:** Anatomy, form, topography, as distinguished from function, physiology.
23. **Synthesis:** The bringing together of elements to form a whole. After a tracing has been analyzed, the parts are rearranged to synthesize an interpretation.
24. **Usurp/usurping:** To take control of aggressively, wrongfully. Usurping mechanisms are abnormal, the result of an ectopic pacemaker functioning at a rate greater than the normal intrinsic one.
25. **Vector/vectorcardiogram:** An arrow representing the three characteristics of a force: magnitude, sense, and direction. The Latin word

means "carrier." In mathematics parlance, a vector value is represented by a line that has two characteristics, magnitude (length) and direction (inclination), as distinguished from a scalar value that has only magnitude and is represented by a point. It is not in conflict with this definition to indicate a third feature (for sense, or polarity, origin and destination) by adding an arrowhead to the line. An EKG expressed as a line connecting the termini of a continuum of instantaneous vectors, all arising from the same point in the center of the chest, is called a vectorcardiogram. (*see* EKG 149)

26. **Volume conductor:** A system that conducts electricity in all directions at once, as distinct from a linear conductor (above). A tank full of Ringer's solution in the Physiology lab is a volume conductor. In electrocardiography, it is a basic premise that the thorax and abdomen comprise a volume conductor; the arms and legs, linear conductors connected to it at the shoulders and symphysis pubis. This volume conductor is assumed to be equally conductive throughout, i.e., there is no difference in the electrically conductive properties of blood, bone, liver, etc., and of infinite extent in all directions with the heart at its center.

Appendix II

Abbreviations Used in This Book

Abn/abns	abnormal/abnormalities
Abn ST-T	ST-T abnormalities, nonspecific
AIMCI	acute inferior myocardial infarct
AF	atrial fibrillation
Ant	anterior
Art	artificial
AAMCI	acute anterior myocardial infarct
AVPM	artificial ventricular pacemaker
AT	atrial tachycardia
AV	atrioventricular
AVB	atrioventricular block
BSTDRA	broad, slurred, terminal forces to the right and anterior
CCW	counterclockwise
Cond	conduction/conducted
Cor insuf	coronary insufficiency
CW	clockwise
Depr	depressed/depression
Diff	diffuse
Dig	digitalis
Dn	down
DSLP	diffuse slur left and posterior
Dx	diagnosis
EKG	electrocardiogram
Enl	enlargement
F	aVF
IHSS	idiopathic hypertrophic subaortic stenosis
In	inferior
Indetin	determinate
Insep	inseparable from
Insuf	insufficiency
IV	intraventricular
IVCD	intraventricular conduction defect
IVCT	intraventricular conduction time
Junc	junctional
L	aVL
LAE	left atrial enlargement
LAFB	left anterior fascicular block
Lat	lateral
LBBB	left bundle branch block
LC	little change
LVH	left ventricular hypertrophy
LVO	left ventricular overload
MCI	myocardial infarct
Mech	mechanism
MFQRS	mean frontal QRS
MFT	mean frontal T
Myo	myocardial
Neg	negative
NR	not remarkable
NSC	no significant change
OAMCI	old anterior myocardial infarct
OIMCI	old inferior myocardial infarct
Occ	occasional
OW	otherwise
OWNL	otherwise within normal limits
PAC	premature atrial contraction(s)
PAT	paroxysmal atrial tachycardia
PM	pacemaker
Pre-ex	pre-excitation
Prob	probable/probably
Prom	prominent
Pt	patient
PVC	premature ventricular contraction(s)
R	aVR
RAE	right atrial enlargement
RBBB	right bundle branch block
Rel T	related to T
Retro	retrograde
RV	right ventricle
RVE	right ventricular enlargement
RVH	right ventricular hypertrophy
SB	see below
S/F	sagging/flattened
S/F/A	sagging/flattened/arched

Sl	slight/slightly	Vent	ventricle/ventricular
ST-T abns	ST-T abnormalities	VT	ventricular tachycardia
SVMR	supraventricular mechanism, rate	VF	ventricular fibrillation
SVT	supraventricular tachycardia	WLM	within the limits of the method
Term	terminal	WNL	within normal limits
Sym	symmetrical	WPW	Wolff-Parkinson-White

Bibliography

1. Blake, TM. *The Practice of Electrocardiography*, 5th ed. Totowa, New Jersey: Humana Press, 1994.
2. Katz, LN. *Electrocardiography*, 2nd ed. Philadelphia: Lea and Febiger, 1946, p. 179.
3. Barker, JM. *The Unipolar Eletrocardiogram, a Clinical Interpretation.* New York: Appleton Ccntury Crofts, 1952, p. 108.
4. Schoolman, HM. The role of the physician as patient advocate *N Engl J Med* 296:103, 1977.
5. Hayakawa, SI. *Language in Thought and Action*, 3rd ed. New York: Harcourt Brace Jovanovich, 1972.
6. Beckwith JR, ed. *Grant's Clinical Electrocardiography,* New York: McGraw-Hill, Blakiston Division, 1970.
7. Hurst JW, *Ventricular Electrocardiography.* Philadelphia: Lippincott, 1991.
8. Wilson FN, Rosenbaum FF, Johnson FD. Interpretation of the ventricuclar complex of the electrocardiogram. Adv Intern Med 2:1, 1947.

Index

The interpretation of every tracing has three components, mechanism, structure, and function, each of which has several elements, and these may be combined in various ways. The vocabulary of the method is almost universal, but definitions of the terms it uses vary widely, and judgment is involved at every step in preparation of a report. The object is to make the information in the tracing as useful as possible.

This index has been compiled with all this in mind, attempting to make major findings, and combinations of findings, easily available. The commitment that each page should be useful by itself imposes limits on the space available for annotation. There are not many cross references, but the index can function in their stead.

With a few exceptions, PACs, PVCs, sinus arrhythmia, borderline values, and common abnormalities, such as those in ST-T, are not indexed.

Bold numbers refer to pages; others, to EKGs.

T

U

V

- W - X - Y - Z -